Women's Health in India
Risk and Vulnerability

Women's Health in India
Risk and Vulnerability

Edited by
MONICA DAS GUPTA
LINCOLN C. CHEN
T. N. KRISHNAN

Bombay
OXFORD UNIVERSITY PRESS
Delhi Calcutta Madras
1995

Oxford University Press, Walton Street, Oxford OX2 6DP

OXFORD NEW YORK
ATHENS AUCKLAND BANGKOK BOMBAY
CALCUTTA CAPE TOWN DAR ES SALAAM DELHI
FLORENCE HONG KONG ISTANBUL KARACHI
KUALA LUMPUR MADRAS MADRID MELBOURNE
MEXICO CITY NAIROBI PARIS SINGAPORE
TAIPEI TOKYO TORONTO
and associated companies in
BERLIN IBADAN

Oxford is a trademark of Oxford University Press

© Oxford University Press 1995

ISBN 0 19 563620 1

Typeset by S.J.I. Services, B-17 Lajpat Nagar Part 2, New Delhi 110024.
Printed at Konam Printers, Tardeo, Bombay 400 034.
and published by Neil O'Brien, Oxford University Press,
Oxford House, Apollo Bunder, Bombay 400001.

To
OUR PARENTS
Renu Das Gupta
Sachindranath Das Gupta
T. K. Narayanan
Subbalakshmi
Samuel and Winifred Chen

Preface

This volume emanates from a collaborative project of the National Council of Applied Economic Research, New Delhi and the Center for Population and Development Studies, Harvard University. A seminar was held in New Delhi on 'Health and Development in India', in which people from a variety of social science disciplines presented papers on critical issues of health.

The seminar papers are now published in two volumes. This volume contains the papers dealing specifically with gender issues. The other volume, entitled 'Health, Poverty and Development in India', contains papers discussing the health situation in India; problems of measurement of health status; the relationship between nutrition, health and socio-economic status, aspects of the political economy of health care; and possible future directions of health policy and health care financing.

We would like to thank the Ford Foundation and Dr S. L. Rao, Director-General of the National Council of Applied Economic Research for their generous support for this seminar. The organization of the seminar owes much to the dedicated efforts of several staff members of the National Council for Applied Economic Research, in particular Shankari Banerji and B. L. Joshi.

Monica Das Gupta
T. N. Krishnan
Lincoln C. Chen

Contents

Preface — vii

Contributors — xi

1. Overview
   Monica Das Gupta and Lincoln C. Chen — 1

Childhood and the Early Years

2. Gender Differentials in Child Mortality: a review of the evidence
   Sunita Kishor — 19

3. Women's Capabilities and Infant Mortality: lessons from Manipur
   A. K. Shiva Kumar — 55

The Reproductive Years

4. Maternal Mortality: estimates from an econometric model
   P. N. Mari Bhat, K. Navaneetham and S. Irudaya Rajan — 97

5. Unsafe Motherhood: a review of reproductive health
   Shireen J. Jejeebhoy and Saumya Rama Rao — 122

6. Women's Roles and the Gender Gap in Health and Survival
   Alaka Malwade Basu — 153

7. Women's Health in a Rural Poor Population in Tamil Nadu
   T. K. Sundari Ravindran — 175

8. Patriarchy and the Risks of STD and HIV Transmission to Women
   Radhika Ramasubban — 212

Old Age

9. Widowhood and Well-Being in Rural North India
   Martha Alter Chen and Jean Drèze — 245

10. The Indian Woman in Later Life: some social and cultural considerations
    Sylvia Vatuk — 289

11. Gender and Health: from research to action
    Adrienne Germain — 307

Index — 317

Contributors

Alaka Malwade Basu, a social demographer, is Visiting Fellow at the Institute of Economic Growth, Delhi, India.

Lincoln C. Chen is Taro Takemi Professor of International Health at the Harvard School of Public Health and Director of the Harvard Center for Population and Development Studies, Harvard University, USA.

Martha Alter Chen is Director of the Program on Non-Governmental Organizations of the Harvard Institute for International Development, Harvard University, USA.

Monica Das Gupta, a demographer and anthropologist, is Associate Director of the National Council of Applied Economic Research, New Delhi, and Senior Fellow at the Center for Population and Development Studies, Harvard University, USA.

Jean Drèze is a development economist with the Centre for Development Economics of the Delhi School of Economics, and also the Department of Economics, London School of Economics, University of London, U.K.

Adrienne Germain is Vice-President of the International Women's Health Coalition, New York, USA.

S. Irudaya Rajan is a demographer at the Population Research Centre, Vidyagiri, Dharwad, India.

Shireen Jejeebhoy is a demographer working as an independent consultant based in Bombay.

Sunita Kishor is WID Analyst, Demographic and Health Surveys at Macro International Inc., Maryland, USA.

T. N. Krishnan, an economist, is Honorary Fellow at the Centre for Development Studies, Trivandrum, India.

P. N. Mari Bhat, a demographer, is Director of the Population Research Centre, Vidyagiri, Dharwad, India.

K. Navaneetham is a demographer at the Population Research Centre, Vidyagiri, Dharwad, India.

Saumya Rama Rao, a demographer, is a Reader at the International Institute for Population Sciences, Bombay, India.

Radhika Ramasubban is a sociologist and Director of the Centre for Social and Technological Change, Bombay, India.

A. K. Shiva Kumar, a demographer, is working with UNICEF, New Delhi.

T. K. Sundari Ravindran is Senior Economist at the National Council of Applied Economic Research, New Delhi, India.

Sylvia Vatuk is a Professor at the Department of Anthropology, The University of Illinois at Chicago, USA.

1
Overview

MONICA DAS GUPTA and LINCOLN C. CHEN

A very simple indication of the level of welfare enjoyed by women in India is that, in large parts of the country, their levels of education are amongst the lowest in the world, and the levels of maternal mortality are amongst the highest in the world. Whether in socio-economic indicators such as education, health and work, or in more subtle processes of power, decision-making and self-esteem, the inferior position of Indian women has been consistently documented. This gender bias is not confined to India alone: it is shared by much of South Asia and is also manifested in some ways in East Asia. Nor is this a recent phenomenon. For well over a century, the low position of Indian women has been of concern to both colonial and indigenous social reformers. The plight of Indian women has also been movingly captured in Indian literature.

Even before the first Indian Census of 1872 and the initiation of vital registration systems, the British were aware of the problem. For example, the highly visible practice of *sati* had attracted great attention, and was officially banned by the colonialists. Subtler forms of discrimination, however, were more difficult to deal with. Investigating the unusual imbalance in the sex ratio of reported births and of the population as a whole, the British concluded that female infanticide was being practised in several regions of Northern India. Unlike an act as public as *sati*, female infanticide is surreptitious and is difficult to prove in any individual case. Thus the measures adopted by the British were more indirect, such as punishing an entire village if its sex ratio at birth, upon investigation, proved to be suspiciously imbalanced.

Actions against blatant abuses such as *sati* and female infanticide were more successful than less visible forms of discrimination. Although reported cases of female infanticide declined, the imbalance in the sex ratio persisted. As the British themselves noted, there was a shift from overt infanticide to covert neglect of female children (Panigrahi 1972; Miller 1981). Child marriage was also prohibited by legal means through the Sharda Act of 1936. Banning child marriage also proved difficult in a society where there was no documentation of age and where traditional marriages were not registered with the civil authorities.

Indigenous social reform movements which swept India from the late nineteenth century also sought to change women's position in society. Although the British efforts were backed by the power of the legal and administrative apparatus, their efforts were often viewed as an alien cultural intrusion by foreigners. The Indian social reform movements were indigenous, closely linked to the emerging political consciousness of Indians, and allied with the incipient nationalist movement. Leaders such as Raja Ram Mohan Roy and Tilak carried cultural and moral legitimacy in their efforts to alter the position of women.

The literature of the period reflects this growing consciousness of the injustice of women's powerlessness in their homes and in the wider society. A moving example is the short story written by Tagore, translated as 'A Wife's Letter'. Reminiscent of Ibsen's 'The Doll's House', the story describes how Mrinal, a beautiful village girl, was chosen by a wealthy urban family as a bride for their son. After marriage, she was treated well by her husband's family but, as Tagore subtly shows us, her material comforts did not extend to her being taken seriously as a person or being given autonomy or authority in the household. Mrinal's desire to leave the 'comfortable' life was sparked by a tragedy which unfolded in the life of another girl, a relative of her in-laws. This girl also belonged to a poor family, but she was considered ugly. She sought desperately to move into Mrinal's household, in any menial capacity, to avoid the threat of an impossible marriage. Mrinal tried to offer this girl some shelter and protection, but was unable to prevent her from being married to a man who turned out to be a lunatic. Unable to cope, the girl killed herself. Mrinal finally decided that she could not live any more with her husband's family. As she put it, she was unfortunately burdened with intelligence as well as beauty.

Mrinal's story rings a chillingly contemporary note, although a century has passed since it was written. This story still strikes a chord in the context of today's social reality, because although important changes have taken place, the majority of Indian women continue to occupy a fundamentally subservient position in their family and society. The root of the problem, as Tagore brought out so clearly, lies in the strongly patriarchal nature of Indian society, where men are defined as being the critical actors in all spheres of life: the family, household and the wider social order.

One dimension of men's pivotal role is that of the *sustainer*, which emanates from their being defined as the appointed breadwinners, regardless of how much contribution women make to the productive process. Another dimension is that of the *reproducer*. This may sound strange, since it is women who bear children. But simply producing children is biological reproduction. Social reproduction requires that children be given an identity as members of an organized social structure. In a patrilineal society, it is the males who form the framework of the social structure. Thus the reproduction of the family, the household and of the society takes place through the male line: it is men who reproduce themselves. This is what underlies the symbolism of the masculine seed and the feminine earth: the woman, like the earth, is merely a necessary accessory for the seed to reproduce itself.

It is easy to see how these structures undervalue women. Their contribution to the household becomes easy to ignore, as there is little that a particular woman provides that another cannot, while a male occupies a clearly defined slot in the social order as the link between different generations of a family, lineage, caste, or other social category. Women's low evaluation in the family and in the society follows from this. As a *category*, women are useful, but it is obviously far less important what happens to an *individual* woman than to a man.

Women's Health: a life-cycle perspective

The subject of this volume is the adverse health outcomes for women. These adverse health outcomes are one of the manifestations of the low value placed on women and their relative powerlessness in patriarchal societies, and are more visible at those points

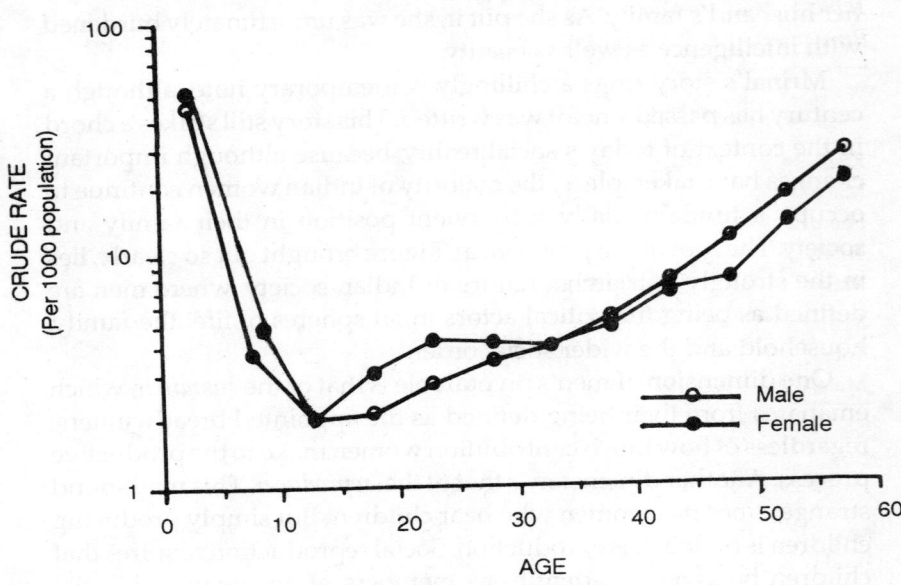

Fig. 1: Age and sex specific death rates in India
(Source: Jain 1982)

of the life-cycle when they are biologically and socially more vulnerable. Early childhood is one such stage, as young children are at high risk to ill health and are more susceptible to dying from their illnesses than at any other time in the life-cycle except extreme old age. Even a little lack of care can cause far more havoc in this age-group than at older ages. Another point in the life-cycle when women are specifically biologically vulnerable is during their peak reproductive years, when the physical drain of pregnancy and lactation increases women's vulnerability to poor health status. Figure 1 shows the divergence between male and female mortality rates at these vulnerable ages, that is during early childhood and during the peak reproductive years. After the peak reproductive years, the female biological advantage shows up again in lower mortality rates for women than for men.

Two other stages of the life-cycle are also important and customarily neglected: adolescence and the older years. Youth and the adolescent period have been relatively understudied. However, this is changing now because of the urgency of understanding adolescent

Table 1: *Infant and child mortality rates by sex, Khanna Study villages in Punjab and Matlab Project area in Bangladesh.*

	Age at death (months)					
	<1	1–11	0–11	12–23	24–59	0–59
Khanna, 1965–84						
Males	50.7	27.1	77.7	9.4	8.2	95.3
Females	43.0	51.3	94.3	18.5	12.6	125.4
Total	47.0	38.6	85.6	13.8	10.3	109.6
Male/Female	1.18	0.53	0.82	0.51	0.65	0.76
Matlab Thana, 1974–77						
Total	73.0	58.2	131.2			
Male/Female	1.16	0.82	1.00			

Source: Das Gupta (1987) for Khanna 1965–84; D'Souza and Chen (1980) for Matlab 1974–77.

sexuality in order to help prevent the spread of AIDS. In the older years, women's biological advantage over men manifests itself in higher survival rates. However, this situation may sometimes be reversed, as in the case of widows.

1. Childhood and the early years

In contrast with most other societies where girls enjoy biological advantages in survival as compared with boys, female children experience higher mortality rates than males in India. The age pattern of sex differentials in mortality is shown in Table 1. Despite strong son preference, the biological advantage of girls keeps their mortality levels lower than that of boys during the first month of life, a phenomenon found in most populations. After the first month, parental preferences and behaviour become more important in child health and survival. As a consequence, the neglect of girls in comparison to boys is manifested in excess female mortality. The consensus amongst those who have studied this phenomenon is that while there is some evidence of poorer nutritional intake, the difference between boys and girls in health care is likely to be the main mechanism whereby sex differentials in child mortality are brought about.[1]

---

[1] See for example Wyon and Gordon 1971; Chen and D'Souza 1981; and Das Gupta 1987.

Existing studies of excess female mortality underscore several issues. For one thing, the sex differentials of mortality demonstrate considerable regional variability. As shown by Dyson and Moore (1983), a distinctive North-South divide exists, with more balanced sex ratios in the South than in the North. They attribute this to differences in the kinship system between the South and the North, with patriliny much stronger in the latter. This regional pattern is not new. Visaria (1969) showed a remarkable constancy in regional differences in sex ratios since the 1881 census. Also, sex differentials in child mortality are not the result of 'benign neglect'; rather, there is evidence of volition in this matter. Excess female child mortality is concentrated among families which already have a daughter (Das Gupta 1987, Muhuri and Preston 1991, Pebley and Amin 1991). The discrimination against girls is not generalized, but is specifically targeted against a subset of 'excess' daughters born into a family.

Kishor's paper reviews much of the literature on sex differentials in mortality in India, focusing especially on the question of how development affects women's status and excess female child mortality. She concludes that, contrary to what might have been predicted by 'modernization' theories, the available evidence in India does not suggest that socio-economic development helps reduce excess female mortality. Even urbanization does not appear to have this effect: indeed, gender equity may even be worsened through greater discrimination in the use of urban medical care facilities.

Based on district-level analysis of all-India data, Kishor analyses how excess female mortality is affected by cultural factors (as indicated by patrilocal exogamy) and by economic factors (as measured by female labour force participation), as well as by a number of demographic, socio-economic and developmental indicators. Among these, cultural factors are apparently more significant than economic factors in explaining excess female mortality. She also finds that development (whether measured in terms of agricultural development, urbanization or industrialization) does not reduce gender biases, but can actually *increase* sex differentials in child mortality. Nor does it seem to be possible to explain discrimination against girls in terms of poverty where families have to make choices about how to allocate limited resources between individual members. Gender discrimination persists and can increase, even when availability of resources is not a constraint.

Shiva Kumar's paper moves from the national level to the study of a distinctive and comparatively under-studied state, Manipur. Along with Kerala, Manipur is an 'outlier' in terms of extremely advanced child health and survival indicators despite low per capita income levels. In considering the reasons for this, Shiva Kumar concludes that the high status of women in Manipur may account for its remarkably low levels of infant mortality. Manipuri society is much more egalitarian in terms of gender relations than most of India. Women have considerable freedom with regard to marriage, divorce, and other aspects of their personal lives. There is also a tradition of active engagement of women in social and political movements.

2. *The reproductive years*

Turning to the adult part of the woman's life-cycle, it is apparent from Figure 1 that the peak childbearing years are associated with excess female mortality. In large parts of India, marriage plunges a woman into a highly vulnerable part of her life-cycle. Especially where exogamy is practised, women find themselves as members of a household in which they are strangers, and their sources of social support are thin. This makes them ill-equipped to protect their health at a stage in their lives when they are most burdened by the reproductive health risks of pregnancy, contraception, abortion and childbirth.[2]

Heavy workloads relative to nutritional intake are common amongst the poor, and for women this nutritional lack is aggravated by the stresses associated with reproduction, Since fertility levels are highest amongst poor women, they suffer the most from maternal depletion. Needless to add, these are a major cause of low birth-weight in children, which in turn contributes to high infant mortality rates.

Reproductive health problems are widely prevalent amongst women, especially amongst poorer women and those living in the rural areas. The available information on these problems is patchy, depending on small-scale studies. Many of these problems are serious in nature. Poor nutritional status during childhood, and

[2] See Das Gupta 1994.

marriage while still physically immature increase women's susceptibility to these problems. Another major source of complications is the fact that a high proportion of births are still attended by poorly-trained women. As a result, complications of delivery are widespread.

As the papers in this volume and other studies indicate, the overwhelming majority of women suffering from reproductive health problems do not seek treatment. Being socially trained to be reticent about sexual matters, lack of interest among other members of the household, creates a situation in which a woman feels alone with her affliction, and feels that it must be borne silently as a 'woman's problem'.

Reliable estimates of these health risks, such as levels of maternal mortality, are scanty at a national level. This is due in large measure to lack of national level data. Something approaching reasonable estimates is available from local studies, which are not necessarily representative of larger regions. The paper by Mari Bhat and his colleagues makes a useful contribution by using a new technique for estimating maternal mortality levels in India. Employing indirect estimation techniques, they estimate that the maternal mortality rate was 555 per 100,000 births for India as a whole in 1982-86. This rate is currently amongst the highest in the world, and the only major regions to show such high rates are South Asia and sub-Saharan Africa. Despite being so high, Mari Bhat and his colleagues conclude that this ratio has shown a substantial decline since the 1960s.

Much of the excess female mortality during the early adult years is due to reproductive stress. With fertility decline the reproductive stress is reduced, and the gap between male and female mortality in these age groups closes and subsequently reverses. This is shown in the case of Sri Lanka by Nadarajah (1983), and is reflected in calculations for India by Dyson (1987).

Not all the excess female mortality during the reproductive ages can be attributed to reproductive stress and maternal mortality. As Mari Bhat points out, 'accidental' fires and suicides are also a major cause of death at these ages. These are the clearest reflection of the vulnerability of women's position in the household and in society during this part of their life. He also points out that men suffer higher death rates from traffic accidents, because they are more exposed to the hazards of travelling than women.

Basu develops this theme of how gender roles influence exposure to different life-threatening situations. She points out that the seclusion of women and the restrictions on their behaviour can also have some positive features from the point of view of health. For example, the fact that they are not allowed to smoke protects them against one source of ill-health, while restrictions on movement protect them from accidents. At the same time, being confined to ill-designed smoke-filled kitchens increases their exposure to domestic pollutants and consequent serious diseases. Thus gender differences in life-styles and roles can affect gender differences in health.

Basu's paper causes us to think about some of the positive aspects of female seclusion and other restrictions on women, which have usually been viewed only in a negative light, as they hamper women's ability to seek health care and more generally to protect themselves from a variety of threats to their physical and psychological well being. Women's vulnerability to these threats, and the constraints they face in dealing with them are brought out in the other papers in this volume.

Reproductive health problems are one manifestation of these threats to women's well-being. Jejeebhoy and Rama Rao's paper is a concise yet wide-ranging review of the scattered literature on women's reproductive health in India. As they put it, maternal mortality is just the tip of the iceberg of reproductive health problems. The World Health Organization estimates that for every maternal death, there are 16 women who suffer morbidities that can last a lifetime. Jejeebhoy and Rama Rao review the available evidence on several aspects of reproductive health: that childhood malnutrition predisposes women to reproductive health problems in adulthood; that adolescent childbearing increases health risks to both mother and child; the poor coverage of antenatal care services; poor diets and heavy workloads during pregnancy; and deliveries under unhygienic conditions unattended by skilled people. Apart from direct childbearing, certain contraceptive services such as sterilization and IUD insertion as well as induced abortion can lead to debilitating and sometimes even fatal health complications if service conditions are poor and follow-up limited. They point out that interest in and concern about women's health has been so limited that even the indicators of reproductive health remain inadequately developed.

Sundari's paper examines women's health in a rural area of Tamil Nadu, bases on a field study. In this population, one-third of the women reported that they currently had a reproductive health problem. Of these, nearly two-thirds had not sought treatment, while one-fifth had tried some form of self treatment. Less than one in four had sought some form of outside medical help. Sundari points out that it is difficult to avoid under-reporting of reproductive morbidity, partly because most surveys probe the respondents insufficiently. Clinical examinations may be required to objectively determine levels and patterns of reproductive morbidity. A clinical study in Maharashtra, for example, found that 92 per cent of women had one or more gynaecological diseases, and only 8 per cent of these women had ever had treatment (Bang et al. 1989).

Ramasubban's paper addresses directly the issue of gender relations and reproductive health, which is touched upon in several papers. She discusses the difficulties that women have in avoiding sexually transmitted diseases (STDs), including AIDS. One example is that of commercial sex workers or prostitutes who are usually unable to impose the use of condoms on paying customers. If infected by an STD, most cannot afford the income loss implied by avoiding sex for the duration of the treatment. Sundari reports that married women also face problems in protecting themselves against STDs. Wives get infected by their husbands and find it difficult to shake off the disease because husbands are often unwilling to cooperate in seeking treatment. Sometimes, husbands end up infecting their wives repeatedly.

A woman's vulnerable position within the household is a factor making not only for difficulty in avoiding being infected by her husband, but also for low levels of treatment of reproductive disorders. Sundari recounts women's reports that they are afraid of being thought to be sickly, in case they are thrown out of their husband's home, or the husband takes another wife. Thus women are inclined to bear their problems in silence. STDs pose yet another kind of problem. Men are more likely than their wives to contract STDs because they are sexually less restricted, and many visit prostitutes, especially if they migrate in search of work. If they infect their wives, the women are placed under the additional risk of becoming infertile or having low-birth-weight children who die. Infertility further reduces a woman's position in the household, and she may well be replaced with another wife. This theme emerges in the papers by Ramasubban, Sundari, and Jejeebhoy and Rama Rao.

Another common theme which emerges from several of the papers is that women's labour force participation may not necessarily have a beneficial effect on the health of women and children. It is frequently assumed in the literature that such a beneficial effect is to be expected, because participating in the labour force should increase women's autonomy in the household, as well as financial capacity: factors which are expected to enable women to look after themselves and their children better. This does not seem to be borne out empirically in the studies in this volume. Kishor points out that female labour force participation is associated with higher child mortality, while Sundari finds that it is also associated with higher maternal morbidity. It is not difficult to understand why this might be the case. It is well known that in India, except in the urban middle classes, a household gains status by withdrawing its women from the labour force. Thus the majority of women who work come from households which are poor and disadvantaged. It is also well known that low socio-economic status is associated with poorer health status. Thus it is not surprising to find a negative association between female labour force participation and health outcomes when factors such as socio-economic status are not taken into account. This relationship is a complex one, and needs to be better understood in the literature.

3. Old age

Women who have successfully reared children, especially sons, gain is strength in the household as they and their children grow older. This is the only point in their lives when the majority of women are able to wield real power within the household. Their greater freedom and autonomy enables them to care better for their own health. This is the only period in the life-cycle when women's natural biological advantage over men manifests itself in lower death rates (Figure 1). However, this situation can be altered by widowhood, in particular if the woman does not have grown sons to support her.

Chen and Dreze's paper presents findings from two field studies carried out in villages in several North Indian states on the situation of widows. Their principal focus is on the question of how widowhood affects a woman's position in the household. Although much is known about the low position of widows in Indian households, little systematic research has been done on this question. Chen and Dreze review the existing studies of widows and health in South Asia. They report on a study in Bangladesh (Rahman et al. 1992) which found that widows have higher mortality than married women of the same age, after controlling for the household's economic status. They point out that the helplessness of widows without grown sons has negative effects not only for their own welfare, but also for that of others in the household and for society as a whole. They face socially determined constraints which makes it difficult for them to be effective economic heads of household, so they can be obliged to withdraw young children from school in order to support the household. Besides, their dependence on sons encourages higher fertility than would be necessarily beneficial for the household or for society as a whole.

Chen and Drèze go on to describe the way in which widows' position is influenced by kinship and inheritance systems, by their ability to earn a living, their social isolation, and the forms of intra- and inter-household support available to them. They examine the effectiveness of the functioning of State support for widows, such as pension schemes. The existing laws protecting widows' access to their husbands' property are often disregarded in practice. The authors conclude that the best way to ensure greater social protection for widows is to recognize them as contributing significantly to the household economy. This could be done, for example, by trying to ensure that their property rights are better protected, and by making it easier for them to be economically active. Unfortunately, as the authors point out, even these relatively straightforward recommendations are difficult to implement, given that women are so marginalized in Indian society.

Vatuk points to the lack of research on older women in India, which is especially surprising given the strong interest in gender studies and the rising interest in social gerontology. Her paper brings out the diversity of women's situation at older ages. She sketches out the changes in activities and position in the household of women as they move from middle age, through early old age, to extreme old age. From middle age to early old age, women are at their peak in terms of power and authority within the household. This situation changes as they age, by which time they may be physically incapacitated and their daughters-in-law are themselves middle-aged. She also points to the diversity in the situation of widows, depending on their age, parental status and the stage of their life-cycle at which they became widowed. It is those who are widowed young who are at greatest risk, while those who have grown sons to support them may suffer relatively little if at all as a result of being widowed.

Moving from an academic to a more activist perspective, Germain takes the discussion into the future by outlining a set of concerns and goals for policy-makers. She reviews the papers in this volume, highlighting the commonalities of theoretical and empirical approaches. She also draws out the potential debates generated by the differences in perspective between some of the papers, especially those dealing with the relationship between the status of women and their health. Focusing essentially on the question of women's reproductive health, Germain stresses the need for wide-ranging policy imperatives, aimed not only at promoting reproductive health directly through specific programmatic efforts, but also at promoting it indirectly by seeking to alter the male-centred nature of most social life and decision-making.

Discussion

Gender is only one dimension of the many pervasive social inequalities in our society which threaten people's health and well-being. Other important inequalities include the gap between the rich and the poor, low and high caste, and the rural-urban divide. Those on the wrong side of these divides suffer from poorer conditions of health and poorer effective access to services which are supposed to be universally available.[3] What distinguishes gender from these other forms of inequalities, though, is that it is an *intra-household* inequality, whereas the others are *between-household* inequalities. The disadvantage that women suffer is *superimposed* on the other disadvantages that the household as a whole suffers. Thus, for example, females in rural households suffer the combined disadvantages of the rural-urban divide as well as the gender divide.[4]

[3] See for example Visaria and Gumber 1995.
[4] This is brought out effectively by Crook 1995.

Although there has been a surge of interest in gender issues in India, the question of women's health has not been studied in a systematic way. To help fill this gap, this volume is structured to take a holistic view of the issue, looking at the health of women from childhood to old age. This helps to highlight at which points of the life-cycle women are the most vulnerable, and what are the sources of vulnerability at these ages. Childhood is perhaps the most systematically researched part of the life-cycle from the point of view of gender and health. Information on health during the reproductive years is scanty and scattered, and the older ages are quite under-researched.

The papers in this volume contribute towards a systematic documentation of the extent and nature of health risks during the reproductive years, which include not only those associated with reproduction but also sexually transmitted diseases, including the looming problem of AIDS. The papers also provide insights into how the status of women affects their exposure to these risks, and the potential ramifications of these health problems for the totality of a woman's life, creating vulnerability which can extend far beyond the immediate problem of ill-health. The older ages appear to be the least vulnerable period in women's lives, which has much to do with the fact that their status within the household rises substantially with age. The papers provide a disaggregated view of the situation of older women, bringing out the circumstances which can increase their vulnerability, and analysing the sources of this vulnerability.

Policy-makers in India have paid much superficial attention to the problems specific to women's health, but neglect it in real terms. The clearest illustration of this is that it is difficult to find reliable estimates even of maternal mortality in this country, let alone of the wider aspects of reproductive health. This indicates that there is a lack of interest in women's health, not only at the household level as is widely accepted, but also at the societal and governmental level. The knowledge base on women's health problems needs to be expanded substantially.

Another problem is that existing programmes related to women's health are designed in the mode of targeting services to passive recipients. Yet it is well known in the field of public health that the most effective way to improve overall levels of health is to improve people's own ability to care for themselves. Female literacy and health education programmes are critical in this regard. For too little effort has been made in India to increase health education. Levels of formal education also continue to be abysmally low in India. An acceleration of efforts in health education and education in general are long overdue in India. These simple and conventional approaches could well be the most effective way of transforming women's lives by empowering them to use the existing health, legal and other infrastructure to protect their own well-being. This is the only way to finally relegate to history the situation of women as portrayed as Tagore.

References

Bang, R. A. et al. 1989. 'High Prevalence of Gynaecological Diseases in Rural Indian Women', *The Lancet*. January 14.

Chen, Lincoln C., E. Huq and S. D'Souza. 1981. 'Sex Bias in the Family Allocation of Food and Health Care in Rural Bangladesh', *Population and Development Review* 7(1):55–70.

Crook, Nigel. 1995. 'Urbanization and health in India' in M. Das Gupta, T. N. Krishnan and L. C. Chen (eds.) *Health, Poverty and Development in India*, Oxford University Press.

D'Souza, Stan and L. C. Chen. 1980. 'Sex Differentials in Mortality in Rural Bangladesh', *Population and Development Review* 6(2):257–70.

Das Gupta, Monica. 1987. 'Selective Discrimination against Female Children in Rural Punjab, India', *Population and Development Review* 13(1):77–100.

Das Gupta, Monica, T. N. Krishnan and Lincoln C. Chen (eds.). 1995. 'Introduction' in *Health, Poverty and Development in India*, Oxford University Press.

Das Gupta, Monica. 1994. 'Lifecourse perspectives on women's autonomy and health outcomes', mimeo.

Dyson, Tim and M. Moore. 1983. 'On Kinship Structure, Female Autonomy and Demographic Behaviour in India', *Population and Development Review* 9(1):35–60.

Dyson, Tim. 1987. 'Excess Female Mortality in India: uncertain evidence on a narrowing differential', paper presented at the Workshop on Differential Female Mortality and Health Care in South Asia, Dhaka, Bangladesh.

Faruqee, Rashid and R. S. S. Sarma. 1983. 'Determinants of Fertility and its Decline' in C. E. Taylor et al. (eds.) *Child and Maternal Health Services in Rural India: the Narangwal experiment*, The Johns Hopkins University Press.

Government of India, Ministry of Health and Family Welfare. 1985. 'Family Welfare Programme in India' *Yearbook 1984–85*, New Delhi.

Government of India, Ministry of Health and Family Welfare. 1987. 'Family Welfare Programme in India' *Yearbook 1986–87*, New Delhi.

Jain, S. P. 1982. 'Mortality Trends and Differentials', *Population of India*, United Nations ESCAP Monograph Series No. 10, ESCAP, Bangkok (for figure 1).

Miller, Barbara D. 1981. *The Endangered Sex*, Cornell University Press.

Muhuri, Pradip K. and S. H. Preston. 1991. 'Effects of Family Composition on Mortality Differentials by Sex among Children in Matlab, Bangladesh', *Population and Development Review* 17(3):415–34.

Nadarajah, T. 1983. 'The Transition from Higher Female to Higher Male Mortality in Sri Lanka', *Population and Development Review* 9(2):317–25.

Panigrahi, Lalita. 1972. *British Social Policy and Female Infanticide in India*, Munshiram Manoharlal.

Pebley, Ann and S. Amin. 1991. 'The Impact of a Public-Health Intervention on Sex Differentials in Childhood Mortality in Rural Punjab, India', *Health Transition Review* 1(2):143–69.

Rahman, Omar, A. Foster and J. Menken. 1992. 'Older Widow Mortality in Rural Bangladesh', *Social Science and Medicine* 34(1):89–96.

Vatuk, Sylvia. 1987. 'Authority, Power and Autonomy in the Life Cycle of the North Indian Woman' in P. Hockings (ed.) *Dimensions of Social Life*, de Gruyter Press.

Visaria, Pravin. 1969. *The Sex Ratio of the Population of India*, Census of India 1961, Vol. 1, Monograph No. 10.

Visaria, Pravin and Anil Gumber. 1995. 'Patterns of Health Care Access and Utilization' in M. Das Gupta, T. N. Krishnan and L. C. Chen (eds.) *Health, Poverty and Development in India*, Oxford University Press.

Wyon, John B. and John E. Gordon. 1971. *The Khanna Study*, Harvard University Press.

*Childhood and the
Early Years*

2

Gender Differentials in Child Mortality: A Review of the Evidence

SUNITA KISHOR

I. Introduction

While males outnumber females at birth, their subsequent higher mortality should rapidly erode their numerical advantage. In fact, male mortality rates exceed female mortality rates today in the majority of both developed and developing countries of the world (Preston and Weed 1976; Hammoud 1977; United Nations 1983) conforming to the biologically expected norm (Waldron 1983).

This broad empirical regularity notwithstanding, in several parts of India, as also in other parts of the subcontinent, the norm appears to be of excess female mortality during childhood. This imbalance in the mortality of female as compared to male children can be directly observed in Indian data on infant and child mortality, as well as indirectly, in the high sex ratios (Visaria 1961, 1967), and more specifically, in the high juvenile sex ratios, that minimize the effects of gender differences in migration (Miller 1981). Such persistent excess female mortality reflects unequal access by gender to the means to sustain life, and suggests that females are undervalued to such an extent that their survival is often jeopardized.

In recent years several researchers have sought to explicate both the *motivations* behind the preference for male children and the discrimination against female children, as well as the actual *mechanisms* which translate such preferences into gender differential childhood mortality. While the under-allocation of food and medical resources to females as compared to males is widely recognized as the *mechanism* responsible for excess female mortality, the *motivations* are still being debated.

In order to enable a comprehensive understanding of the nature of excess female mortality in India this paper draws together information from several different sources on the extent and variation in this phenomenon, and the mechanisms and motivations which bring it about. The paper also attempts to identify the impact on excess female mortality of factors such as the level of economic development and patterns of demographic change. Our review of the literature finds that although both economic and cultural motivations for gender discrimination are discussed, most empirical research has in the past focused almost exclusively on either one or the other. In order to assess the simultaneous contribution of both economic and cultural factors, as well as of the interaction between them, this survey also presents the results of recent research which allows for both sets of factors.

The paper is organized as follows: Section II examines the extent and variation in gender differences in mortality across India, using community, state, and district level data from different sources. In Section III are discussed the mechanisms by which preference for sons appears to be transformed into excess female childhood mortality. The underlying economic and cultural bases of gender discrimination are discussed in Section IV, and in Section V we review the available evidence examining the impact of socio-economic development and demographic factors on gender differences in mortality. Section VI summarizes the results from a recent study which has attempted a comprehensive all-India district-level analysis of excess female mortality. Finally, in Section VII we draw conclusions.

II. Evidence of Gender Differences in Mortality

In reviewing evidence for gender differences in mortality during infancy and childhood it is profitable to differentiate between mortality at the different stages of child development: perinatal, neonatal, post-neonatal and beyond infancy.

The little evidence that is available on perinatal and neo-natal mortality in India derives mainly from localized in-depth studies of mortality. In 18 villages of Ludhiana district, in north India, the Narangwal study (Kielmann et al. 1983a) found that between 1970 and 1973, male mortality was 58 per cent of total perinatal mortality. However, beyond the first 7 days, female mortality consistently exceeded male mortality, the former being 53 per cent of neonatal deaths and 59 per cent of total post-neonatal deaths. Also, for the total period of 0–3 years, male deaths constituted only 41 per cent of deaths. The Khanna study (Wyon and Gordon 1971) which was also conducted in Ludhiana district, found that during 1957–59, there were 114.6 male deaths as compared to 168.4 female deaths per 1000 live births before the age of 1 year; between the ages of 1 and 4, there were 19.4 male deaths as compared to 36.9 female deaths per 1000 population per year. Simmons et al. (1982), using survey data from rural Uttar Pradesh, also report higher male than female neonatal mortality, but greater female childhood mortality thereafter. Evidence reported by Miller (1981, p. 81), and from a project in Vellore city, Chingleput District in the South of India (Sundar Rao 1978), on the other hand, shows higher female neonatal mortality but greater male post-neonatal mortality. While these studies are not necessarily representative of the whole of India, they do highlight the regional variation to be found in gender differences in mortality throughout India, even within the first year of life, and suggest that the mortality disadvantage of females increases beyond early infancy.

While all-India data are not available on perinatal and neonatal mortality, we do have such data for infant and child mortality. Table 1 presents data on male and female mortality by age 1 and age 5, per 1000 live births ($q(1)^m$, $q(1)^f$ and $q(5)^m$, $q(5)^f$ respectively), by state, from two different sources: the 1981 Census of India (Census of India 1988) and the Sample Registration Scheme (SRS) of the office of the Registrar General, India. The mortality rates from the Census are estimates derived from census data on children ever born and children surviving, cross-classified by the age of the mother.

Although there is little consistency between the Census and the SRS figures, they do appear to be telling the same story of excess female mortality in most parts of India. Factors worth noting are:

(a) While females have a mortality advantage in some states during infancy, this advantage is lost by the age of 5 in all states except Andhra Pradesh and Kerala. However, even in Kerala and Andhra Pradesh the male advantage is greater during infancy than it is by age 5. The pattern of greater female mortality is revealed consistently by both the Census and SRS data for states other than Haryana and Rajasthan. For Rajasthan and Haryana, data from at least one source (the SRS for Haryana and the Census for Rajasthan) are consistent with this finding. Excess female mortality thus

Table 1: *All-India and state level male and female mortality at ages 1 year and 5 years based on the Census and the SRS data.*

State		Mortality at age 1		Mortality at age 5	
		Census	SRS (IMR 1980)	Census	SRS (1976–1980)
NORTH and NORTH-WEST					
Bihar	M	95	n.a.	131	n.a.
	F	94		153	
	M/F	1.01		0.86	
Gujarat	M	81	112	119	193
	F	84	114	129	212
	M/F	0.96	0.98	0.92	0.91
Haryana	M	87	95	125	150
	F	119	113	153	202
	M/F	0.73	0.84	0.82	0.74
Himachal Pradesh	M	101	n.a.	142	132
	F	89		136	163
	M/F	1.13		0.96	0.81
Jammu & Kashmir	M	78	n.a.	114	123
	F	78		117	135
	M/F	1.00		0.97	0.91
Madhya Pradesh	M	158	144	193	223
	F	140	139	201	241
	M/F	1.13	1.04	0.96	0.93
Punjab	M	74	89	104	132
	F	79	94	118	167
	M/F	0.94	0.95	0.88	0.79
Rajasthan	M	114	105	166	206
	F	114	105	186	200
	M/F	1.00	1.00	0.89	1.03
Uttar Pradesh	M	131	152	174	242
	F	128	168	208	317
	M/F	1.02	0.90	0.84	0.76
SOUTH					
Andhra Pradesh	M	100	102	143	173
	F	82	82	135	170
	M/F	1.22	1.24	1.06	1.02
Karnataka	M	87	71	143	136
	F	74	71	140	147
	M/F	1.18	1.00	1.02	0.93
Kerala	M	55	44	85	71
	F	48	36	76	69
	M/F	1.18	1.22	1.12	1.03
Maharashtra	M	96	73	146	137
	F	89	78	144	150
	M/F	1.08	0.94	1.01	0.91

Contd.

State			Mortality at age 1		Mortality at age 5	
			Census	SRS (IMR 1980)	Census	SRS (1976–1980)
Tamil Nadu		M	89	94	134	167
		F	82	91	131	171
		M/F	1.09	1.03	1.02	0.98
EAST						
Orissa		M	119	143	181	193
		F	111	143	176	207
		M/F	1.07	1.00	1.03	0.93
West Bengal		M	103	n.a.	123	n.a.
		F	87		125	
		M/F	1.18		0.98	
ALL INDIA		M	122	113	147	181
		F	108	115	157	206
		M/F	1.13	0.98	0.93	0.88

Source: *Child mortality estimates of India*, Census of India 1981, Occasional Papers #5 of 1988.

appears to be greater in later childhood than in infancy throughout India.

(b) There is a clear regional patterning of gender differences in mortality: excess female mortality being greatest in the northern states. While both the SRS and Census data indicate that all the northern states (with the exception of Rajasthan) have a sex ratio of mortality at age 5 of less than 1, they also reveal that in two of the five southern states the ratio is greater than 1. For the remaining three southern states, the Census data yield a ratio greater than 1, and the SRS data a ratio less than 1.

(c) There is not only large variation in gender differences in mortality across states, but also in the actual levels of female and male mortality. The highest rates of both female and male mortality are also found in the northern states.

Although state level data do suggest a large range in gender differences in mortality across India, the highly aggregated nature of these data masks the true extent of inter- as well as intra-state variation. While the state level ratio of male to female mortality taken from the Census varies from 0.73 in Haryana to 1.22 in Andhra Pradesh at age 1 and from 0.82 in Haryana to 1.12 in Kerala at age 5, the corresponding ranges at the district level are from 0.53 in a

Table 2: *Cross-classification of districts by male and female mortality rates at ages 1 and 5 according to whether female mortality is greater than less than or equal to male mortality.**

Frequency Percent. Row Percent. Column Percent.	$q(5)^f > q(5)^m$	$q(5)^f \le q(5)^m$	Total
$q(1)^f > q(1)^m$	113 30.87 94.96 51.36	6 1.64 5.04 4.11	119 32.51 100.00 --
$q(1)^f \le q(1)^m$	107 29.23 43.32 48.64	140 38.25 56.58 95.89	247 67.49 100.00 --
Total	220 60.11 -- 100.00	146 39.89 -- 100.00	366 100.00 -- --

*Calculations based on Census data in the India District Development Database (Vanneman and Barnes 1992).

district in Kerala to 1.96 in a district in the Punjab at age 1 and from 0.69 in a district in Uttar Pradesh to 1.23 in a district in Himachal Pradesh at age 5. Thus clearly, to fully understand the variation and the regional patterning of gender differences in mortality at both ages 1 and 5, we need to examine data at the district level.

For this purpose we use the 1981 district level census mortality data as available in the Indian District Development Database (Vanneman and Barnes 1992). This database is the most accurate of all census data sources. The total number of districts is 366 because the smaller states and union territories are all treated as single districts and the districts of Assam, a state not included in the 1981 Census, are excluded.

Table 2 cross-classifies districts according to whether their female mortality rates at ages 1 and 5 are either greater than, or equal to or less than their male mortality rates at ages 1 and 5 respectively. From this table we see that female mortality exceeded male mortality in one-third of all districts by age 1, and in 60 per cent of all districts by age 5. Interestingly, of the 220 districts in which female mortality was in excess of male mortality by age 5, only half were those in which female mortality also exceeded male mortality at age 1; the other half were those in which male mortality was in excess of female mortality at age 1. Thus, while 31 per cent of all 366 districts had excess female mortality at both ages 1 and 5, 29 per cent started with a female advantage in mortality at age 1 and lost it by age 5, and 38 per cent displayed no excess female mortality at either age. Notably, the number of districts that had no excess female mortality at either age 1 or 5 was greater than the number of districts that did have excess female mortality at both ages. Clearly, the problem of excess female mortality is the severest where females do not have a mortality advantage even at age 1. Consequently, it has been suggested (Census of India 1988) that the problem of excess female mortality should be tackled first in districts where females have a mortality advantage at least at age 1.

To examine the regional dispersion of gender differences in mortality in more detail, in Table 3, each of the cell totals of Table 2 has been broken down by region. It is evident from this table that female mortality exceeded male mortality predominantly in districts in northern India. Northern districts accounted almost entirely (95 per cent) for all the districts that had higher rates of female than male mortality at both ages 1 and 5; they accounted for 92 per cent of the

Table 3: Cross-classification by region of male and female mortality rates at ages 1 and 5 according to whether female mortality is greater than, or less than or equal to male mortality.*

	Region	$q(5)^f > q(5)^m$	$q(5)^f \leq q(5)^m$	Total
$q(1)^f > q(1)^m$	All	113	6	119
	North	107 (94.7%)	2 (33.3%)	109 (91.6%)
	South	3 (2.7%)	1 (16.7%)	4 (3.4%)
	East	3 (2.7%)	3 (50.0%)	6 (5.0%)
$q(1)^f \leq q(1)^m$	All	107	140	247
	North	79 (73.8%)	40 (28.6%)	119 (48.2%)
	South	21 (19.6%)	76 (54.3%)	97 (39.3%)
	East	7 (6.5%)	24 (17.1%)	31 (12.6%)
Total	All	220	146	366
	North	186 (84.5%)	42 (28.8%)	(100.0%)
	South	24 (10.9%)	77 (52.7%)	--
	East	10 (4.5%)	27 (18.5%)	--

* Calculations based on Census data in the India District Development Database (Vanneman and Barnes 1992).

districts that had greater female than male mortality by age 1 and for 85 per cent of all districts that had excess female mortality at age 5. Nonetheless, it is also worth noting that districts in the north accounted for almost 29 per cent of all the districts in which male mortality exceeded female mortality by age 5 compared to districts in the south which accounted for over half.

Thus, the evidence on gender differences in mortality in India is unambiguous: female mortality exceeds male mortality during early childhood in large parts of India. Such excesses in female mortality are more likely to occur by age 5 than they are in the first year of life. There is great intra- and inter-state variation in gender differences in mortality. Regions where female mortality is greater than male mortality by ages 1 and 5 are predominantly, though not exclusively, in the north of India. Similarly, although a majority of districts where male childhood mortality exceeds female childhood mortality are found in the south and east of India, almost one-third of districts in the north also have greater male mortality by age 5.

III. The Basis for Gender Differences in Mortality: Evidence of gender biases in allocation of food and medicine

In the influential Mosley and Chen (1984) framework for the study of child survival in developing countries, maternal factors, environmental contamination, nutrient deficiency, injury, and personal illness control have been identified as proximate determinants. Of these, the influence of maternal factors and environmental contamination are not likely to be gender-specific. However, survival risks due to nutrient deficiency and personal illness control, as well as injury, may differ by gender to the extent that the allocation of food and medicine is found to be differentiated by gender.

While some ethnographic evidence garnered by Miller (1981) suggests that differential allocation of food may begin with breast milk, no such discrimination is found in rural Bangladesh (Koenig and Wojtyniak 1987). Also, the age at start of 'other' milk was not found to differ significantly by gender in the Ludhiana villages of the Narangwal study (DeSweemer et al. 1983): the means for 237 males and 198 females being 8 months and 7.3 months, respectively. The lack of significant gender differences in early nutrition of infants is consistent with the earlier finding that excess female mortality is more common in the years beyond infancy.

A review of studies done in the Punjab on weanling-diarrhoea and implied malnutrition of infants, is more conclusive. Both the Khanna study (Gordon, Singh and Wyon 1965) and the Morinda study (Levinson 1972) found infantile diarrhoeal diseases and associated nutritional deprivation to be more widespread among female than male infants. The latter study also finds that males were given more supplementary nutrition than girls. In Matlab, Bangladesh, male children were found to receive both more and higher quality supplementary foods than girls of the same age (Brown et al. 1982).

There is more evidence for the discrimination against females in the allocation of food beyond infancy. In the Narangwal study, females at all ages received only 86 per cent as many calories as males, while receiving 84 per cent as much protein, 69 per cent as much calcium, 88 per cent as much iron and 78 per cent as much vitamin A (DeSweemer et al. 1983). Several other regional studies also reveal imbalances in the caloric intake of women as compared to men (Horowitz and Kishwar 1982), and as compared to their estimated needs (Batliwala 1985; Gulati 1978). A definitive study documenting under-allocation of food to females in Bangladesh is that of Chen, Haq and D'Souza (1981). This study meticulously measured individual food intake in 130 families twice a month for three months. It found the food intake of males to exceed that of females in each age group. Despite adjustments made for the observed differentials for body weight, extra caloric needs of lactating or pregnant women, and assumed activity levels, the gender differentials persisted for the 0–5 and the 45+ age groups.

The under-allocation of food to females is also suggested by studies based on malnutrition data. Sen and Sengupta (1983) find females below 5 years of age to be more malnourished than males in two villages in West Bengal. Malnutrition was found to be more widespread among female children 0–6 years of age than males of the same ages following the 1978 floods in many parts of rural West Bengal (Kynch and Sen 1983; Sen 1988). The greater nutritional disadvantage of rural female children during the 1974–75 famine in Bangladesh is also documented (Bairagi 1986). Discrepancies in weight relative to height, irrespective of socioeconomic class, are found to favour males in rural Punjab

Table 4: Clinical impressions of nutritional status of rural Punjabi children by gender, July 1970.

	Marasmus[a]		Under-nourished[b]		Subtotal		Normal		Total
	No.	%	No.	%	No.	%	No.	%	No.
Male	19	1.7	149	13.4	168	15.1	940	84.9	1108
Female	23	2.5	210	22.7	223	25.2	691	74.8	924
No information	--	--	2	14.4	2	14.4	12	--	14

[a] A child was classified as marasmic when it had little or no subcutaneous fat and wrinkled skin over the buttocks.
[b] This represents mild–moderate protein calorie malnutrition (PCM) including nutritional dwarfing, pre-kwashiorkor.
Source: DeSweemer et al. (1983).

(Horowitz and Kishwar 1982). The relatively greater malnutrition of females in the Narangwal study area is also evident from the data presented in Table 4.

Data on nutritional status at death also indicate that at each level of malnutrition below 80 per cent of Harvard weight median, girls significantly outnumbered boys amongst those that died. However, in the highest category of nutrition (80+ per cent of Harvard weight median) 55 per cent of those that died were males (Kielmann et al. 1983a).

Thus, it appears that female children are at a greater risk both of being malnourished, and of dying when there is malnutrition, than male children. If there is no malnutrition, the mortality rates by gender are more likely to be consistent with the biological expectation of male mortality exceeding female mortality when all else is the same.

Access to medical care in India also appears to be differentiated by gender. In fact, wider sex differentials have been found in medical care than in the allocation of food (Das Gupta 1987; Wyon and Gordon 1971; Chen, Haq and D'Souza 1981). Some research even suggests that differences in the use of health care, are sufficient, even without differences in the allocation of food, to explain gender differences in mortality (Basu 1989). This latter research finds, in a sample of poor households, originally from two contiguous districts of Uttar Pradesh and four contiguous districts in Tamil Nadu, that more girls than boys get no treatment, or non-professional treatment, for illnesses, and that boys are more likely to be seen by a physician. Basu finds no link in her data between malnutrition and gender differences in mortality.

Kelly (1975), in a detailed study of mortality differences of females in the Punjab and Kerala, also attributes the greater survival of females in Kerala mainly to differences in medical care. Miller (1981), using hospital admissions data, reports that two or more boys are admitted to hospitals in the north for every one girl. In the south, the corresponding ratio is 1.2 to 1. Longitudinal data from two Bombay hospitals reveal significant urban differentials in male to female treatment ratios for adults as well as for children (Kynch and Sen 1983). For the villages of the Khanna study in the Punjab, Das Gupta (1987) finds that in the first year of life, expenditure on medical care for sons is 2.34 times higher than for daughters. For these villages Singh, Gordon and Wyon (1962) had earlier found that fewer females than males had medical care during severe illnesses, and that males had a higher quality of care. In the Narangwal study (Kielmann et al. 1983a) 48 per cent of the female children who died had received care in the first 24 hours of their illness, as compared to 64 per cent of boys.

An important aspect of bias in the allocation of both food and medicine is that it appears to be parity-linked. Daughters born into families which already have one daughter are found to be at greater risk of mortality in the Punjab (Das Gupta 1987). In the Narangwal study villages, the average weights and average heights were found to be lower for those children that had two or more male siblings than those with fewer male siblings (Kielmann et al. 1983b). These differences were found to be even higher for those who had two or more male as well as two or more female siblings. In rural Uttar Pradesh, Simmons et al. (1982) find that females born into families with a male less than three years older, are more likely to die. In Bangladesh, Muhuri and Preston (1991) estimate that girls with older sisters are 5.8 times more likely to die than those with no sisters.

IV. The Economic and Cutural Bases of Gender Discrimination, and the Role of Poverty

The existence of bias in the allocation of critical life-sustaining resources has micro-foundations in the household-level evaluations of the relative worth of female versus male children. To the extent that the worth of male children is perceived to be greater than that of female children, scarce life-sustaining resources are likely to be disproportionately allocated to male rather than female children.

The potential worth of a child to a household has both an economic and a cultural dimension, and any analysis of gender differences in mortality which ignores either one remains incomplete. In addition, the question arises whether the availability of resources to the household, i.e. the socio-economic status of the household, will influence their allocation. Greater access to critical life-sustaining resources, by making such resources less scarce, will diminish the economic *need* to discriminate in their allocation. Nonetheless, if the economic and cultural worth of females is found to be inversely related to the socio-economic status of the household, discrimination may be greater in richer households where there is no scarcity of resources. Thus, it is important to examine the economic and cultural rationales for discrimination against females, and how these interact with the scarcity-driven need to discriminate along lines of gender in the allocation of limited life-sustaining resources.

(a) The economic dimension of child worth

Simply put, the under-investment of resources in females can be explained, at least in part, by the low expected economic returns to such investment (Bardhan 1974, 1984, 1988; Rosenzweig and Schultz 1982; Miller 1981). Since females are less likely than males to participate in the labour force, and are consequently less likely than males to contribute to the economic resources of the household, they receive a smaller share of household resources. Hence, female survival will be relatively low whenever women's labour force participation is relatively low. Accordingly, the lower gender differences in mortality in the south, where rice is the major crop, have been explained in terms of the typically female-labour-intensive nature of rice cultivation, and the higher excess female mortality found in the north has been explained in terms of the exclusion of women in the plough-based or mechanized production of wheat (Sen 1990; Bardhan 1974, 1988; Miller 1981).

Empirical support for the economic worth explanation of gender differences in mortality is found by Rosenzweig and Schultz (1982).

They estimate that a rise in the adult female employment rate of 37 per cent would erase the mean survival difference at the household level; alternatively, an increase in female employment by one-half would erase differentials at the district level. However, this research does not allow for the contribution of cultural worth to relative female survival. In addition it fails to test for the level effect of overall mortality rates. This omission may bias the results, especially at the district level, since overall mortality conditions differ greatly across districts.

Miller (1981) finds that 1961 district juvenile sex ratios are never high where female labour force participation is low, although female labour force participation is not necessarily high where the juvenile sex ratio is high. Also, the regression of 1961 district level juvenile sex ratios on male/female disparity in work levels is unable to explain the north/south variation in the juvenile sex ratio. Miller concludes that while there does not appear to be a one-to-one relationship between female work and female survival in rural India, the two are 'clearly related' (p. 121).

Sen (1990) also equates excess female mortality to low female rates of labour force participation. However, as distinct from other proponents of the economic worth perspective, he sees female labour force participation as a means by which women can gain more bargaining power within intra-household 'cooperative conflicts'. The 'gainful' employment of women is likely to make their position less vulnerable, improving their status within the household, as well as in society.

The relative expected earnings of females will, along with expected rates of female labour force participation, determine the expected *value* of returns. One study of six villages in the north and south of India (from Rajasthan to Tamil Nadu), reveals that, on average, female wages are 56 per cent lower than male wages (Ryan and Ghodake 1984), whereas another study found that women earned 70 to 80 per cent of the male wage (Parthasarthy and Rao 1975, as quoted in Harris and Watson 1987). Thus it would seem that the economic worth of females is low not only because they are not expected to participate in income-earning activities, but when they do they can be expected to earn less than men.

The economic worth of females is further reduced, and may even become negative, wherever non-reciprocal marriage payments have to be made. Marriage costs, especially dowry payments, increase the economic burden of having a daughter. In recent years the pressures to pay dowry, its incidence, and costs, all appear to be increasing (Caldwell, Reddy and Caldwell 1988; Billig 1991). In this connection, Miller's (1981) ethnographic evidence shows a strong correlation between regions of high dowry payments and very adverse juvenile sex ratios; where marriage costs are low, juvenile sex ratios are not so adverse. In addition, regions of high marriage costs and regions with low female labour force participation, are positively correlated.

Note that the concept of 'economic worth' ignores the non-wage 'invisible' contributions of women to household consumption and reproduction. Most women in rural areas, with the exception of women in very rich households, do pre- and post-harvest 'indoor' (using a distinction made by Chakravarthy 1977) work (as is clear from the list of agricultural tasks done by women, provided by Kala 1976). However, 'indoor' work appears not to be accorded the same economic worth as 'outdoor' work, even though 'outdoor' work, which takes women beyond the immediate environs of the home, is often culturally taboo for higher caste women. In fact, the importance of domestic and reproductive contributions of females is specifically used by Harris and Watson (1987) in altogether rejecting an exclusively 'economic worth' explanation of gender differences in mortality. They argue that differences in female labour force participation cannot be used to explain variations in the sex ratio, since 'women throughout India are important not only as unvalorized domestic producers and biological reproducers but also as socially responsible for the reproduction of productive labour' (p. 106). In addition, as pointed out by Kalpana Bardhan (1985), productive labour may not be a sufficient or even a necessary condition for female autonomy and voice in a class and hierarchy ridden society.

Thus while the relative level of female labour force participation will be an important determinant of gender differences in mortality, its effect cannot be evaluated independent of the cultural context.

(b) The cultural dimension of child worth

The culturally prescribed power and prestige associated with having male children forms the basis of the relative 'cultural worth' of the sexes. Such power and prestige are conceptualized as net of the perceived economic worth of the two sexes, and derive essentially from the associated kinship structure.

The more patriarchal and male-centred the kinship structure, the more that sons are seen to be the major source of social and political power. Differentiating between the north and the south Indian kinship systems, Dyson and Moore (1983) find that the northern kinship system undermines the cultural worth of females much more than the kinship system of the south. It is in the northern kinship system that (a) cooperation and help are sought only from male blood relatives; (b) rules of marriage dictate patrilocal village exogamy, requiring women to reside with their husband's family outside their natal villages, and consequently, preventing daughters from providing even emotional support to their natal families; (c) inheritance rules specify that women play no role in the inter-generational transfers of fixed property and dowry payments place great burdens on the parents of daughters; (d) family honour depends on the purity of patriarchal descent that should be ensured by enforcing strict controls over women's sexuality by secluding them, curtailing their activities outside the home, and by marrying them off at very young ages. By contrast, in the southern states, the descent group tends to be endogamous, affinity is as important as descent in social, political and economic cooperation, and women sometimes inherit property. Accordingly, Dyson and Moore find that regions of excess female mortality and sex ratios unfavourable to women, high fertility, low ages at marriage of females, and high infant and child mortality, coincide with regions where kinship arrangements approximate those of the north Indian kinship system stereotype.

Miller views kinship arrangements and female labour force participation as 'emic' and 'etic' aspects, respectively, of the same phenomenon of female worth. Her analysis suggests the need to combine the economic and cultural dimensions of child worth in any analysis of gender differences in mortality. This need is also emphasized by research on Kerala which finds the low sex ratio there to be associated with the historical prevalence of the 'southern' kinship system, declining fertility, and the increasing rate of female labour force participation there (Kumar 1989). In rural Punjab, too, the selective discrimination against females has been explained in terms of the strong patriarchal traditions which marginalize women and prevent them from making both economic and non-economic contributions to their natal family (Das Gupta 1987).

However, too much emphasis on the contrast between north and south Indian kinship systems may be misplaced. For one thing, there are likely to be variations in kinship systems within regions as also across regions. For another, as Caldwell and Caldwell (1990) suggest, it is not on contrasts between north and south Indian kinship systems that emphasis should be placed, but on the degree of moderation between them. In fact, as Harris and Watson (1987) have done, emphasis can be equally well placed on the similarity of patrilineal descent and patrilocal residence after marriage for females across regions. They suggest that explanations for excess female mortality need to be sought in the practice of patrilocal exogamy which increases female vulnerability while limiting female autonomy and, following Clark (1983), in caste endogamy mediated by the supply of women.

Cultural worth also derives from religious worth. Children are imbued with religious worth to the extent that roles are prescribed for them by their religion in the fulfilling of earthly tasks. If these roles are sex-specific, and one sex has a larger and more critical role to play than the other, that sex will have relatively greater religious worth. Thus, amongst Hindus, it is the son (preferably the eldest), and not the daughter, who must light the funeral pyre of the parent so as to secure the latter's after-life, and sons who make offerings to give strength to the souls of ancestors. This imbues the male child with greater religious significance. In this context, a daughter appears to be valued by parents only because the giving of a daughter in marriage earns 'punya' (religious merit) for a Hindu (Srinivas 1989). However, significant differences have not been found at least between Hindu and Muslim survival rates by gender (Sopher, 1980; Rosenzweig and Schultz, 1982).

This review of literature on the motivations underlying excess female mortality, reveals that both economic and cultural factors are important. This emphasizes the need to evaluate their simultaneous contribution to excess female mortality.

(c) The impact of socio-economic status on gender discrimination

It has been suggested that it is economic pressures that force households to discriminate in the allocation of scarce resources along lines of culturally determined preference for male offspring (Koenig and D'Souza 1986), i.e. gender discrimination is essentially poverty-driven. Most empirical evidence does not appear to support such a conclusion. In addition, this argument must assume that the economic and cultural worth of children is either independent of or positively associated with the socio-economic status of the household. Such an assumption appears to be untenable in the Indian context where both the extent of cultural controls over women and the sexual division of labour are found to vary by two important dimensions of socio-economic status—caste and land-ownership.

Strict rules of conduct separate castes, especially the upper castes from the lower ones; and, in fact, lower castes are forbidden from the life-styles of the upper castes (Liddle and Joshi 1986). The northern kinship system described above is most typical of the upper castes and often involves the enforcement of strict seclusion of women in the form of 'purdah', forcing their restriction to the domestic sphere. The payment of dowry is also a more common practice amongst the higher castes; by contrast, lower caste marriages often involve bride-price payments. In fact, economically mobile lower castes, aspiring to raise their standing in the caste hierarchy, do so, in part, by increasing controls over their women and by moving from the payment of bride-price to the payment of dowry, as well as by emulating other essential cultural attributes of ritual purity of the upper castes. This process, called 'Sanskritization' by Srinivas (1989, 1962), has the effect of culturally and economically devaluing the women of these castes.

Thus the economic and cultural value of women is likely to differ by caste: women of lower castes having greater economic and cultural value since there are fewer restrictions placed on their autonomy, their mobility, and their activities in the productive sphere. In this context, Rosenzweig and Schultz (1982) find that the proportion of scheduled castes affects gender differences in mortality only through its effect on adult employment rates of females and males. Note however that they find female employment to be lower in districts with a higher share of scheduled caste population. Given that scheduled castes constitute only a minority of district population (on average about 16 per cent), this result is probably a contextual effect arising from the impact that the presence of scheduled castes has on the behaviour of non-scheduled castes.

Although scheduled caste women are likely to be in the labour force in greater numbers than non-scheduled caste women, the fact of the increased presence of lower caste women may lead to a withdrawal of the non-scheduled caste women from the labour force. This withdrawal may be due both to the greater need of upper caste women to distinguish themselves from lower castes, and because of the lesser need for upper caste women to do 'outdoor' work if there are scheduled caste men and women to do it. It is relevant that wealthier districts appear to have more scheduled castes (Schuth 1980).

Among the propertied there is a greater pressure to have sons to inherit land (Miller 1981) and a lesser need for women to enter the labour force. Krishnaji (1987), using data from the Rural Labour Enquiries for 1964–65 and 1974–75, finds that labour households without land contain a higher proportion of females than those with some land. Also, based on 1961 state-wise data for persons of all ages classified by land size, he finds that in all states, with the exception of Assam, Rajasthan and Bengal, a landholding size of less than 1 acre is associated with a sex ratio which favours females. Even in the Punjab (including Haryana) and Uttar Pradesh, which on average have very masculine sex ratios, females outnumber males in the smallest landholding class. In the south, which has relatively low sex ratios, the upper end of the land scale reveals relatively masculine sex ratios. These results are due to narrower mortality differentials between males and females in families with little land, and not due to sex differential emigration.

Support is also found for the positive relationship between landholding and gender differences in mortality by Rosenzweig and Schultz (1982) but only at the district level; at the household level, land-ownership is positively associated with greater female survival when controlling for estimated female labour force participation. Miller (1981) does not find a clear association between property ownership and juvenile sex ratios. In the North, the propertied have more masculine sex ratios, and the non-propertied have sex ratios that tend to favour females; by contrast, in the south, she finds little distinction in the sex ratios of the unpropertied and propertied classes.

Research on gender differences in malnutrition does not find richer households to be necessarily less discriminatory. For example, during famine in Bangladesh, Bairagi (1986) finds the gender difference in malnutrition to be greater among children of the higher socio-economic status group. In research in West Bengal, Sen and Sengupta (1983) report that male-female differentials in undernourishment were greater in agricultural labourer and Harijan households as compared to the households of higher socio-economic status where there was no external food supplementation; but, where there was food supplementation, the gender difference was larger among children from the more economically well-off households. Further, using data from the Calcutta Metropolitan Development Authority, Sen (1988) finds that while health conditions of both male and female residents improved with income, females remained disadvantaged in each expenditure group.

From this discussion two facts emerge: (a) the economic and cultural worth of females is likely to be greater in landless and lower caste households rather than in landed and upper caste ones; and (b) in most empirical analyses, either the relative mortality (or malnutrition) of females is found to be greater in higher caste and landed households, or else it is found not to differ significantly by socio-economic status. As such, there is little evidence that higher socio-economic status actually *increases* the survival chances of females relative to males.

So does this mean that poorer households are less discriminatory? Not necessarily. While the higher economic and cultural worth of women among lower castes and landless, noted above, is likely, it remains a testable hypothesis. In addition, of relevance to the question of discrimination against females is not just the absolute worth of females but their worth relative to males. The relative worth of females in poorer households, though higher than in richer ones, may still not be enough to make males and females equally 'valuable'. Especially, given the increasing pressures towards Sanskritization (Srinivas 1989) and dowry payments (Billig 1991; Caldwell, Reddy and Caldwell 1988) the lower castes and landless may not be immune to the impact of the dominant cultural preference for sons. Nonetheless, any discriminatory allocation of resources between males and females in poorer households may not get reflected in gender differences in mortality since such households may be too poor to have effective control over survival of any of their children, male or female. Thus, while it is probably safe to say that gender discrimination is not poverty-driven, we do not as yet have conclusive evidence that poorer households are necessarily less discriminatory.

Another important aspect of the socio-economic status of a household is its education level. Increasing literacy, Caldwell (1990) has argued, has two multiplicative impacts: (a) it changes the behaviour of individuals in relation to society, and (b) it changes society as a whole by bringing about shifts in the belief system itself. To the extent that increasing literacy exposes individuals to more gender egalitarian Western ideals, greater gender equality may result.

Specifically, literacy of women, marriage patterns, female labour force participation and fertility are all related to one another and to female autonomy: the more literate a woman, the higher the age at marriage and, in general, the lower the required dowry and associated marriage costs. Most of these variables, in turn, have reciprocal relationships with female autonomy (Mason 1987). These manifestations of female autonomy are likely to be reflective of a higher worth of females with consequent results for female survival.

Nonetheless, the empirical evidence even for a positive association between literacy and greater survival of females is mixed. Rosenzweig and Schultz (1982) do not find a significant effect of female education, controlling for employment, on relative female survival at either household or district level. Nonetheless, at least at the household level, the effect of male education on the relative survival of females is significant and negative.

Interestingly, Cleland and Ginneken (1988), using cross-national data, find that although maternal education significantly improves the life chances of children especially beyond infancy, more egalitarian treatment of the sexes does not contribute to this outcome. On comparing women with some education and those with no education in the Punjab, Das Gupta (1987) finds that uneducated women have experienced 50 per cent more child mortality than 'educated' women; however, when the mortality of girls born to mothers who have one or more surviving daughters in the two groups is compared, the rates are found to be similar. Thus the relative risk of mortality for daughters born into households with a daughter(s) already present, may actually be greater, when the mother is educated. In Bangladesh, the risks of mortality are found to fall for both boys and girls with increases in literacy; however, the reduction in risk for boys is much greater than for females (Bhuiya and Streatfield, 1991). On the other hand, in their sample taken from rural Uttar Pradesh, Simmons et al. (1982) find that girls are more likely to survive in relatively more educated households than in uneducated ones; by contrast, the education level of the household does not affect male survival.

One possible explanation for the often contradictory or limited impact of education on female survival is that low levels of education may not be indicative of increased female worth or status in the short run, and may be seen as only a means to attaining traditional goals for women/daughters. For example, some education of females may be necessary to ensure the marriage of a daughter. Educated men, the most desirable husbands, prefer their wives to have some (but less than their own) education. Thus moderate levels of education may be 'optimal' for a daughter's marriageability. Under these circumstances women's literacy may serve the purpose of increasing the domestication of women rather than of empowering them, at least in the short run.

Thus we see that the socio-economic status of the household, whether measured in terms of caste, land-holdings or education, is, in general, not found to increase the survival chances of female children compared to those of male children.

V. The Dynamic Context: Development, demographic change and gender differences in mortality

While the proximate determinants of gender differences in mortality have been identified above to be the relative economic and cultural worth of females, such worth is not independent of the developmental and demographic contexts within which households live and exercise their gender preferences.

Boserup's (1970) pioneering work first revealed that, at least at the initial stages of economic development, women experienced a decline in their status mainly due to the devaluation of their traditional work roles. Indeed, cross-national analysis suggests a curvilinear relationship between female labour force participation and development levels (Pampel and Tanaka 1986). Female labour force participation is high in both the least and the most developed countries, and lowest at medium levels of development.

Within the Indian agricultural context, research suggests that increase in wealth may be associated with lower female labour force participation. Bina Agarwal (1984) on examining the impact of High Yielding Variety (HYV) rice technology on female labour force participation in two southern and one eastern state, finds that while the adoption of HYV rice increases the use of both female and male labour, 'the effect on female family labour use on the farm is found to vary by state, being the net effect of two contradictory tendencies, one relating to the increased requirements for labour on the farm with HYVs and the other relating to family prestige considerations which cause women to withdraw from manual work in the fields as family income increases' (p. A-50). In Rosenzweig and Schultz's (1982) research, female employment at the household level falls as gross cropped area increases, and at the district level it falls as the proportion of irrigated land increases. Further, the response of rural households to both higher male and higher female wage rates appears to be to reduce female labour force participation.

The impact of industrialization on female employment is however not clear. Rosenzweig and Schultz (1982) find that the smaller the scale of industry the higher is female labour force participation and the presence of a factory in a village reduces household level female labour force participation; but the greater the number of factories per household at the district level, the higher is female employment. Note that in this research, all of the various indicators of development are found to affect gender differences in mortality only through their effects on female and male labour force participation.

In the context of kinship arrangements and religion, modernization literature implies that with economic growth, traditional attitudes would be replaced by 'modern' ones (Inkeles and Smith 1974; Lerner 1958; Moore 1979). Industrialization especially has been considered a motor of social change. The break with the land and associated traditional values, the exposure to new technologies and ways of doing things, the need to obtain specialized skills and be literate, and the process of rising expectations, all make for a break with the past, and a need and readiness for innovative behaviour (Lerner 1958; Inkeles and Smith 1974). Further, industrialization draws investment away from land into forms which are more fluid and divisible and can be more easily spread among progeny, irrespective of gender and residence. Thus, while on the one hand, industrialization, if it is heavy and capital intensive, may lower the economic worth of females by leaving them out of this process of development, on the other, it may very well be that it changes attitudes, thereby leading to greater gender equality. Such changes will be reflected in changing family structures which to a large extent index female autonomy in society.

Such an argument implies that higher levels of economic growth will be associated with less discrimination against females on the basis of their sex alone. Indeed, there is cross-national evidence that a lower proportion of primary sector employment and increased urbanization may be related to the increased relative survival of females (Preston and Weed 1976), and urbanization is also found to decrease son preference (Williamson 1973).

Nonetheless, in India, important anthropological work (Srinivas 1962, 1989) suggests (as mentioned earlier) that increasing wealth and upward socio-economic mobility (especially in the context of the caste system) is associated with increasing Sanskritization, i.e. the adoption of the customs of the upper castes derived from Brahmanic culture. As already noted, Brahmanic customs regarding marriage emphasize dowry payments, patrilineal lineage, and the deification of the husband. 'In short, Sanskritization results in increasing the importance of having sons by making them a religious necessity. (Srinivas 1962).

Also, Kynch and Sen (1983) find that urbanization does not appear to significantly improve female life chances and may even decrease them. Based on Sample Registration System data the percentage excess of female mortality for ages between 5 and 20 years, is higher in urban areas than in rural areas. Gender discrimination in the use of urban medical care facilities is also found to be particularly high in this research. However, Rosenzweig and Schultz (1982) do not find that urbanization significantly affects either the relative survival of females or their employment rates.

Development can also act directly, as a determinant of female survival at young ages, because it affects the degree of scarcity of resources. Even when there is discriminatory allocation of resources, such discrimination may not show up in terms of differential mortality if the female share, even if it is well below the share of males, is still enough to sustain life. By increasing resources, development may have the effect of decreasing excess female mortality even when there is no change in discrimination (Ware 1986).

Accordingly, development appears to have the potential to reduce gender differences in mortality directly by increasing the availability of resources, and indirectly by striking at the very roots of the value system which underlies gender discrimination. However the limited amount of empirical evidence available for India does not reveal a negative relationship between development and excess female mortality. This may be partially due to the fact that the specification of the relationship between development and gender differences in mortality in most empirical work has been linear when it may actually be non-linear. Indeed Lenski's (1966) comparative work on social stratification revealed a curvilinear relationship between societal complexity and social inequality, and later research (Martin and Voorhies 1975) suggested that a similar relationship may apply to the specific case of gender inequality.

Gender differences in mortality are also likely to be affected by the prevailing levels of fertility and infant mortality. The most obvious influence will be through the impact of fertility and mortality on the per capita availability of resources. Further, research suggests that mortality may sometimes be a response to high fertility (Scrimshaw 1978) and that the relative degree of unwantedness of a child may be a factor in both mortality and fertility (Taylor, Newman and Kelly 1976). When mortality is high, the female advantage in mortality (which could be expected on biological grounds) is found to be 'relatively small' (UN Population Division 1983, p. 20). Further, female children are most likely to die in families where no additional children or no additional daughters are desired (Simmons et al. 1982).

The fact that higher parity has been found to be associated with greater risk of death for females in the Punjab (Das Gupta 1987), Uttar Pradesh (Simmons et al. 1982) and Bangladesh (Muhuri and Preston 1991) makes high fertility a factor in sex-selective mortality. Interestingly, the excess mortality of higher order females is even higher when the mother is young and educated (Das Gupta 1987). Das Gupta suggests that the falling fertility of the more educated women, in combination with a desire for one to two sons in a completed family size of fewer than three children, may underlie this excess female mortality. It is educated young mothers who are the ones most likely to control their fertility and 'through a better ability to manipulate both their fertility and their children's mortality, educated women are better equipped than others to achieve the family size and sex composition that they desire' (Das Gupta 1987, p. 95).

Also, as already noted, high fertility appears to be another aspect of kinship arrangements associated with the devaluation of women: lower fertility being more characteristic of areas with more gender-neutral practices (Dyson and Moore 1983). In addition, lower fertility is likely to permit higher rates of women's labour force participation.

High fertility combined with falling infant mortality has the effect of broadening the base of the population pyramid. This fact in combination with the socially-culturally constructed customary age difference between wife and husband is creating a 'marriage squeeze' because eligible females greatly outnumber the available males in the appropriate age group. This marriage squeeze, and not increasing 'Sanskritization', has been cited in some recent research, as the critical factor in the substitution of bride-price payments by dowry (Caldwell, Reddy and Caldwell 1988). The shortage of eligible men is further aggravated by the need for caste and status hypergamy in addition to age hypergamy (Billig, 1991). Thus while the relative importance of demographic factors needs to be determined, it does appear that demographic factors are interacting with socio-cultural ones to increase the costs of having daughters.

VI. Explaining District-level Excess Female Mortality: Results from a comprehensive model of gender differences in childhood mortality

Based on the discussion in Sections IV and V it is possible to generate a theoretical model explaining excess female mortality. Such a model is outlined in Figure 1.

We see from Figure 1 that the proximate determinants of excess female mortality in India are hypothesized to be the cultural and economic undervaluation of daughters as compared to males. While cultural undervaluation is the result of male-centred kinship arrangements, economic undervaluation stems mainly from the expectation of low labour force participation by women. Kinship arrangements and female labour force participation are both likely to differ by socio-economic stratification of the population. The cultivation of rice should enhance relative female survival mainly

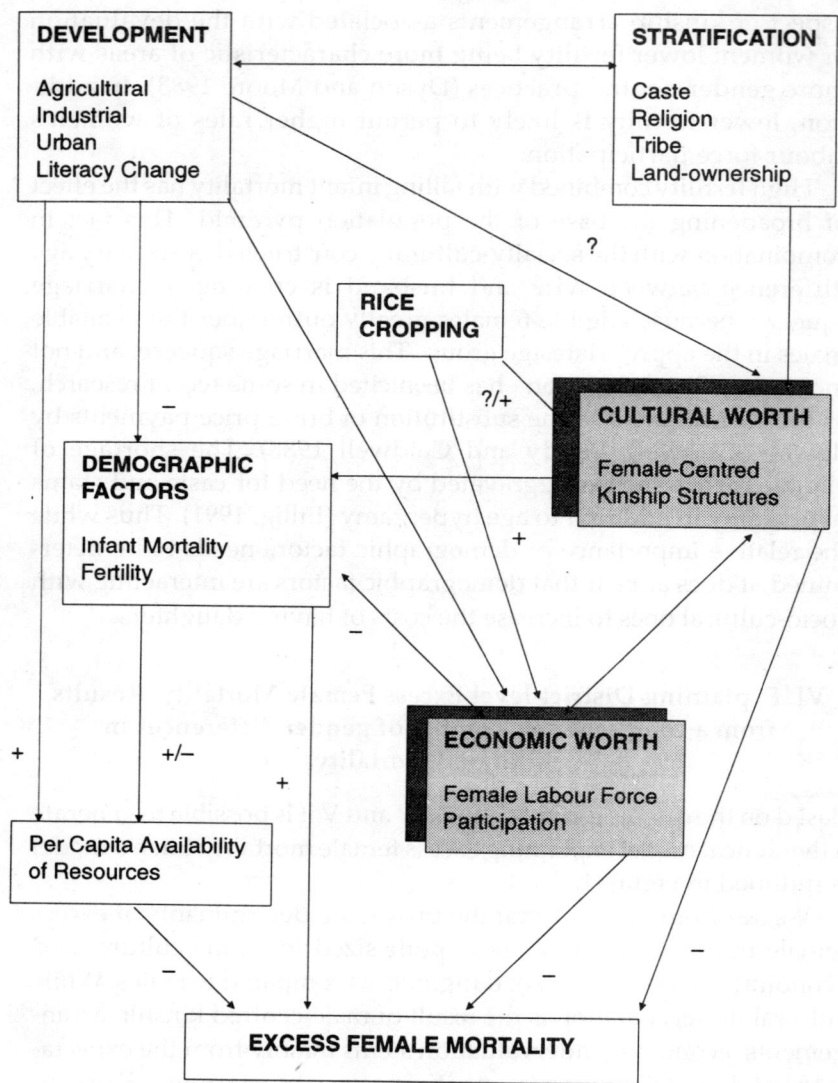

Fig. 1: A model for the analysis of excess female mortality

due to its greater demand for female labour. The level of economic development will influence excess female mortality directly by increasing the overall availability of scarce resources, and indirectly, through its impact on kinship arrangements and female labour force participation. Fertility and infant mortality levels are likely to affect gender differences in mortality directly, as well as indirectly by altering per capita availability of resources. Finally, if regional differences in excess female mortality are due to the corresponding variation in female labour force participation and kinship structures, this model is expected to effectively explain the observed variation.

Recent research (Kishor 1993) has empirically tested this model using all-India district level data from the Indian District Development Database (Vanneman and Barnes 1992) described earlier. While gender differential intra-household distribution of resources is accepted in this research as the basis of gender differences in mortality, the influence of cultural practices, female labour force participation, rice cropping, socio-economic stratification of the population, fertility and mortality levels, development levels and region of the country on the district level gender differences in mortality is sought to be evaluated. The indicators used for the dependent and each of the independent variables are defined in Table 5. The model was tested first for D_j, the measure of gender differences in mortality between ages 0 and 5, and then separately for male and female mortality between the same ages. The most important findings of this research are summarized below.

(1) Gender differences in early childhood mortality are best modelled by simultaneously taking into consideration both kinship structures and female labour force participation. While male-centred kinship arrangements, especially as manifested in the practice of patrilocal exogamy of females, are associated with higher gender differences in mortality, higher female rates of labour force participation are associated with lower gender differences in mortality. Of the two sources of worth, economic and cultural, this research finds that cultural factors may contribute more to explaining excess female mortality across India than does female labour force participation.

(2) Further, cultural and economic factors appear to interact to determine the level of gender differences in mortality. As noted, the higher the level of exogamy, the greater are gender differences in mortality; however, the higher is female labour force participation,

Table 5: *Description of dependent and independent variables used in the analysis of gender differentials of mortality.*

Variables	Definitions
Dependent Variables	
D_j	Log of the ratio of female to male mortality for ages 0–5
Male mortality ratio	Log ratio of male mortality for ages 0–5
Female mortality ratio	Log ratio of female mortality for ages 0–5
Economic-worth Indicator	
Labour force participation ratio	Log of the ratio of female to male labour force participation
Kinship-structure Indicators	
Exogamy	Log of the ratio of female to male migrants
Early marriage ratio	Log ratio of females 15–20 yrs not married
Development Indicators	
Agricultural Product	Log of agricultural product per farm worker
Industrial Product	Log of industrial product per capita
Male literacy ratio	Log ratio of literate males
% Urban	Percent. of population in urban areas
Rice Cropping	
% Rice	Percent. of cropped area under rice
Stratification Indicators	
% Landless	Percent. of agricultural population that is landless
% Castes	Percent. of population that is scheduled caste
% Tribes	Percent. of population that is scheduled tribe
% Muslim	Percent. of population that is Muslim
Mortality Level Control and Fertility	
Male mortality ratio[1]	Log ratio of male mortality for age 0–5
Child–woman ratio	Log of the child–woman ratio
Region Dummies	
East	Eastern states
South	Southern states
North	Northern states

Note: The analysis was based on the Indian districts (a total of 357) as defined in the Indian District Development Database.

[1]This variable is used as a control for mortality in the analysis of D_j, and is also analysed separately as a dependent variable.

the weaker is the impact of exogamy. Conversely, the greater the female labour force participation, the higher is the relative survival of females and this association is weaker for lower exogamy, and is insignificant if there is no exogamy (Exogamy = 0). Thus, in combination, low economic and low cultural worth reinforce one another to produce especially higher levels of excess female mortality. However, this result also implies that in the reduction of excess female mortality, women's economic activity may substitute for male-centred kinship arrangements, especially where such arrangements are very unfavourable; and female-centred kinship arrangements can substitute for especially low female economic participation.

(3) The separate analysis of male and female mortality also reveals that wherever patrilocal exogamy is practised, irrespective of the level of women's labour force participation, the probability of male survival is always enhanced; by contrast, that of females is actually lowered at mean levels of female labour force participation, and at best, is left unaffected when rates of female labour force participation are exceptionally high. Contrary to most hypotheses, female labour force participation is associated with higher, not lower, male and female mortality. The negative relationship observed between female labour force participation and gender differences in mortality is due to the fact that female labour force participation increases male mortality more than female mortality.

(4) Regions where rice is a major crop do reveal much lower gender differences in mortality. However, this effect is not explained by either higher rates of female labour force participation or variations in kinship structures.

(5) Districts with high proportions of Muslims, scheduled castes or landless, do not appear significantly different from other districts with respect to gender differences in mortality. While a greater proportion of tribals in a district is associated with lower gender differences in mortality, this effect is explained by variations in kinship practices.

(6) With higher development, female children do not experience an improvement in their survival chances relative to male children. In fact, high levels of agricultural development decrease the life chances of females while leaving those of males unaffected, while urbanization increases the life chances of males more than females.

Industrialization, too, is associated with higher gender differences in mortality. Only increases in male education do not affect gender differences in mortality because they tend to decrease both male and female mortality equally. Clearly, gender-based discrimination in the allocation of resources does not decrease with development. Such discrimination persists, and can increase, even when availability of resources is not a constraint.

(7) While higher fertility is associated with significantly greater gender differences in mortality, no association is found between male mortality (the indicator for the mortality level) and excess female mortality.

(8) Neither cultural variation in kinship structures nor differences in agricultural ecology and the associated demand for female labour, are able to explain the average difference in excess female mortality between the north and the south of India. The results suggest that a higher mortality of girls as well as a lower mortality of boys in the north as compared to the south comprise this difference.

VII. Conclusions

State and district level data presented early in this paper affirm that the considerable excess female mortality found in large parts of India is regionally patterned and that excess female mortality is, in general, greater in the north of India than in the south or east. Nonetheless, district level data reveal large amounts of intra-state variation. This implies that states that on average have low gender differences in mortality may very well have districts with high gender differences in mortality; as also, states that on average have high gender differences in mortality do contain districts with low gender differences in mortality.

We also found that while more districts had excess female mortality by age 5 than by age 1, one-third of all districts had higher rates of female than male mortality even by age 1. It is notable that, of these districts, only 5 per cent did not have excess female mortality by age 5. Clearly, discrimination against female children starts early, and is maintained as the female child grows.

A critical manifestation of this discrimination is the under-allocation of medicine and food to female offspring. This gender bias in the allocation of critical life-sustaining resources appears to be the mechanism that gives rise to gender differences in mortality.

Both theoretical and empirical evidence supports the cultural and economic bases of gender differences in childhood mortality. In fact, cultural and economic undervaluation of females interact giving rise to especially high levels of excess female mortality. This suggests that excess female mortality can be decreased, either by increasing women's economic activity, especially where male-centred kinship arrangements predominate, or by introducing female-centred kinship arrangements where female economic participation is especially low.

While the survival of both male and female children appears to rise with the socio-economic status of the household, there is no evidence of a corresponding decline in gender discrimination as manifested in gender differences in mortality or malnutrition. Nonetheless, we know little about whether poorer, lower caste, and landless households actually *discriminate* less against females than do richer, higher caste, and landed households. Without appropriate data, we can only speculate. It may be that households of lower socio-economic status discriminate less than those of higher socio-economic status, or else it may be that due to lack of resources, gender discrimination in such households makes no difference to the relative survival of males and females. By contrast, in high caste and landed households both the means and the motivations are likely to exist to effectively manipulate mortality differences.

Most literature has emphasized the role of rice cultivation in enhancing female status. Indeed, relative female survival does appear to be greater where rice is the major crop. However, neither female labour force participation nor kinship practices are able to explain this effect. At the minimum this belies any simplistic explanations of the relationship between rice-based agriculture and gender inequality in terms of the greater demand for female labour in rice cultivation. Similarly, no facile explanation of the north-south differences in mortality is possible either in terms of agricultural ecology or variation in rates of female labour force participation in the two regions.

The effect of fertility and infant mortality on excess female mortality has not been adequately researched. While excess female mortality appears to be positively associated with fertility, little is conclusively known about its relationship with infant mortality. In addition, we need a dynamic analysis to determine what impact the combination of falling fertility and falling infant mortality has on the relative survival of females.

Although the general expectation based on the assumptions of modernization theory, as well as the mortality experience of the West, has always been that gender differences in mortality will diminish with development, there appears to be little empirical evidence supporting such a conclusion for India. Indeed, in the Kishor research, agricultural development, industrialization and urbanization are all associated with higher, not lower, excess female mortality. Only higher literacy levels appear to benefit both males and females equally. However, the impact of development on relative female survival over time remains to be evaluated.

Finally, we conclude that the unequal access to life of girls in India is widespread and has both economic and cultural roots. Although development appears to affect these roots, it is too slow, or too little, to better the life chances of little girls and, at least, in cross-sectional analysis actually appears to decrease them. The proximate economic and cultural variables determining female discrimination need to be manipulated *directly* to reduce gender inequality and ensure the survival of young girls. It is suggested that this can be quite effectively done by attempting to increase the economic worth of females where their cultural worth is particularly low, or by raising their cultural worth where their economic worth is particularly low.

References

Agarwal, Bina 1984, 'Rural women and high yielding variety rice technology'. *Economic and Political Weekly* 19: A39–A52.

Bairagi, Radheshyam 1986, 'Food Crisis, nutrition, and female children in rural Bangladesh', *Population and Development Review* 12, #2 (June).

Bardhan, Kalpana 1985. 'Women's work, welfare and status'. *Economic and Political Weekly* XX, #51 and 52 (21–28 December).

Bardhan, Pranab K. 1974. 'On life and death questions'. *Economic and Political Weekly* 9: 1293–1304.

———1984, *Land, Labor, and Rural Poverty*. New York: Columbia University Press.

———1988. 'Sex disparity in child survival in rural India'. Pp. 472–82 in *Rural Poverty in South Asia* edited by T. N. Srinivasan and P. K. Bardhan. Oxford University Press.

Basu, Alaka Malwade 1989. 'Is Discrimination in food really necessary for explaining sex differentials in childhood mortality?' in *Population Studies* 43: 193–210.

Batliwala, S. 1985. 'Women in poverty: The energy, health and nutrition syndrome' in Devaki Jain and Nirmala Banerjee (eds.) *Tyranny of the Household: Investigative Essays on Women's Work*. New Delhi: Shakti Books.
Bhuiya, Abbas and Kim Stretfield 1991. 'Mothers' education and survival of children in a rural area of Bangladesh', *Population Studies*, 45: 253–64.
Billig, Michael S. 1991. 'The Marriage Squeeze on High-Caste Rajasthani Women', *The Journal of Asian Studies* 50, #2: 341–60.
Boserup, Ester. 1970. *Women's Rule in Economic Development*. New York: St. Martin's.
Brown, K.H., R.E. Black, S. Becker and J. Sawyer 1982. 'Consumption of foods and nutrients by weanlings in rural Bangladesh', in *American Journal of Clinical Nutrition*, 36, 878.
Caldwell, John C. 1990. 'Cultural and social factors influencing mortality levels in developing countries', *Annals of the American Academy of Political and Social Science* 510 (July): 44–59.
Caldwell, John C., P.H. Reddy and P. Caldwell 1988. *The Causes of Demographic Change: Experimental Research in South India*. Wisconsin: University of Wisconsin Press.
Caldwell, Pat and John C. Caldwell 1990. 'Gender implications for survival in South Asia'. Health Transition Working Paper #7. National Centre for Epidemiology and Population Health, Australian National University.
Census of India 1988. *Child Mortality Estimates*. Census of India, Occasional Papers, No. 5 of 1988. Demography Division, Office of the Registrar General, Ministry of Home Affairs, New Delhi, India.
Chakravarthy, Kumaresh 1977. 'Regional Variations in Women's Employment: A Case Study of Five Villages in Three Indian States'. Programme on Women's Studies ICSSR (mimeo).
Chen, L.C., E. Huq, and S. D'Souza 1981. 'Sex bias in the family allocation of food and health care in rural Bangladesh', *Population and Development Review* 7: 55–70.
Clark, Alice W. 1983 'Limitations on female life chances in rural central Gujarat', *Indian Economic and Social History Review* 20: 1–25.
Cleland, J. G. and J. K. van Ginneken 1988. 'Maternal education and child survival in developing countries: The pathways of influence', *Social Science and Medicine* 27, #12: 1357–68.
Das Gupta, Monica 1987. 'Selective discrimination against female children in rural Punjab, India', *Population and Development Review* 13: 77–100.
DeSweemer, Cecile, A. A. Kielmann and Robert L. Parker 1983. 'Indicators of Nutritional Risk' in A.A. Kielmann and Associates (eds.) *Child and Maternal Health Services in Rural India: The Narangwal Experiment* Vol. 1. Baltimore: The Johns Hopkins Press.
Dyson, Tim and Mick Moore. 1983. 'On kinship structure, female autonomy and demographic balance', *Population and Development Review* 9: 35–60.
Gordon, John E., Sohan Singh and John B. Wyon 1965. 'Causes of death at different ages by sex and by season in a rural population of Punjab 1957–59', *Indian Journal of Medical Research*, Sept.: 906–17.
Gulati, Leela 1978. 'Profile of a female agricultural labourer', *Economic and Political Weekly* (Review of Agriculture) 13, #12, 25 March.
Hammoud, E. I. 1977. 'Sex Differentials in Mortality', *World Health Statistics Report*, #3, 30: 170–206.

Harris, Barbara and Elizabeth Watson 1987. 'The Sex Ratio in South Asia' in J. H. Momsen and J. G. Townsend (eds.) *Geography of Gender in the Third World*. State University of New York Press.

Horowitz, B. and Madhu Kishwar 1982. 'Family Life–The unequal deal: Women's condition and Family life among agricultural labourers and small farmers in a Punjab village', *Manushi* No. 11.

Inkeles, Alex and David H. Smith 1974. *Becoming Modern: Individual Change in Six Developing Countries*. Cambridge, Mass.: Harvard University Press.

Kala, C.V. 1976. 'Female Participation in farm work in Kerala', *Sociological Bulletin* 25, #2.

Kelly, Narinder, O. 1975. 'Some socio-cultural correlates of Indian sex ratios: Case studies of Punjab and Kerala'. Unpublished doctoral dissertation, University of Pennsylvania.

Kielmann, Arnfried A., Cecile DeSweemer, Robert L. Parker and Carl E. Taylor 1983a. 'Analysis of Morbidity and Mortality' in A.A. Kielmann and Associates (eds.) *Child and Maternal Health Services in Rural India: The Narangwal Experiment* Vol. 1. Baltimore: The Johns Hopkins Press.

——, Cecile DeSweemer, William Blot, Inder S. Uberoi, A. Douglas Robertson, and Carl E. Taylor 1983b. 'Impact on Child Growth, Nutrition and Psychomotor Development' in A. A. Kielmann and Associates (eds.) *Child and Maternal Health Services in Rural India: The Narangwal Experiment* Vol. 1 Baltimore: The Johns Hopkins Press.

Kishor, Sunita 1993. 'May God Give Sons to All: Gender and Child Mortality in India', *American Sociological Review*, Vol. 58, #2: 247–65.

Koenig, Michael A. and Stan D'Souza. 1986. 'Sex Differences in Childhood Mortality in Rural Bangladesh', in *Social Science and Medicine* 22, #1: 15–22.

—— and B. Wojtyniak 1987. 'Excess female mortality during infancy and early childhood: Evidence from rural Bangladesh', paper presented at BAMANEH-SSRC Workshop on Differential Female Mortality and Health Care in South Asia (Dhaka, 4–8 January 1987).

Krishnaji, N. 1987. 'Poverty and sex ratio: some data and speculations', *Economic and Political Weekly* 22: 892–97.

Kumar, Gopalkrishna. 1989. 'Gender, differential mortality and development: the experience of Kerala', *Cambridge Journal of Economics* 13: 517–39.

Kynch, Jocelyn and Amartya Sen 1983. 'Indian women: Well-being and survival', *Cambridge Journal of Economics* 7, #3/4, Sept–Dec.

Lenski, Gerhard 1966. *Power and Privilege: A theory of social stratification*. New York: McGraw-Hill.

Lerner, Daniel 1958. *The Passage of Traditional Society: Modernizing the Middle East*, Glencoe: The Free Press.

Levinson, Franklin J. 1972. *Morinda: An Economic Analysis of Malnutrition among Young Children in Rural India*. MIT/Cornell University Press.

Liddle, Joanna and Rama Joshi 1986. *Daughters of Independence: Gender, Caste and Class in India*. Zed Books Ltd.

Martin, M. Kay and Barbara Voorhies 1975. *Female of the Species*. New York: Columbia University Pres.

Mason, Karen Oppenheim 1987. 'The impact of women's social position on fertility in developing countries', *Sociological Forum* 2, #4: 718–45.

Miller, Barbara D. 1981. *The Endangered Sex: Neglect of Female Children in Rural North India*. Ithaca: Cornell University Press.
Moore, Wilbert E. 1979. *World Modernization: The limits to convergence*. New York: Elsevier.
Mosley, W. Henry and L.C. Chen 1984. 'An analytical framework for the study of child survival in developing countries' in W. Henry Mosley and Lincoln C. Chen (eds.) *Child Survival: Strategies in Research*. Population and Development Review, Supplement, Vol. 10.
Muhuri, Pradip K. and Samuel H. Preston 1991. 'Mortality Differentials by sex in Bangladesh', *Population and Development Review* 17, #3 (Sept.).
Pampel, Fred C. and Kazuko Tanaka. 1986. 'Economic development and female labor force participation: A reconsideration', *Social Forces* 64: 599–619.
Parthasarthy G. and G.D. Rama Rao 1973. 'Employment and unemployment among rural labour households: a study of west Godavari', *Economic and Political Weekly* Review of Agriculture, 8(52) A118–32 (December).
Preston, Samuel H. and J. A. Weed 1976. 'Causes of Death Responsible for International and Intertemporal Variation in Sex Mortality Differentials', *World Health Statistics Reports*, #4, 30: 144–88.
Ramachandran, K. V. and V. A. Deshpande 1964. 'The Sex Ratio at Birth in India by Regions', *The Milbank Memorial Quarterly* 42 #2: 84–95.
Rosenzweig, M. R. and T. P. Schultz 1982. 'Market opportunities, genetic endowments and the intrafamily distribution of resources: child survival in rural India', *American Economic Review*: 803–15.
Ryan, J. G. and R. D. Ghodake 1984. 'Labor market behaviour in rural villages in south India: effects of season, sex and socioeconomic status' in H. P. Binswanger and M. R. Ronsezweig (eds.) *Contractual Arrangements. Employment and Wages in Rural Labor Markets in Asia*. New Haven: Yale University Press.
Schuth, Sister Katarina 1980. 'Village Literacy and its Correlates: A Mysore Case Study' in Sopher (ed.) *An Exploration of India*. Cornell University Press.
Scrimshaw, Susan C. M. 1978. 'Infant mortality and behaviour in the regulation of family size', *Population and Development Review* 4, #3.
Sen, Amartya K. 1988. 'Family and food: Sex bias in poverty.' Pp. 453–80 in T. N. Srinivasan and P. K. Bardhan (eds.) *Rural Poverty in South Asia*. Delhi: Oxford University Press.
──────1990. 'More than 100 million women are missing', *New York Review of Books*, 20 December.
──────and Sunil Sengupta 1983. 'Malnutrition of rural children and the sex bias', *Economic and Political Weekly* Annual Number, May.
Simmons, George B., Celeste Smucker, Stan Bernstein and Eric Jensen 1982. 'Post-neonatal mortality in rural India: Implications of an economic model', *Demography* 19, #3: 371–389.
Singh, Sohan, John E. Gordon and John B. Wyon 1962. 'Medical care in fatal illnesses of a rural Punjab population', *Indian Journal of Medical Research* 50, #6 (November): 865–80.
Sopher, D. E. 1980. *An Exploration of India: Geographical Perspectives on Society and Culture*. Cornell University Press.
Srinivas, M. N. 1962. *Caste in Modern India and other Essays*. Bombay: Asia Publishing House.

———— 1989. *The Cohesive Role of Sanskritization and Other Essays*. Delhi: Oxford University Press.

Sunder Rao, P. S. S. 1978. Unpublished finding of the Vellore Project. Vellore, Madras.

Taylor, C. E., Jeanne S. Newman and Narindar U. Kelly. 1976. 'The Child Survival Hypothesis,' *Population Studies* 30, # 2.

United Nations Population Division 1983. 'Patterns of Sex Differentials in Mortality in Less Developed Countries' in Alan D. Lopez and L.T. Ruzicka (eds.) *Sex differentials in mortality: Trends, determinants and consequences*. Canberra: Australian National University.

Vanneman, Reeve and Douglas Barnes. 1992. *Indian Development District Database*. Unpublished Codebook available from Center for Population, Gender and Social Inequality, University of Maryland, College Park, Maryland.

Visaria, Pravin M. 1961. *The Sex Ratio of the Population of India*, 1961 Census of India, Vol. I Monograph 10 New Delhi: Office of the Registrar General.

————1967. 'The sex ratio of the population of India and Pakistan and regional variation during 1901–1961', in A. Bose (ed.), *Pattern of Population Change in India 1951–61*. New Delhi: Allied Publishers.

Waldron, Ingrid. 1983. 'The Role of Genetic and Biological Factors.Sex Differences in Mortality', in Alan D. Lopez and L.T. Ruzicka (eds.), *Sex differentials in mortality: Trends, determinants and consequences*. Canberra: Department of Demography, Australian National University.

Ware, H. R. 1986. 'Differential mortality decline and its consequences for the status and roles of women', in *Consequences of Mortality Trends and Differentials*, Population Studies, No. 95 United Nations, New York.

Williamson, Nancy E. 1976. *Sons or Daughters: A cross-cultural survey of parental preferences*. Beverly Hills: Sage Publications.

Wyon, John B. and John E. Gordon 1971. *The Khanna Study*. Harvard University Press.

3

Women's Capabilities and Infant Mortality: Lessons from Manipur

A. K. SHIVA KUMAR

1. Introduction

It has been customary to examine the relationship between levels of per capita incomes and infant mortality rates (IMRs), with the expectation that lower levels of infant mortality will be associated with higher levels of incomes.[1] Empirical evidence from a number of 'low income' countries and regions of the world, such as China, Costa Rica, Cuba, Jamaica, Kenya, Zimbabwe, Botswana and Sri Lanka indicates, however, that high levels of incomes need not be a prerequisite for low IMR.[2] In these countries and regions, governments with a strong political commitment to social development, and a mix of appropriate policy interventions in the health sector, have been able to record impressive gains in health and welfare indicators. In this context, Kerala in India has frequently been cited as an example of a 'positive' outlier: a state whose IMR is much lower than is predicted by its level of per capita income.

Figure 1 plots the IMRs of 25 Indian states against their per capita state domestic products (SDPs). India's overall IMR in 1981 was 110 per 1000 live births and the per capita level of income was Rs 1627. The IMR in the country varied from 32 per 1000 live births

---

[1]See, for instance, Preston (1976), Cochrane (1980), Gwatkin and Brandel (1981), and World Bank (1984).
[2]See, for example, Caldwell (1986); Drèze and Sen (1989); and Rockefeller Foundation (1985).

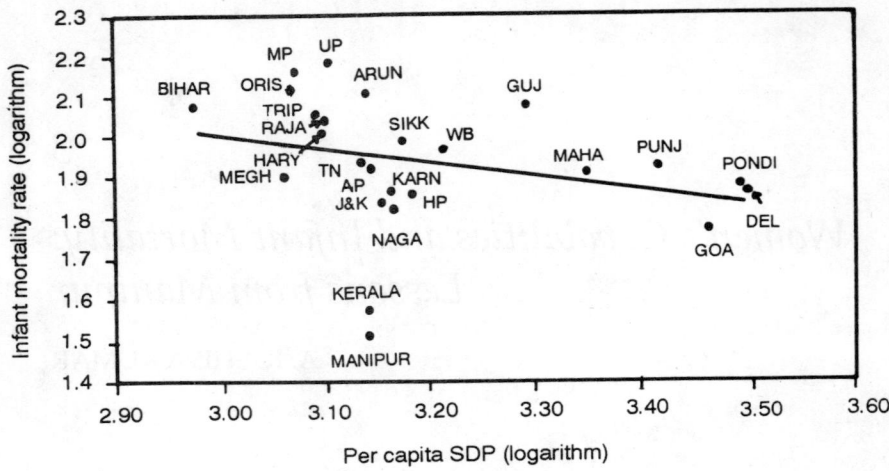

Fig. 1: Infant Mortality Rate and Per Capita SDP for 25 Indian States and UTs, 1981.

log (IMR) = 3.1281 − 0.3758 log (SDP); R Square = 0.11

Code: AP = Andhra Pradesh: Arun = Arunachal Pradesh; Del = Delhi; Guj = Gujarat; Hary = Haryana; HP = Himachal Pradesh; J & K = Jammu and Kashmir; Karn = Karnataka; MP = Madhya Pradesh; Maha = Maharashtra; Megh = Meghalaya; Naga = Nagaland; Oris = Orissa; Pondi = Pondicherry; Punj = Punjab; Raja = Rajasthan; Sikk = Sikkim; TN = Tamil Nadu; Trip = Tripura; UP = Uttar Pradesh; WB = West Bengal

Source: Ministry of Health and Family Welfare (1990) and Census of India (1988)

in Manipur to 150 in Uttar Pradesh. Two prominent positive outliers, however, emerge: Manipur and Kerala, both states recording low IMRs at low levels of incomes. Only a weak negative relationship exists between SDP and IMR. This should, however, not come as a surprise as several factors intervene in the income–infant mortality linkage. Sen (1981a, 1984, 1985, 1989), for instance, points out that access to health care may be constrained, not so much by a shortage of incomes, but by a shortage of services, and by socio-cultural factors and other considerations of race, class and gender that restrict people's access. Again, factors such as levels of environmental pollution, maternal skills, and personal hygiene that are known to have an impact on the health of children may not be correlated with income in any predictable manner.

Table 1 presents salient demographic features for two groups of Indian states: for Manipur and Kerala, the low IMR states, and for Bihar, Madhya Pradesh, Rajasthan and Uttar Pradesh, the four high IMR 'BIMARU' states.[3] Analysis of the experience of 'good-health-at-low-cost' countries and regions point to four common elements in the strategies: political and social will, equitable distribution of public health facilities, assurance of adequate calorie intake, and an emphasis on education, particularly among women.[4] Table 2 presents basic data for the two sets of states on some of these variables.[5] Kerala and Manipur are similar in that both have a better availability and more equitable distribution of health facilities, though the physical provisioning in Kerala is far better than in Manipur. Manipur currently, and Kerala in the past, have also apportioned a higher-than-average percentage of their expenditures to the health sector. On the other hand, per capita calorie intake is higher in Manipur than in Kerala. But the most striking difference is that unlike in Kerala, the levels of female literacy in Manipur are not high in absolute terms.

Considerable attention has focused on Kerala, but much less is known about the Manipur phenomenon.[6] This paper examines the case of Manipur, and in attempting to explain the state's low IMR, suggests that greater women's freedoms, higher levels of maternal advancement, increased political participation, stronger social organization, and an overall system of entitlement protection operate synergistically to lower infant mortality in Manipur.

---

[3] The reference to the high IMR states as BIMARU states is attributed to Prof. Ashish Bose who coined the term by using the first letters of each state. BIMARU in Hindi means 'suffering from ill health'.
[4] See Rockefeller Foundation (1985) and in particular, Warren (1985).
[5] In addition to the generally poor quality of data on the health sector, there are several problems with the definition and measurement of many of these factors, such as social and political will, per capita calorie intake, non-inclusion of indigenous systems of health, and so on. Discussions on problems of data can be found in Kumar (1992) and Murray (1987).
[6] There is an extensive body of literature on Kerala that has grown since the mid-1970s, when the state gained recognition for its welfare successes. For a discussion on health-related aspects, see in particular, United Nations (1975), Krishnan (1984, 1985), Panikar and Soman (1984), Panikar (1985), Nag (1985), and Bhat and Irudayarajan (990).

Table 1: Salient demographic features: Manipur, Kerala and the BIMARU states

	Area in sq. km	Population (millions)	Density persons per sq. km	Females per 1000 males	Proportion of urban population %	Infant mortality rate	Child-Woman ratio*	Dependence ratio**	Total fertility rate	Crude birth rate	Crude death rate	State domestic product (Rs.)
	1991	1991	1991	1991	1991	1981	1981	1981	1981	1981	1981	1981
	[1]	[2]	[3]	[4]	[5]	[6]	[7]	[8]	[9]	[10]	[11]	[12]
Manipur	22,327	1.9	82	961	28	32	534	827	4.7	27	7	1382
Kerala	38,863	29.0	747	1040	26	37	409	741	2.8	26	7	1385
Bihar	173,877	86.3	497	912	13	118	597	935	5.7	37	14	943
Madhya Pradesh	443,446	66.1	149	932	23	142	611	901	5.2	39	14	1181
Rajasthan	342,239	43.8	128	913	23	108	656	946	5.2	38	17	1220
Uttar Pradesh	294,411	138.7	471	882	20	150	629	946	5.8	40	16	1272
India	3,287,263	843.9	267	929	26	110	546	854	4.5	34	13	1627

* Child-woman ratio is the ratio of children in the age group 0-4 to 1000 women in the age group 15-49.
** Dependency ratio has been calculated as the number of persons in age groups 0-14 and 60 and above per 1000 persons in the age group 15-59.

Source: Columns [1], [2], [3] and [4] from Census of India (1991a); Column [5] from Census of India (1991b); Column [6] from Ministry of Health and Family Welfare (1989); figure of Manipur is from Census of India (1988). Columns [7], [10], [11], [12] from Ministry of Health and Family Welfare (1989). In column [9], the figure for Manipur is from Office of Registrar General (1987); all other figures are from Office of Registrar General (1985a).

Table 2: Basic data on health expenditure allocations, availability and utilization of health services, and female literacy

	Health expenditure as a % of annual state expenditure 1980–81	Hospital beds per 100,000 population early 1980s	Hospital beds in rural areas as % of total 1987	% distribution of sample births by beds in type of medical attention at birth, 1981			Per capita daily calorie intake in rural areas (cal) 1983	Adult female literacy rate (15 plus) % 1981
				Institutions	Delivery conducted by trained personel	Delivery conducted by untrained personel		
	[1]	[2]	[3]	[4]	[5]	[6]	[7]	[8]
Manipur*	16.5	89	28	2	5	93	2296	29
Kerala	13.1	169	51	53	17	30	1844	71
Bihar	11.1	32	9	8	5	86	2189	13
Madhya Pradesh	11.9	33	6	11	7	82	2323	16
Rajasthan	17.4	53	6	3	13	84	2433	12
Uttar Pradesh	9.4	42	5	6	23	71	2399	14
India	11.7	73	14	18	19	63	2221	26

Note: Figures have been rounded.
* Data for Columns 5–7 for Manipur are from UNICEF (1983), and do not relate to 1981 alone; they include deliveries in earlier periods as well.

Source: Column [1] has been computed from Reserve Bank of India (1982).
Column [2] is from the Census Atlas, 1981, for each state.
Column [3] from Ministry of Health and Family Welfare (1987).
Column [4], [5] and [6] are from Office of Registrar General (1985a).
Columns [7] is from Sarvekshana (1939).
Column [8] is from Census of India (1981a).

2. The Female Literacy–Infant Mortality Linkage

There is strong evidence to show that levels of child mortality are negatively correlated with women's education.[7] It has been much more difficult, however, to establish the pathways of influence. Several hypotheses have been put forward. Caldwell (1979), for instance, suggests that education empowers women by leading to (a) reduced fatalism in the face of children's ill health and a more ready acceptance of 'western' medicine; (b) greater capability for manipulating the world resulting from better awareness, greater confidence in seeking out and gaining access to quality care, and enhanced self-esteem; and (c) a shift in the traditional intrafamily balance of power away from the patriarch and the mother-in-law such that children become beneficiaries of a better allocation of domestic resources. Cleland and van Ginneken (1988) point out that higher levels of female literacy could lead to favourable changes in reproductive behaviour (namely, its influence in delaying marriages, leading to early cessation of childbearing, and better spacing of children), enhanced socio-economic status of families, better use of health services, and improved domestic care of children, all of which contribute to lowering infant mortality rates.

Figure 2 plots IMRs for 30 Indian states against the levels of adult female literacy. While the inverse relationship between female literacy and IMR is generally true, two features are striking. The first, as already pointed out, is the co-existence of low IMR with a low level of absolute literacy in Manipur. If we look at the age group of 15 to 34 years, less than 34 per cent of women in Manipur were literate against the corresponding figure of 86 per cent for Kerala in 1981 (Table 3).

The second feature about the literacy–infant mortality relationship is that for the same band of female literacy, say 15 to 20 per cent, we observe a wide range of infant mortality rates from 70 per 1000 live births in Jammu & Kashmir to 150 in Uttar Pradesh. The feature about Indian states that different levels of IMR correspond to more or less similar levels of female literacy should not come as a surprise. It is conceivable, particularly in the Indian context, for several factors

---

[7]See, for instance, Caldwell (1979, 1985, 1986); Cochrane et al. (980); Hobcroft et al. (1984, 1985); United Nations (1985). Ware (1984) and Cleland and van Ginneken (1988) provide an extensive review of literature on the subject. For additional related readings, see Caldwell, Santow and Gigi (1989).

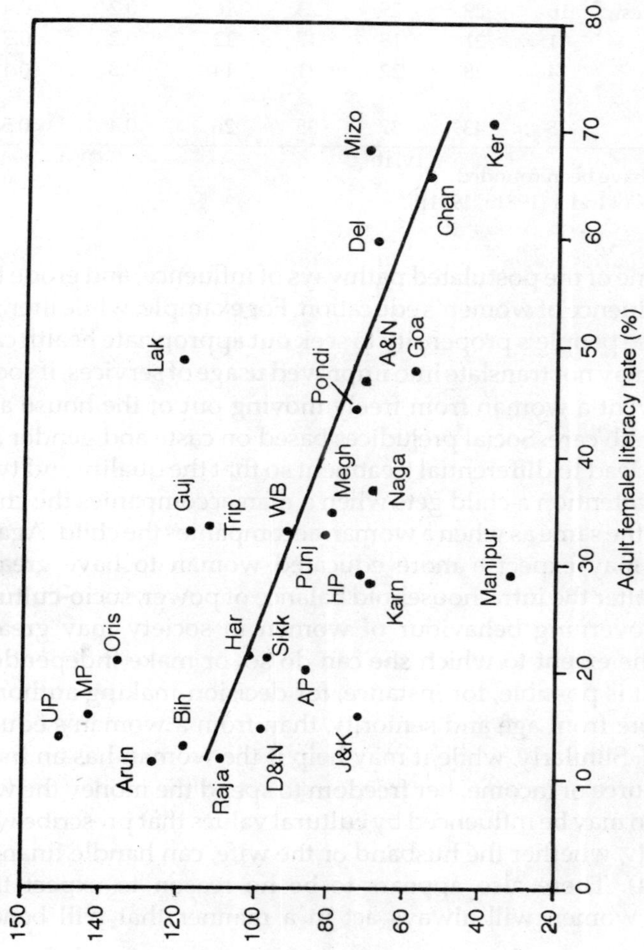

Figure 2: Adult Female Literacy and IMR in 30 Indian States and UTs, 1981

IMR = 124.13 − 1.064 (fem lit); R square = 0.38

Code: AP = Andhra Pradesh; A&N = Andaman & Nicobar Islands; Arun = Arunachal Pradesh; Bih = Bihar; Chan = Chandigarh; D&N = Dadra and Nagar Haveli; Del = Delhi; Guj = Gujarat; HP Himachal Pradesh; Har = Haryana; J&K = Jammu & Kashmir; Karn = Karnataka; Ker = Kerala; Lak = Lakshadweep; MP = Madhya Pradesh; Megh = Meghalaya; Mizo = Mizoram; Naga = Nagaland; Oris = Orissa; Pondi = Pondicherry; Punj = Punjab; Raja = Rajasthan; Sikk = Sikkim; Trip = Tripura; UP = Uttar Pradesh; WB = West Bengal

Source: Census of India (1988); Ministry of Health and Family Welfare (1990).

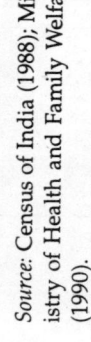

Table 3: Literacy levels in selected states, 1981

	Female literacy rate (%)					Ratio of rural to urban literacy rates	Ratio of female to male literacy rates
	All	15-19	20-24	15-34	15+		
	[1]	[2]	[3]	[4]	[5]	[6]	[7]
Manipur	29	54	45	43	29	0.6	0.5
Kerala	66	91	88	86	71	0.9	0.9
Bihar	14	24	19	18	13	0.3	0.4
Madhya Pradesh	16	29	25	23	16	0.2	0.4
Rajasthan	11	21	18	17	12	0.2	0.3
Uttar Pradesh	14	28	22	21	14	0.3	0.4
India	25	43	37	35	26	0.4	0.5

Note: Figures have been rounded.
Source: Census of India (1981a, 1981b).

to block some of the postulated pathways of influence, and erode the positive influence of women's education. For example, while literacy may increase people's propensity to seek out appropriate health care services, it may not translate into improved usage of services, if social norms prevent a woman from freely moving out of the house and seeking health care. Social prejudices based on caste and gender are reported to lead to differential treatment so that the quality and type of medical attention a child gets when a man accompanies the child may not be the same as when a woman accompanies the child. Again, while one may expect a more educated woman to have greater abilities to alter the intra-household balance of power, socio-cultural practices governing behaviour of women in society may greatly influence the extent to which she can do so, or make independent decisions. It is possible, for instance, for decision-making authority to stem more from age and seniority, than from a woman's educational level. Similarly, while it may help if the woman has an independent source of income, her freedom to spend the money the way she wants to may be influenced by cultural values that prescribe who in the family, whether the husband or the wife, can handle finances (Ware 1984). There also appears to be no reason to expect that 'educated' women will always act in a manner that will benefit children. There are several examples of discrimination against the female child, and the second born daughter particularly, in the north Indian states, which appears to persist despite higher levels of education among women (Das Gupta 1987). Finally, there appears to be no convincing evidence to show that education leads to favourable shifts in maternal behaviour, since factors such as age at marriage, child spacing, family size, and so on appear to be strongly influenced by socio-cultural norms of society (Ware 1984, Cleland 1990). All this in no way reduces the significance of literacy. On the contrary, it only suggests that we ought to focus on other factors as well which may combine with education to effectively enhance a woman's capabilities. In this context, there are at least two other factors which are known to strongly influence infant survival: women's occupational status and marital choices.

3. Women's Occupational Status and Marital Choices

Women's Work and Child Survival
According to the 1981 Census of India, 'main workers', namely those who work for more than six months of the year, accounted for 35 per cent of Manipur's female population, a figure significantly higher than the corresponding figure of 14 per cent for India.[8] Women's work participation rates in Manipur are high across all age groups, and reach a maximum between the ages of 35 and 49, when more than two-thirds of the women are employed. The state has a high proportion of women (63 per cent) engaged as 'cultivators', and a relatively small proportion (only 7 per cent) engaged as 'agricultural labourers'. This is in sharp contrast to many other states where women often work predominantly as 'agricultural labourers' (46 per cent for India), and a much smaller proportion work as 'cultivators' (33 per cent for India). Of all Indian states, Manipur also reports the highest proportion of women engaged in household industry, 20 per cent, which is substantially higher than the national average of 5 per

---

[8]There are several problems relating to the recognition of women's work, definition, and measurement of 'economic' activities. It has been pointed out that if appropriate adjustments are made to recognize fuel and fodder collection, domestic poultry keeping, etc. as economic activities, then there is a marked increase in female work participation rates (Sen and Sen 1985). In the Indian context, the Census which provides the most comprehensive and disaggregated data on work participation excludes all non-market activities with the exception of cultivation.

cent. Most of the women are engaged in handloom weaving, and in petty trade. A unique feature of the handloom sector in the state is that all activities, from the procurement of raw materials to the production and marketing of fabric, are undertaken almost exclusively by women, unlike in many other parts of the country where men often operate the loom, and nearly always market the product.[9] Another striking feature of the state is the high proportion of women who work alongside men. 731 females per 1000 males were employed as main workers in Manipur; the corresponding figure for India was 253, and for Kerala, 101 (Table 4).

Women's work has been postulated to have both a negative and a positive impact on the well-being of children. The negative relationship is often hypothesized on the grounds that maternal employment, by reducing the time that mothers devote to child care, and by possibly reducing the duration of breast-feeding, adversely affects infant and child survival. There is, however, little conclusive evidence to this effect.[10] It is recognized that much depends not on employment per se, but on the nature of the work, the level of earnings, the flexibility and conditions of work, post-partum leave of absence from work, access to arrangements for child care, the location of the work, and the overall circumstances of the family.

Several features of women's work in Manipur seem to suggest a greater compatibility with caring for the child than in other states of India. Unlike agricultural labourers who face the threat of irregular employment, most women in rural areas of Manipur work as cultivators on owned or leased land. The home-based activity of handloom weaving that predominates in the valley is also not particularly incompatible with child safety. It does not require the worker's continuous attention; it can be stopped and resumed at any time. These features of employment give women greater flexibility, and

---

[9]The phenomenon of high levels of women's participation in Manipur's 'economic' activities is not new, but was noted even at the turn of the century. Allen (1905), for instance, wrote: 'Women exceed men in numbers. They enjoy a position of considerable importance, and most of the trade of the valley is in their hands.... The internal trade of the State is carried on at markets which are held in the neighbourhood of the larger village.... Almost all the business is transacted by women, who are shrewd and capable, the men thinking it below their dignity to come and traffic at the bazaar.'

[10]Leslie (1989) presents a useful summary of the various studies examining the relationship between women's work and child welfare.

Women's Capabilities and Infant Mortality 65

Table 4: Features of women's employment in selected states, 1981

	Proportion of women who are			Female main workers in 15–59 years age group	Females per 1000 males by category of main workers					Ratio of rural to urban work participation rates
	main workers	marginal workers	non-workers		Main workers	Cultivators	Agricultural workers	Household industry	Others	
	[1]	[2]	[3]	[4]	[5]	[6]	[7]	[8]	[9]	[10]
Manipur	35	5	61	57	731	721	1610	7316	225	1.71
Kerala	13	4	83	21	321	101	599	1014	240	1.40
Bihar	9	4	87	15	174	298	1028	527	172	2.33
Madhya Pradesh	22	8	69	36	393	345	896	458	128	3.10
Rajasthan	9	12	79	15	172	189	456	145	84	2.38
Uttar Pradesh	5	3	92	9	95	76	236	139	49	1.97
India	14	6	80	23	253	192	598	365	121	2.20

Notes:
1. Figures may not add due to rounding.
2. Main workers are defined as those who had worked for at least 6 months (183 days) or more during the year; marginal workers are those who had not worked for at least 6 months.
3. A person is considered a cultivator, if he or she is engaged either as employer, single worker or family worker in cultivation of land owned or held from Government or held from private persons or institutions for payment in money, kind or share. Cultivation includes supervision or direction of cultivation.
4. A person who works on another person's land for wages in money, kind or share is regarded as an agricultural labourer.
5. Household industry is defined as an industry conducted by the head of the household himself or herself and/or by the members of the household at home or within the precincts of the house where the household lives in rural areas and only within the village in rural areas and only within the precincts of the house where the household lives in urban areas. The main criterion of a household industry is the participation of one or more members of the household.
6. All workers, i.e. those who have been engaged in some economic activity during the year preceding enumeration who are not cultivators or agricultural labourers or household industry workers are 'other workers'.

Source: Census of India (1981a).

also an opportunity to adjust more easily to unforeseen situations that may require special attention to be paid to the child. Most of the domestic and agricultural work is often shared between the households.[11] There also exist strong informal associations of women in Manipur that provide valuable support to mothers. At the same time, these characteristics of the work environment do not appear to impose any serious strains on breast-feeding. On the contrary, women's engagement in income earning activities yields additional resources which could facilitate purchase of food supplements for the child.

While there appears to be no conclusive evidence for the negative impact of women's employment on child survival, there are several ways in which women's engagement in the workforce and their participation in the market can strengthen their position in society, and contribute to the well-being of children. To the extent the women's employment brings additional income, the resources of the household are augmented. Sen (1990) emphasizes, for instance, that outside employment for wages makes women less vulnerable by making access easier; it also improves their standing in the family, and offers a valuable 'educational' experience of the outside world. What, however, increases the likelihood of women's work in Manipur having a more favourable impact on child survival than in other parts of the country is also the tradition of strong collective action that accompanies the high rates of women's work participation in the state. Most prominent are the women's agitation of 1939, known locally as *Nupi Lan* (Women's War), and the major campaign launched in the mid-1970s by women to check misbehaviour by men under the influence of alcohol.[12]

Age at Marriage and Infant Survival

In most societies, marriage and particularly the age at marriage, becomes an important intervening variable in the educational and occupational choices open to women. In societies with virtually no

---

[11]Descriptions of the functioning of such groups providing free, voluntary and exchange labour for cultivation and harvesting, building houses for widows and the aged, helping during marriages and social occasions can be found, for instance, in Chaki-Sircar (1984), Das (1986), Hodson (1911), Thaimei (1976), Singh (1990) and Burman (1989).

[12]See descriptions of socio-political movements in Chaki-Sircar (1984), Jain (1980), Kabui (1991a, 1991b, 1991c), and Singh (1991c).

contraception, early marriages also increase the probability of early childbearing, and childbearing by women is then likely to continue longer than would be the case if marriages were delayed. While these events may restrict a woman's options to study further, or pursue her vocational interests, it also increases the risks of infant deaths which are known to be high among very young (below 19 years) mothers.

In Manipur, the mean age at marriage among women, 23.3 years, is higher than even in Kerala, where it is around 21.8 years.[13] In both the states, the mean age at marriage is significantly higher than the age at marriage among women in the BIMARU states, where it is around 16.5 years (Table 5). In 1981, only 12 per cent of the women in the age group 15 to 19 were married in Manipur as against over 60 per cent in the BIMARU states. In both Kerala and Manipur, only 38 per cent of currently married women had ages below the statutory minimum of 18 years; in the BIMARU states, the corresponding figures were between 74 and 82 per cent.

Some of the explanations for the delayed age at marriage among women can be found in the socio-cultural context in Manipur which is characterized by the significant presence of populations classified as 'Scheduled Tribes' (27 per cent of the state's population) and Christians (30 per cent of the state's population). Interestingly, the majority of the non-Scheduled Tribe population is Hindu (referred to locally as the *meitheis*), and 95 per cent of the Scheduled Tribe population is Christian (Table 6). Historians point out that Hinduism in Manipur gained formal recognition only in AD 1703 when Charairongba, the *meithei* king of Manipur was initiated into the religion. In 1714, Hinduism was declared the state religion by his son, Panheiba, who succeeded him to the throne, changed his name to Garib Nawaz, and also adopted Hinduism. Until then, there do not appear to have been major differences in the religious affiliations of the people, all of whom were broadly labelled 'animists'. The interaction between Hinduism and the traditional religion has led to the emergence of a hybrid form of Hinduism which even today retains many of the elements of the traditional religion without reflecting some of the negative features of classical Hinduism. Child marriages were never practised, *sati* was unheard of, divorce was

---

[13] This is the singulate mean age at marriage which indicates the average number of years spent single before marriage.

Table 5: Selected nuptiality indicators, 1981

	Proportion married in each age group (%)			Singulate mean age at marriage (years)		Couples per 1000 population	Proportion of women married before 18 years[a]	Rural to urban ratio of married women below 18[b]
	15–19	20–44	15–44					
	[1]	[2]	[3]	[4]	[5]	[6]	[7]	[8]
Manipur	12	49	59	27.2	23.3	130	38	0.98
Kerala	14	58	61	27.3	21.8	146	38	1.14
Bihar	64	94	89	21.5	16.6	180	77	1.09
Madhya Pradesh	62	92	87	20.6	16.6	176	82	1.17
Rajasthan	64	95	89	20.3	16.1	175	79	1.09
Uttar Pradesh	61	94	88	21.0	16.7	171	74	1.29
India	43	84	81	23.3	18.2	169	68	1.24

Notes:
[a] Column 7 gives the proportion of currently married women with age at marriage below the statutory minimum of 18 years.
[b] Column 8 gives the rural–urban ratio of the currently married proportion of women below 18 years.

Source: Census of India (1981b) for Columns [1] to [6]; Census of India (1981c) for Column [7].

Table 6: Religious composition of population, 1981

	Religious Composition (percentage)			Scheduled Tribe population that is Christian
	Hindus	Muslims	Christians	
	[1]	[2]	[3]	[4]
Manipur	60	7	30	95
Kerala	58	21	21	6
Bihar	83	14	0.2	12
Madhya Pradesh	93	5	0.7	2
Rajasthan	89	7	0.1	0
Uttar Pradesh	83	16	0.2	0
India	80	11	2	

Source: Census of India (1981b) for columns [1] to [3]. Column [4] has been computed from Census of India State Reports, 1981, Part-ix, Special Tables for Scheduled Tribes, ST-7.

allowed, and widow remarriage was permitted. Little pressure from parents existed for an early marriage. Women enjoyed the freedom to choose their partners, and seldom were marriages 'arranged' by the parents against the wishes of the daughter.[14] Women did not face social disapproval for inter-community marriages. Chaki-Sircar (1984) also points out that among the *meitheis*, the independent rights of women to their economic assets and earnings were recognized.

People in the hills had practically no contact with Hinduism.[15] Child marriages were unheard of, and women had the freedom to chose their partners. 'Marriage by elopement' in many communities was the popular form of marriage. Wife-giving lineages were often considered superior to wife-taking lineages, and bride-price was

---

[14] A popular form of marriage is referred to as 'marriage by elopement', where following their decision to get married, the young couple leave their parents' home without the knowledge of the elders. The alliance is later recognized and legitimized by a proper marriage ceremony without any form of social disapproval.

[15] Several studies discuss the cultural practices among the hill communities and the impact of the Christian influence on communities in Manipur. Useful descriptions can be found in Allen (1905), Burman (1989), Das(1985), Dena (1991a), Gori (1984), Hodson (1911), Horam (1990), Johnstone (1896), Roy and Rizvi (1990), and Singh (1991d).

paid in all marriages.[16] Both patrilocal and matrilocal residences were found, and even after her marriage, a woman retained close ties with her family. This was often facilitated by the preferred practice for a woman to marry her mother's brother's son. Divorce was permitted in practically all the hill communities. If divorce was sought by the husband, or when it was sought by the wife and agreed to by the husband, properties given by her parents, and also those earned out of her own labour, were returned to the wife. Polygamous unions were very rare, and widow remarriages were permitted.

Christianity made its entry into the hills of Manipur towards the end of the 19th century, when in 1896, permission was granted to Father Pettigrew of the American Baptist Mission to work among the Tanghkhul Nagas. According to the Census reports, there were only 45 Christians in the state in 1901. Their numbers grew slowly until 1951, and more rapidly thereafter with increasing conversions of the local population to Christianity. Between 1961 and 1981, there was almost a threefold increase in Christian population. While the proportion of Hindus in Manipur's population has remained around 60 per cent since the beginning of the century, the proportion of Christians in the population has continued to increase.

Many of these features of Manipur that suggest greater freedoms for women should not be taken to imply that there is no discrimination against women. Both in the valley and in the hills, communities are essentially patriarchal and patrilineal. Among the Scheduled Tribe population, no share of the immovable property is inherited by daughters. In case there are no sons in the family, immovable property goes to the brother of the deceased, though movable property is distributed among women. There are dietary and other taboos that apply exclusively to women. While women's rights to maintenance are recognized, these are conditional. Daughters receive maintenance as long as they are unmarried, and widows receive support *dum sola et casta*. It is the father or the husband who represents his family in clan meetings and in courts; women do not have equal rights to public office. Polygynous marriages were common in the valley, and there are still such cases to be found in urban areas.[17]

---

[16] Among some groups, the son-in-law had to work for three years in the girl's parents' house before gaining eligibility to marry the daughter.

[17] An equally disturbing feature is that while the female-to-male ratio in Manipur, 971 in 1991, is much higher than India's corresponding figure of 929, there has been a steady decline in the sex ratio since 1921. This trend suggests that all may not be well with women; and requires careful analysis.

4. Assessing Women's Capabilities and Levels of Maternal Advancement

While there is little doubt that the role and position of women in society strongly influence infant survival, characterizing or assessing levels of women's achievements is by no means an easy task. Some form of measurement is nonetheless useful to compare differentials across communities. Building on the significance of women's educational, occupational and marital status for infant survival, an attempt is made here to use these three variables to construct an Index of Maternal Advancement (IMA).

The first component relates to a woman's level of knowledge. In the absence of more specialized data, *adult literacy* rates among women have been taken as a measure of the knowledge component.

The second component relevant for infant survival relates, in a sense, to a woman's degree of control over reproduction in terms of her ability to avoid high risk pregnancies. Inability to postpone such pregnancies could arise due to a number of factors, such as ignorance, lack of access to appropriate birth control technologies, and socio-cultural practices and norms that dictate early marriages. It is difficult to directly assess the extent of control a woman has on these matters. Nonetheless, indirect measures could provide some useful clues. Of the various such indicators, *the proportion of women not married in the age group 15 to 19* is suggested as a preferred indicator. While use of this indicator assumes that marriage is a pre-requisite for childbearing, and that the recording of the age at marriage is done accurately, it has the advantage of directing attention to a high risk age group of young mothers. To the extent that women who get married at a young age are often less capable of exerting an influence on their families and husbands, using this indicator also provides some indication of the freedoms that women have in marital matters. It also conveys an idea about the extent to which early marriages may restrict women's educational and occupational choices.

The last component of women's achievements relevant to child survival relates to women's 'gainful' employment. Ideally, this should reflect both paid and unpaid employment, regardless of whether it is at home or outside. In spite of the various problems associated with work participation rates for 'economic' activities, *the proportion of working women in the age group 15 to 60*, is recommended as an indicator that reflects 'gainful' employment.[18] A major problem with these data is the exclusion of several activities which are not often perceived as 'gainful' economic activities. To the extent that this arises due to the limited recognition of women's economic contribution, the underestimate offers additional insights into society's perceptions of women in society.[19]

Focusing on only these three dimensions of women's achievements is intended to give an indication of the 'levels of maternal advancement' using elements that are directly relevant to infant survival. This, however, does not imply that other dimensions of women's achievements are not relevant for child survival. The restriction to these three variables suggests the overwhelming importance of these factors.

Data on the three indicators are available for all the states, and the range of values within India is quite stunning. For 1981, adult female literacy rates varied from 12 per cent in Rajasthan to 68 per cent in Kerala. The proportion of women not married in the age group 15 to 19 years ranges from 36 per cent in Bihar and Rajasthan (i.e., 64 per cent of girls get married before 19) to 86 per cent in Kerala, 88 per cent in Manipur, and 93 per cent in Goa, Daman and Diu. Punjab reported the lowest women's work participation rate of 4 per cent, and Arunachal Pradesh reported 67 per cent. While the range of values gives an indication of the differences in the levels of women's achievements across the states, it is quite likely that, qualitatively speaking, the actual situation could be much worse than what the figures suggest.

Having identified the main components of maternal advancement, and the indirect measures, a composite Index of Maternal Advancement (IMA) is constructed by focusing on deprivation of three types: maternal deprivation in knowledge, in control over reproduction, and in 'gainful' employment.[20] To construct the composite index for the Indian states, each state is placed on a scale of

---

[18] Ideally, one should consider women in the age group 15 to 45, rather than 15 to 60 years. Data on women employed between 15 and 45 years of age are not readily available.

[19] An example of this could be the surprisingly low female work participation rates reported for 1981 in Haryana (8 per cent) and Punjab (4 per cent), two states that are known for having sex ratios that are extremely adverse to women (870 females per 1000 males in Haryana, and 879 in Punjab).

[20] IMA is similar in its construction to the Human Development Index (HDI) developed by UNDP (1990). See Kumar (1992) for a discussion on the technical considerations in IMA's construction.

0 to 1, where 0 represents the worst performance and 1 represents best performance. A minimum value and a desirable or achievable value are specified for each of the three deprivation type indicators, X_i. The next step is to define the deprivation indicator, I_{ij} for the jth state with respect to the ith variable as:

$$I_{ij} = \frac{(\max_j X_{ij} - X_{ij})}{(\max_j X_{ij} - \min_j X_{ij})}$$

An average deprivation indicator, I_j, is then defined by taking the simple average of the three indicators:

$$I_j = \frac{1}{3} \sum I_{ij}$$

The final step is to arrive at the Index of Maternal Advancement (IMA) as:

$$(IMA)_j = 100 \, (1 - I_j)$$

Using the above methodology and data for 1981, India's overall value of IMA works out to 33 (Table 7).[21] Mizoram had the highest IMA, 76, and Uttar Pradesh the lowest, 18, indicating more than a fourfold difference in the levels of maternal advancement between the two extremes. Haryana, a state with higher than average per capita incomes, along with Madhya Pradesh, Bihar, Rajasthan and Uttar Pradesh, was among the five poorest states in terms of IMA. These states also accounted for nearly 40 per cent of the country's population. Kerala, and four other states from the north-eastern region, Mizoram, Nagaland, Manipur and Meghalaya, are the top five states in terms of the IMA. These five high IMA states, however, represent around 4.3 per cent of India's population, and Kerala alone accounts for 3.7 per cent of the country's population.

5. IMA and IMR: A contextual interpretation

IMA combines a set of endogenous factors into an index that gives an idea of the levels of women's maternal advancement in the states.[22] The

---

[21] The IMA for Indian states has been constructed using the minimum and the maximum district-level values for the three indicators.
[22] Incidentally, the word 'ima' in Manipuri, and in Hebrew, means 'mother'.

Table 7: Index of Maternal Advancement (IMA) for 30 Indian States and Union Territories, 1981

States and Union Territories		Female literacy rate (%) in the 15+ age group	% women NOT married in age group 15-19 %	Female work participation rate (%) in age group 15-59	Index of deprivation			Average index of deprivation	Composite index of maternal advancement (IMA)
					Literacy	Marriage	'Gainful' Employment		
		[1]	[2]	[3]	[4]	[5]	[6]	[7]	[8]
1	Mizoram	68	89	57	0.32	0.08	0.33	0.24	76
2	Nagaland	37	90	65	0.65	0.07	0.23	0.31	69
3	Manipur	29	88	57	0.73	0.09	0.33	0.38	62
4	Kerala	71	86	21	0.30	0.12	0.76	0.39	61
5	Meghalaya	35	79	56	0.67	0.21	0.34	0.41	59
6	Goa, Daman & Diu	48	93	24	0.54	0.03	0.72	0.43	57
7	Chandigarh	66	83	14	0.35	0.16	0.83	0.45	55
8	Sikkim	21	76	57	0.81	0.24	0.32	0.46	54
9	Arunachal Pradesh	12	71	67	0.91	0.31	0.21	0.48	52
10	Tamil Nadu	35	77	34	0.67	0.23	0.60	0.50	50
11	Delhi	60	76	11	0.41	0.24	0.87	0.51	49
12	Pondicherry	44	79	18	0.57	0.20	0.79	0.52	48
13	Maharashtra	35	62	39	0.67	0.41	0.54	0.54	46
14	Himachal Pradesh	29	68	30	0.73	0.33	0.64	0.57	43
15	Dadra & Nagar Haveli	15	66	43	0.88	0.36	0.49	0.58	42
16	Gujarat	33	73	18	0.69	0.27	0.79	0.58	42
17	Lakshadweep	49	68	10	0.53	0.34	0.89	0.58	42

Contd.

Table 7 (contd):

		[1]	[2]	[3]	[4]	[5]	[6]	[7]	[8]
18	Punjab	33	87	4	0.69	0.11	0.96	0.59	41
19	Karnataka	28	64	31	0.74	0.39	0.64	0.59	41
20	Tripura	34	74	15	0.68	0.27	0.83	0.59	41
21	A & N Islands	46	66	9	0.56	0.37	0.89	0.61	39
22	Orissa	21	69	17	0.81	0.32	0.80	0.64	36
23	Andhra Pradesh	20	44	42	0.82	0.63	0.51	0.65	35
24	West Bengal	33	63	10	0.69	0.40	0.88	0.66	34
25	Jammu & Kashmir	16	72	9	0.86	0.29	0.89	0.68	32
26	Madhya Pradesh	16	38	36	0.86	0.70	0.57	0.71	29
27	Haryana	21	52	8	0.81	0.53	0.91	0.75	25
28	Bihar	13	36	15	0.89	0.73	0.82	0.81	19
29	Rajasthan	12	36	15	0.90	0.73	0.82	0.82	18
30	Uttar Pradesh	14	39	9	0.88	0.69	0.90	0.82	18
	India	26	54	23	0.76	0.51	0.73	0.67	33
	minimum value	2.8	13.6	0.2					
	maximum value	100.0	95.7	84.5					

Note: Out of 402 districts, East Kameng in Arunachal Pradesh reports the lowest adult female literacy rates (2.76%); Sultanpur in U.P. reports the lowest percentage of women not married in the age group 15–19 (13.57%); and Aligarh in UP reports the lowest work participation rates for women (0.24 per cent). Kottayam in Kerala reports the highest adult female literacy rate (86.67%); however, the maximum desirable has been taken to be 100%. Kottayam also reports the highest percentage of women not married in the age group 15–19 (95.7%). Tamenglong, a hill district in Manipur, reports the highest work participation rates among women (84.51%). For details on the construction of IMA, see Section 4.

Source: Census of India, 1981.

three factors combine to act independently and interdependently to influence infant survival favourably as well as negatively. For instance, the benefits of a higher level of education may be reduced by social customs that dictate early marriages. On the other hand, the benefits of delayed marriages, like in Manipur, may be offset by deprivation in literacy. Similarly, early marriages and social norms regulating the behaviour of women may deprive them of the opportunity to pursue their vocational or educational interests. It therefore becomes necessary to understand how these factors operate independently and synergistically to either enhance or limit women's achievements, and their capacity to act, before linkages can be established with child survival.

Generally speaking, a low level of IMR will tend to be associated with a high IMA value. Figure 3 shows the levels and composition of IMA in the high and low IMR states. The two low IMR states, Kerala and Manipur, have significantly higher IMA values than the four high IMR states. However, while the IMA values for Kerala and Manipur are similar, there is a marked difference in the composition of IMA in the two states. In Kerala, the high rates of female literacy and the proportion of women not married in the age group 15 to 19 years dominate the composition of the index. In Manipur, on the other hand, while the absolute level of female literacy is much lower than in Kerala, and the proportion of women not married more or less the same, the female work participation rates are much higher than in Kerala. In sharp contrast, one finds that the benefits of work participation rates (which are higher than even Kerala's) are weighed down by the low levels of literacy and the high proportion of girls getting married in the age group 15 to 19.

While the above analysis does suggest an inverse relationship between IMA and IMR, the linkages are not obvious. Hence, in attempting to explain inter-state IMR differentials, the differentials in IMA need to be related to differences that may exist across the states in household entitlements, family and social structures, and the availability of and access to services and commodities necessary for promoting the well-being of children. It also becomes necessary to examine the levels of IMA in relation to women's capabilities, the level of entitlements in the community, and the levels of provisioning of public health and related services necessary for ensuring child survival. It is only through such a contextual analysis that one can

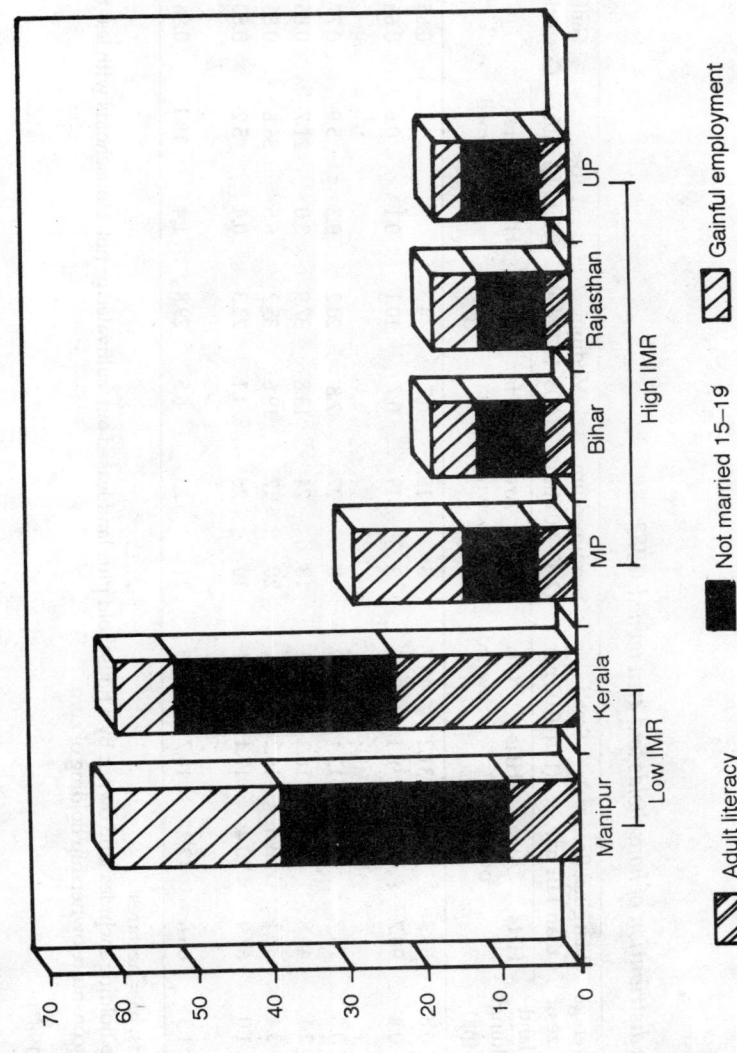

Figure 3: Index of Maternal Advancement (IMA) in low and high IMR States, 1981.

Table 8: Percentage distribution of households and area owned, 1982

	Average size of land holdings (ha)	Marginal (less than 1.01 ha)		Small (1.01–0.02 ha)		Semi-medium (2.03–4.04 ha)		Medium (4.05–10.12 ha)		Large (10.13 ha plus)		Gini Coefficient
		HHs	Area owned	HHs	Area owned	HHs	Area owned	HHs	Area owned	HHs	Area owned	
Manipur	0.8	63.3	31.7	31.2	48.7	5	15	0.7	4.3			0.65
Kerala	0.4	90.7	45.7	6.1	23.5	3	19	0.7	10.1	0.1	0.6	0.66
Bihar	0.8	76.7	23.9	12.4	22.9	8	27	2.8	20.2	0.3	5.9	0.77
Madhya Pradesh	2.1	48.8	5.0	16.2	11.1	18	24	13.8	37.9	3.0	21.7	0.86
Rajasthan	3.4	37.1	3.6	16.2	7.3	20	17	19.6	35.2	6.5	36.6	0.85
Uttar Pradesh	1.0	67.9	20.4	17.4	24.1	10	28	4.1	22.3	0.4	5.2	0.80
India	1.3	66.6	12.2	14.7	16.5	11	23	6.5	29.8	1.4	18.1	0.86

Note: HH = households; ha = hectares.
Household ownership holding includes land owned by a household plus land leased out, cultivated or not. Households with less than 0.002 hectares of land constitute ownership holding of zero.

Source: Sarvekshana (1987).

identify factors that may be contributing to a positive relationship between IMA and IMR. Some of the dimensions of Manipur's economic life that tend to suggest a greater freedom for women to effectively utilize their higher levels of achievements are discussed below.

Wealth and Income Distribution

An indication of the patterns of income and wealth distribution in the state is obtained from data on land ownership patterns.[23] Both Manipur and Kerala have a far more equitable distribution of landholdings than the poorly performing states, which is revealed by the gini coefficient for land holdings. 94 per cent of rural households in Manipur own 80 per cent of land in the 'marginal' and 'small' categories (less than 2.02 hectares). This pattern of landholdings is somewhat similar to Kerala's where 97 per cent of households own 68 per cent of land in the 'marginal' and 'small' categories. Both states have negligible 'large' (more than 10.12 hectare) holdings. In sharp contrast are the four BIMARU states. In Rajasthan, for instance, we find that over a third of the area is in the 'large' category, and is owned by 6.5 per cent of the households. Over 50 per cent of the households own less than 11 per cent of the area in the 'marginal' and 'small' categories (Table 8).

According to the National Sample Survey data, Manipur reports the lowest percentage of population below the poverty line among all Indian states.[24] More recently, Minhas et al. (1991) have adjusted for price level changes in the states, and have worked out state-wise estimates of headcount ratios of population below the poverty line. With such an adjustment, in 1987–8, Manipur had a headcount ratio of 16.80 per cent, followed by Punjab, a high per capita income state, with 17.97 per cent. In the two groups of states that we are examining, the headcount ratio is far lower in Manipur than in the four BIMARU states (Table 9). These figures, and the figures on land ownership do suggest that the income and asset distribution are more equitable in Manipur than in many other states.

[23]Land ownership includes both owned land, as well as land leased in on a long-term basis.
[24]These estimates are derived by using the poverty line of Rs 49.09 per capita per month at 1973–4 prices corresponding to a daily calorie requirement of 2400 calories per person in rural areas, and the poverty line of Rs. 56.64 per capita per month corresponding to a daily calorie requirement of 2100 calories in urban areas. Osmani (1990) and Harris (1990), in particular, discuss many of the problems associated with the use of these criteria for determining poverty levels.

Table 9: Statewise headcount ratios of population below the poverty line in 1970–71, 1983 and 1987–88: Rural, urban and entire state population

	Rural			Urban			Entire State		
	1970–71	1983	1987–88	1970–71	1983	1987–88	1970–71	1983	1987–88
Manipur	73	30	20	37	13	9	68	26	17
Kerala	69	47	44	62	48	44	68	47	44
Bihar	69	70	66	54	51	57	67	68	65
Madhya Pradesh	62	54	50	58	52	46	62	54	49
Rajasthan	55	42	42	46	37	42	53	41	42
Uttar Pradesh	51	50	48	54	48	42	52	49	46
India	57	49	45	46	38	37	55	46	43

Source: Minhas, Jain and Tendulkar (1991).

Government and Public Provisioning

As reported earlier, the proportion of the annual budget allocated for 'medical, public health, family planning, and related items' in Manipur is higher than the national average, and the allocations by a number of other states. It was also observed that Manipur has a far more equitable spatial distribution of health facilities between rural and urban areas than the high IMR states. This is an important feature given the extremely strong urban bias in the location of government facilities that is noticed in most other states. Another striking feature of the state relates to the levels of per capita government expenditure on health. In Kerala and Manipur, the two exceptional states with respect to IMR, per capita health expenditures by governments have been higher than the national average. In Manipur particularly, per capita public sector health expenditure in 1980–1 was almost four times higher than the national average of Rs 24. By contrast, in Bihar, Uttar Pradesh and Madhya Pradesh, the per capita health expenditures by government have been below the national average (Figure 4).

Drinking Water and Sanitation

Two other aspects of community life are striking about Manipur. The first relates to the levels of personal and environmental hygiene. Anecdotal evidence tends to suggest that the *meitheis* maintain an 'exceptionally clean' household. Shoes and other forms of footwear are never brought into the house. Entry into the kitchen, and handling of food containers is carefully monitored. While this may indicate lower levels of environmental contamination, it is, however, difficult to establish a direct linkage with infant mortality. Some indication of a possibly cleaner environment is provided by National Sample Survey data on the access of households to latrine facilities. Of all the states, rural Manipur had the lowest percentage of households with no latrine facilities (27 per cent). Even in Kerala, 60 per cent of rural households did not have such facilities (Table 10). The situation in these two states is far better than the position for the country as a whole where 91 per cent of rural households had no access to latrines. In the four high-IMR states, nearly 95 per cent of rural households had no latrine facilities connected to their place of dwelling (Figure 5).

The second feature is the practice of drinking 'boiled' water reported in many parts of the hill districts of the state. Water is not

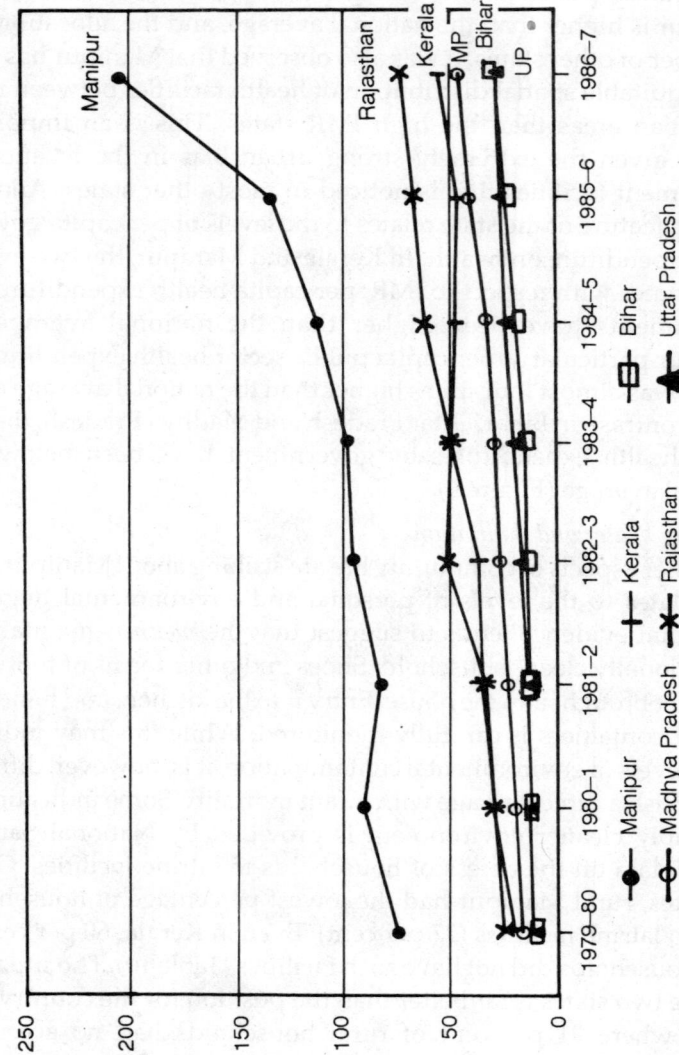

Figure 4: Per Capita Public Sector Health Expenditures
Source: Ministry of Health and Family Welfare (1984, 1987, 1989)

Table 10: Percentage distribution of rural households with latrines, 1983

	No latrine	Shared latrine	Exclusive	Breakdown of shared and exclusive latrines			
				Service latrine	Septic tank	Flush system	Others
Manipur	27	29	44	12	0.1	0.0	62
Kerala	60	5	35	1	13.1	0.3	25
Bihar	95	2	3	2	1.6	0.0	2
Madhya Pradesh	96	1	3	1	0.6	0.1	2
Rajasthan	96	1	3	1	0.8	0.2	2
Uttar Pradesh	94	2	3	4	0.6	0.2	0
India	91	3	6	2	2.2	0.3	4

Note: Figures have been rounded, and so may not add up to 100.

Source: Sarvekshana (1988).

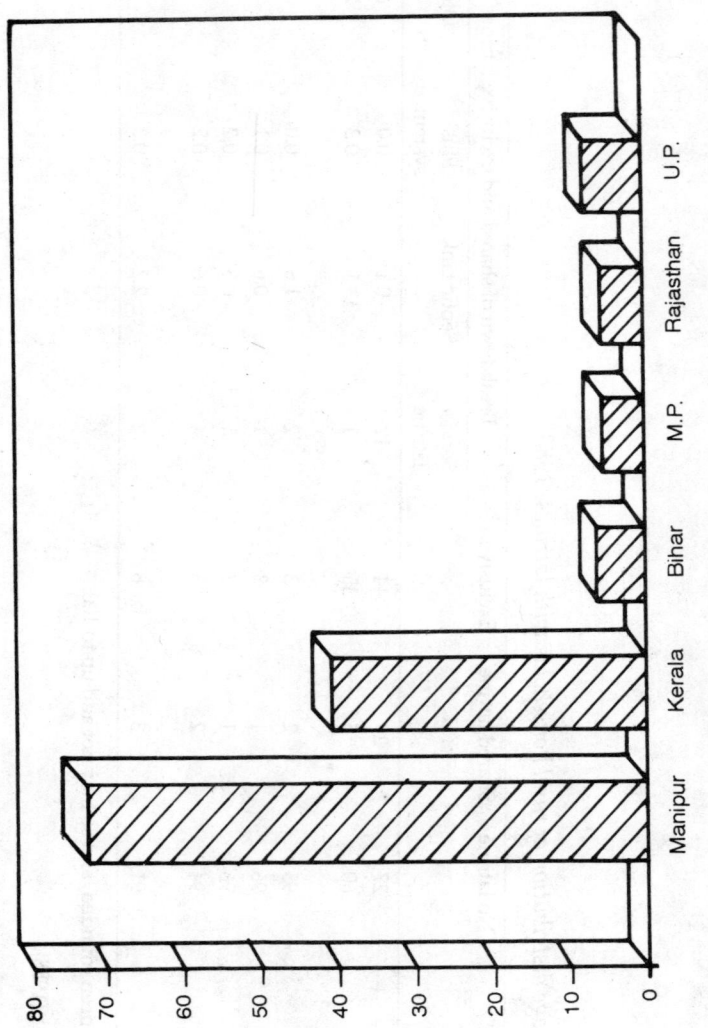

Figure 5: Percentage of Rural Households with Latrines, 1983
Source: Sarvekshana (1988).

consciously boiled, but it is the practice in most of the households in the hills to leave a pot of water on the cooking stove especially after the cooking is done. It is this water that is usually used for drinking and for making tea. The significance of drinking 'boiled' water for improving child survival conditions has been pointed out earlier. Such a practice is found in Kerala too, and has been advanced as an important factor responsible for lower infant mortality in the state (Nagraj 1985). Interviews with families belonging to Manipur hills revealed that newborn children are often given either the 'boiled' water, or sometimes a boiled and very diluted rice-based solution (*kanji*). Such a practice is also reported by communities in Darjeeling (in West Bengal) and the surrounding hill regions. While it is difficult to assess the extent to which this practice is likely to influence child survival, it could well be a significant feature explaining the low IMR among the hill communities.

Role of Community Action

Women in the valley have had a tradition of collective action, organized around the market place, and at home. Several informal organizations, locally known as *marups* (friendship associations), have been formed by both men and women at the village level.[25] A commonly formed friendship association is the marriage *marup*. When a son or daughter of any of the members gets married, each member of the association makes a small pre-determined contribution to cover part of the marriage expenses. In some cases, members agree to contribute a fixed amount of money as well as a fixed amount of rice. Savings associations also exist for the purchase of specific commodities, such as brass buckets, bicycles, gold, and so on. While membership of the *marups* is usually open to both men and women, there are also certain exclusive women's *marups* where members offer wage labour to collect money for the association to be used for different occasions and purposes. There are trade *marups* organized around a common product (example, fish *marups*, rice *marups*, etc.) to provide mutual assistance. Similar *marups* exist to cover funeral costs, and to meet expenses incurred on religious ceremonies and cultural events. Particularly impressive are the informal credit organizations that exist for making consumption and emergency loans.

---

[25]Chaki-Sircar (1984) describes the functioning of several of these *marups*; the examples cited here draw on her case studies.

Table 11: Voter turnout in Vidhan Sabha elections in selected states

Election year	Manipur	Kerala	Bihar	Madhya Pradesh	Rajasthan	Uttar Pradesh
1952			41	46	36	38
1957		78	43	37	39	48
1960		84				
1962			47	45	53	51
1965		75				
1967	69	76	52	53	58	55
1970		75				
1971			49			46
1972	78			55	58	
1974	85					
1977		79	61	53	54	56
1980	82	72	52	49	52	50
1982		74				
1984	87			59		56
1985				50	55	
1987		81				
1989			60			51
1990				55	57	
Lowest	69	72	41	37	36	38
Highest	87	84	61	59	58	56

Source: Butler, Lahiri and Roy (1991)

Levels of Electoral Participation

Further evidence of women's freedoms and social recognition is provided by data on women's participation in electoral politics. Electoral statistics reveal that Manipur and Kerala have among the highest female voter turnout rates in the country, significantly higher than in the four low IMA states in both state-level elections (Table 11) and in national elections (Figure 6).[26]

Summing up

In general, while one can expect a higher level of IMA to be associated with a lower level of IMR, the relationship is not obvious. Clearly a number of social, cultural, economic, political and other factors in Manipur operate simultaneously to exert a positive influence on child survival. The IMA is a useful instrument to assess

---

[26] As with all data, errors are likely in the reporting of electoral statistics. There are however few arguments why data for Manipur should be more unreliable than that for the other states. For a discussion, see Kumar (1992).

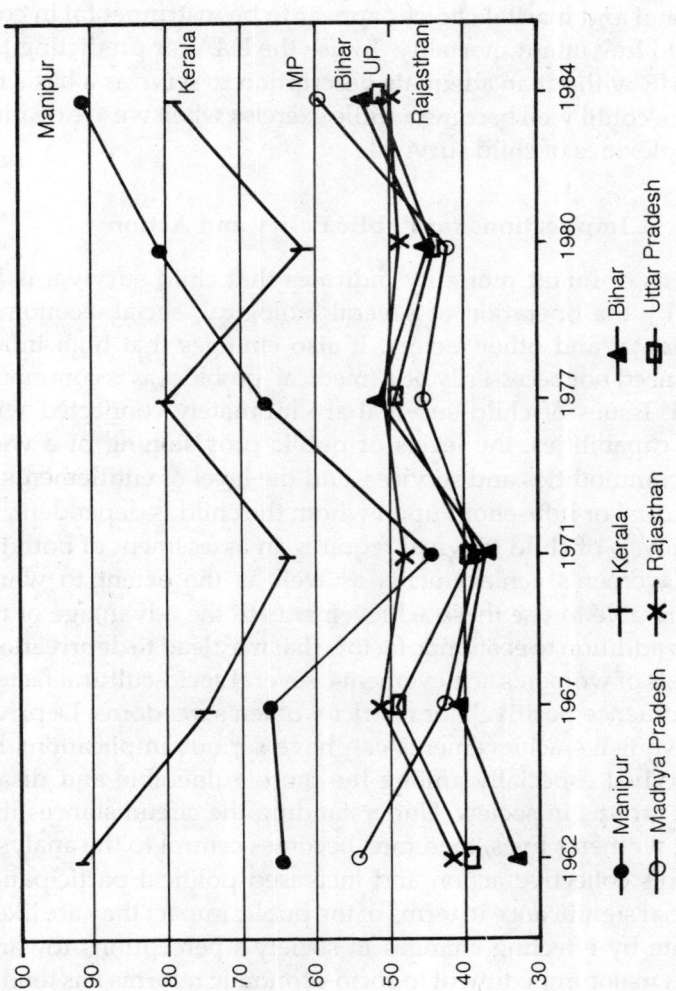

Figure 6: Female Voter Turnout Rates in Lok Sabha Elections
Source: Election Commissioner of India

differentials in maternal advancement, but it does not do away with the detailed descriptive analysis that is required before evaluating the impact on child survival. In the case of Manipur, the greater freedoms enjoyed by women in matters relating to their educational, occupational and marital choices appear to be instrumental in contributing to low infant mortality. To use the IMA for predicting the level of IMR without an adequate description to serve as a basis for evaluation, could well become a futile exercise when we are dealing with complexities of child survival.

6. Implications for Public Policy and Action

An analysis of infant mortality indicates that child survival is influenced by the operation of several biological, social, economic, environmental and other factors. It also emerges that high infant mortality need not necessarily be a 'medical' problem as is commonly perceived. Issues of child survival are intimately connected with maternal capabilities, the levels of public provisioning of a wide range of commodities and services, and the level of entitlements of the individual or household upon whom the child is dependent.

An analysis of child survival requires an assessment of both the levels of women's achievements as well as the extent to which women are able to use these achievements to the advantage of the child.[27] In addition to economic factors that may lead to deprivations in the levels of women's achievements, several socio-cultural factors tend to influence positively or restrict women's freedoms. Deprivations in women's achievements can have serious implications for infant survival especially among the more vulnerable and disadvantaged groups in society. Understanding the circumstances that dominate women's lives, therefore, becomes central to the analysis.

Women's collective action and increased political participation have special significance in terms of the public impact they are likely to generate by effecting changes in society's perceptions towards women. A major impediment to socio-economic reforms has tended to be society's perceptions about women's roles and their contribution to society. Such perceptions and attitudes are extremely slow to

---

[27] There is also evidence to suggest that, as in Kerala, lower levels of anti-female bias prevail in Manipur than in many other states. For a discussion, see Kumar (1992).

change, and without interventions, the gender-biases that dominate society are likely to persist. Government mediation through legislative and other means can help in bringing about changes in such perceptions and opening up opportunities for women. While such measures definitely facilitate the process, the example of women in Manipur highlights the importance of visible public action by women themselves in effecting changes and becoming instrumental in ensuring a better deal for themselves.

Social relations play an important role in providing 'extended entitlement' especially in low-income regions where both income and support services for child care are limited. Many of the reciprocal arrangements for child care and domestic help, for example, become extremely important especially for the more vulnerable and disadvantaged groups in society. Several factors may contribute to the emergence of such arrangements, and the formation of informal alliances between women. Ties to the natal home, compactness of the the community, more face-to-face contact, and common economic interests appear to be significant in the case of Manipur. Organization by women around the work place, and at home has the advantage of providing relatively 'costless' social insurance.[28] Given that, in most societies, women have the primary responsibility for looking after the child, the concept of 'economic' security for women extends well beyond an independent source of earnings, or getting wage employment. The concern becomes one of finding ways by which women can balance their work and family obligations better. While collective action and recognition of their contribution do provide women with an extra economic and social leverage, a unique feature of Manipur is women's access to market plots, over which they have hereditary rights. While most of the property is handed down to the sons, women have exclusive rights over the market plots, which are transferred only to other women in the family. While there is no formal legal provision for such an arrangement, the rights of women in this matter are legitimized by strong social sanctions.

The active participation of government, community organizations, the press and other forms of public media, and public agencies are essential for effectively addressing issues of child survival. In Manipur and Kerala, the two low IMR states, the public has played

---

[28]For a discussion on the role of informal security systems and concerted action in extending people's entitlements, see Drèze and Sen (1989).

an important role in demanding appropriate service, and in influencing the public agenda. In Kerala, the initiative of the government was sustained by an education-led mobilization of people making demands on a responsive state apparatus. In Manipur, we find collective action, a high level of political awareness and participation by the people, responsible for making demands on the government system. Such active public participation is not apparent in the other states where the process of organizing the public for making demands on the system have been relatively weak and diffused.

There can be no excuses for high levels of avoidable infant mortality in India, or for that matter, in several parts of the world today. Given how closely issues of infant survival are linked to the well-being and capabilities of the mother, it reflects the lack of seriousness with which society tends to address issues of primary concern to women. Technical and medical interventions do help; but many of the solutions call for social change which is often slow, and difficult to bring about. There is an urgent need for policy-makers to promote strengthened people's involvement and public action to bring about an enhancement in women's capabilities for better child survival in India.

Acknowledgements

I am grateful to the participants at the Workshop on 'The Future of Health and Population in India' held in New Delhi in January 1992 for their comments and suggestions. I would also like to thank David Bell, Lincoln Chen, Michel Garenne, T. N. Krishnan, V. K. Ramachandran and Amartya Sen for very valuable comments at different stages.

Bibliography

Allen, B.C. (1905), *Naga hills and Manipur: Socio-economic history* (reprinted 1980), Gian Publications, Delhi.
Bhat, Mari and S. Irudaya Rajan (1990), 'Demographic Transition in Kerala Revisited', *Economic and Political Weekly*, 18 September.
Boserup, E. (1970), *Women's role in economic development*, St Martin's Press, New York.
Burman, B.K. Roy (1989?), *Community Land and Institutional Finance*', Council for Social Development, New Delhi.
Butler, D., A. Lahiri and P. Roy (1991), 'India Decides: Elections: 1952–1991', Living Media India Ltd., New Delhi.

Caldwell, John C. (1979), 'Education as a factor in mortality decline: An examination of Nigerian data, *Population Studies*, 33.

Caldwell, John C and P. Caldwell (1985), 'Education and Literacy as factors in Health' in Rockefeller Foundation, *Good Health at Low Cost*, 1985.

Caldwell, John C. (1986), 'Routes to Low Mortality in Poor Countries', *Population and Development Review*, 12, No. 2., pp. 171–220, June.

Caldwell, John C. and Gigi Santow (eds.) (1989), *Selected Readings in the Cultural, Social and Behavioural Determinants of Health*, Health Transition Series No. 1, Highland Press, Canberra, Australia.

Census of India (1981a), *Primary Census Abstract*, General Population, Series-1, India: Part II-B (i), .

Census of India (1981b), *A Handbook of Population Statistics*, Office of Registrar General and Census Commissioner (published in 1988), New Delhi.

Census of India (1981c), Series-1, *Census Abstract, General Population*, India; Part II-B (i), Office of Registrar General and Census Commissioner, New Delhi.

Census of India (1981d) *Female Age at Marriage: an analysis of 1981 census data*, Occasional Paper No. 7 of 1988, Demography Division, Office of the Registrar General, New Delhi.

Census of India (1988), 'Child Mortality Estimates of India, Census of India (1991a), *Provisional Population Totals: India, 1991*, New Delhi.

Census of India (1991b), *Provisional Population Totals: workers and their distribution*, Series-1, India; Registrar General and Census Commissioner, New Delhi.

Chaki-Sircar, Manjusri (1984): *Feminism in a Traditional Society: Women of the Manipur Valley*, Shakti Books, Vikas Publishing House, New Delhi.

Cleland, John G. and Jerome K. Van Ginneken (1988), 'Maternal Education and Child Survival in Developing Countries: The Search for Pathways of Influence', *Social Science and Medicine*, 27(12): 1357–68.

Chelland, John (1990), 'Maternal Education and Child Survival: further evidence and explanations' in John C. Caldwell, Sally Findley, Pat Caldwell, Gigi Santow, Wendy Cosford, Jennifer Braid and Daphne Broers-Freeman (eds.), (1990), *What we know about Health Transition: The social, cultural and behavioural determinants of health*, Health Transition Series No. 2 (Volume I), Health Transition Centre, The Australian National University, Canberra.

Cochrane, S.H. (1980), 'The socioeconomic determinants of mortality: The cross national evidence' in Susan H. Cochrane, Donald O'Hara and Joanne Leslie, '*The Effects of Education on Health*, World Bank Staff Working Paper No. 405, The World Bank, Washington, D.C.

Cochrane, Susan H., Donald O'Hara and Joanne Leslie (1980), *The Effects of Education on Health*, World Bank Staff Working Paper No. 405, The World Bank, Washington, D.C.

Das, R.K. (1985), *Manipur tribal scene: Studies in Society and Change*, Inter-India Publications, New Delhi.

Das, S.T. (1986), *Tribal life of north-eastern India*, Gian Publishing House Delhi.

Das Gupta, Monica (1987), 'Death Clustering, mother's education and the determinants of child mortality in rural Punjab, India' in John C. Caldwell, Sally Findley, Pat Caldwell, Gigi Gantow, Wendy Cosford, Jennifer Braid and Daphne Broers-Freeman (eds.), (1990), *What we know about Health Transition: The social, cultural and behavioural determinants of health*, Health Transition Series No. 2

(Volume I), Health Transition Centre, The Australian National University, Canberra.
Dena, Lal (ed.) (1991a), *History of Modern Manipur (1826–1949)*, Orbit Publishers, New Delhi.
Dena, Lal (1991b), 'Anglo-Manipur Relations, 1762–1834' in Dena, Lal (1991a).
Dena, Lal (1991c), 'Some anomalies of colonial rule, 1891–1919' in Dena, Lal (1991a).
Dena, Lal (1991d), 'INA Movement' in Dena, Lal (1991a).
Drèze, Jean and Amartya Sen, (1989), *Hunger and Public Action*, Oxford: Clarendon Press.
Gori, G.K. (1984), *Changing Phase of Tribal Area of Manipur*, B.R. Publishing Corporation, Delhi.
Gwatkin, Davidson R. and Sarah K. Brandel (1981) *Reducing Infant and Child Mortality in the Developing World, 1980–2000*, Working Paper No. 2, Overseas Development Council, Washington, D.C.
Harris, Barbara (1990), 'The intrafamily distribution of hunger in South Asia' in Jean Drèze and Amartya Sen (eds.), *The Political Economy of Hunger: Volume 1*, Oxford: Clarendon Press.
Hobcroft, J.N., R.W. McDonald and S.O. Rutstein (1984), 'Socioeconomic factors in infant and child mortality: a Cross-national comparision, *Population Studies*, 38.
Hobcroft, J.N.. R.W. McDonald and S.O. Rutstein (1984), 'Demographic determinants of infant and early child mortality: comparative analysis;, *Population Studies*, 39.
Hodson, T.C. (1911), *The Naga Tribes of Manipur*, Low Price Publication, Delhi (1989 reprint).
Horam, M (1990), *North East India: A Profile*, Cosmo Publications, New Delhi.
Jain, Devaki (1980), 'The night patrollers of Manipur' in Devaki Jain, et. al., *Women's quest for Power: Five Indian Case Studies*', Vikas Publishing House Pvt. Ltd., New Delhi.
Johnstone, Sir James (1896), *Manipur and the Naga hills*, (reprinted in 1983) Cultural Publishing House, Delhi.
Kabui, Gangmumei (1991a), 'Anglo-Manipur War of 1891', in Dena, Lal (1991a).
Kabui, Gangmumei (1991b), 'Socio-religious Reform Movement', in Dena, Lal (1991a).
Kabui, Gangmumei (1991c), 'Zeliangrong movement under Jadonang and Rani Gaidinliu', in Dena, Lal (1991a).
Krishnan, T.N. (1984), 'Infant Mortality in Kerala State, India: A Preliminary Analysis', pp. 293–308, UNICEF *Assignment Children*, vol. no. 65/68.
Krishnan, T.N. (1985), 'Health Statistics in Kerala State, India', pp. 39–46 in Rockefeller Foundation, *Good Health at Low Cost*.
Kumar, Shiva A.K. (1991), 'The UNDP's Human Development Index: A computation for 17 Indian States', *Economic and Political Weekly*, 17 October.
Kumar Shiva A.K. (192), 'Maternal Capabilities and Child Survival in Low Income Regions: An Economic Analysis of Infant Mortality in India', Ph.D. Dissertation, Harvard University.
Leslie, Joanne (1989), 'Women's work and child nutrition in the third world' in Joanne Leslie and Michael Paolisso (eds.) *Women, Work, and Child Welfare in the Third World*, Westview Press Inc., Boulder, Colorado.

Minhas, B.S., L.R. Jain and S.D. Tendulkar (1991), 'Declining Incidence of Poverty in the 1980s: Evidence versus Artefacts', *Economic and Political Weekly* 6–13 July.

Ministry of health and Family Welfare (1987), *'Health Information of India, 1987*, Central Bureau of Health Intelligence, Directorate General of Health Services New Delhi.

Ministry of Health and Family Welfare (1989), *Family Welfare Programme in India, Year Book 1987–88*, New Delhi.

Murray, Christopher (1987), 'The Determinants of Health Improvements in Developing Countries', unpublished Ph.D dissertation.

Nag, Moni (1985), 'The Impact of Social and Economic Development on Mortality: Comparative Study of Kerala and West Bengal' in Rockefeller Foundation, *Good Health at Low Cost*.

Nagraj, K. (1985), 'Infant mortality in Tamil Nadu', Working Paper of the Madras Institute for Development Studies, Madras, India.

Office of Registrar General (1985), *Sample Registration System, 1981*, Ministry of Home Affairs, New Delhi.

Office of Registrar General (1987), *Recent Fertility Trends in North Eastern India*, Office of the Registrar General, India.

Office of Registrar General (1988), *Sample Registration System, 1986*, Ministry of Home Affairs, New Delhi.

Osmani, S.R. (1990), 'Nutrition and the economics of food: Implications of some recent controversies' in Jean Drèze and Amartya Sen (eds.) (1990), *The Political Economy of Hunger: Volume 1*, Oxford: Clarendon Press.

Panikar, P.G.K. (1985) 'Health Care System in Kerala and Its Impact on Infant Mortality' in Rockefeller Foundation, *Good Health at Low Cost*, 1985.

Panikar, P.G.K., and C.R. Soman (1984), *Health Status of Kerala*, Centre for Development Studies, Trivandrum, Kerala.

Preston, S.H. (1976), 'Causes and Consequences of Mortality Declines in Less Developed Countries during the 20th Century', Edited by R.A. Easterlin, *Population and Economic Changes in Less Developed Countries*, NBER Conference, Philadelphia, Chicago: University of Chicago Press, 1976.

Reserve Bank of India (1982), *Reserve Bank of India Bulletin*, September 1982, New Delhi.

Rockefeller Foundation (1985), *Good Health at Low Cost*, Rockefeller Foundation, New York.

Roy, Shibani and S.H.M. Rizvi (1990), *Tribal Customary Laws of North-East India*, B.R. Publishing Corporation, Delhi.

Sarvekshana (1989), *A note and survey results on monthly per capita consumption of cereals for various sections of the population: NSS 38th round*, Vol. XIII, No. 2, issue No. 41, Oct–Dec.

Sarvekshana (1987), *A note on some aspects of household ownership holding: NSS 37th Round (Jan–Dec. 1992)*, October.

Sarvekshana (1988), *Survey results on sources of drinking water and energy used for cooking and lighting: NSS 38th round (Jan–Dec 1983)*, Issue No. 37, Vol. XII, No. 2, October.

Sen, Amartya (1984), 'Goods and people' in Amartya Sen: *Resources, Values and Development*, Harvard University Press, Cambridge, Mass.

Sen, Amartya (1985), *Commodities and Capabilities*, Oxford University Press, Delhi.

Sen, Amartya (1989), 'Development as Capability Expansion' in 'Human Development in the 1980s and Beyond', *Journal of Development Planning*, United Nations, No. 19.
Sen, Amartya (1990), 'More Than 100 million women are missing', *The New York Review of Books*, 20 December.
Sen, Gita and Chiranjib Sen (1985), 'Women's domestic work and economic activity, *Economic and Political Weekly*, Vol xx, No. 17, 27 April.
Singh, M. Bokul (1990), 'Tribal culture of Manipur' in Kabui, Gangmumei (ed.), *Tribal Profile of Manipur*, Centre for Tribal Studies, Manipur University, Imphal.
Singh, Joykumar N. (1991a), 'First women's agitation, 1904' in Dena, Lal (1991a).
Singh, Joykumar N. (1991b), 'Women's agitation of 1939' in Dena, Lal (1991a).
Singh, Joykumar N. (1991c), 'Political Agency, 1835–1919' in Dena, Lal (1991a).
Singh, K.M. (1991d), *History of Christian Missions in Manipur and Other Neigbouring States*, Mittal Publications, New Delhi.
Thaimei, Mangthoi (1976), 'The Kabuis (or the Rongmeis)' in K.B. Singh (ed), *An Introduction to Tribal Language and Culture of Manipur*, Manipur State Kala Akademi, Imphal.
United Nations (1975), *Poverty, Unemployment and Development Policy: A Case Study of Selected Issues with Reference to Kerala*. St\ESA\29, United Nations Publication, New York.
United Nations (1985), *Socio-economic differentials in child mortality in developing countries*, ST/ESA/SER.A/97, United Nations Publications, New York.
UNDP (1990), *Human Development Report 1990*, Oxford University Press.
Ware, Helen, (1984), 'Effects of Maternal Education, Women's Roles, and Child Care on Child Mortality' in Henry W. Mosley and Lincoln C. Chen (ed), *Child Survival Strategies for Research*, Population and Development Review Supplement to Volume 10, 1984.
Warren, Kenneth S. (1985), 'Remarks' pp. 245–46, in Rockefeller Foundation's *Good Health at Low Cost*.
World Bank (1984), *Population Change and Economic Development*, reprinted from the *World Development Report 1984*, published by Oxford University Press.

The Reproductive Years

4

Maternal Mortality: Estimates from an Econometric Model

P. N. MARI BHAT, K. NAVANEETHAM and
S. IRUDAYA RAJAN

I. Introduction

Complications of pregnancy and childbirth are believed to be the leading cause of death among women in most parts of South Asia. In his landmark study on the sex ratio of India's population, Visaria (1971) singled out maternal mortality as the main culprit for the deficit of females found in this part of the world. Ironically, no one knows exactly how many women die in India from this cause. Perhaps the neglect of the subject is itself an indicator of the position accorded to women in our society. However, the situation appears to be slowly changing with the advent of the Safe Motherhood Initiative. However, in their zeal to promote the movement further, a rather exaggerated picture of the problem is being painted in the media, and even in scientific conferences, which could have a not entirely positive effect.

In order to bridge the data gap, we first outline in this paper a method of estimating maternal mortality indirectly from information on age-specific death rates by sex, and fertility rates classified by age of mother. We then apply this method to data from the Sample Registration System and National Sample Surveys to derive estimates of maternal mortality levels in different states, and over time. It is hoped that the estimates presented in this paper would help in a realistic assessment of the problem, and in targeting intervention programmes.

Before proceeding to a discussion of the method, it is helpful to briefly review the present state of knowledge on maternal mortality levels in India. Visaria (1971) has presented a comprehensive review of studies carried out before the 1970s. These suggested a maternal mortality of 15 to 20 per thousand live births in the early part of this century in urban areas of India. Visaria also reviewed evidence from health research stations at Poonamalle near Madras, Singur near Calcutta, and Ramnagaram near Bangalore, that indicated a steady fall in maternal mortality. A probable cause for the decline, he suggests, was the fall in the incidence of malaria, as pregnant women were especially susceptible to malarial infection and had higher fatality. But the evidence of declining maternal mortality at a time when India's population was becoming increasingly masculine seems odd, and begs further investigation.

Since the mid-1960s, data on maternal mortality began to be collected as a part of the Registrar General's survey on cause of death in rural areas. Data on live births and maternal deaths collected for the years 1970, 1971 and 1972 from this source suggest a maternal mortality of 4 per 1000 live births for rural India.[1] Unfortunately, the level of maternal mortality for the years since 1974 cannot be assessed directly from this source because the Office of the Registrar General, for reasons best known to itself, has ceased publishing data on live births from this source. It is these estimates for the early 1970s that form the basis for the official claim of 4 maternal deaths for 1000 live births in India.[2] Despite being 20 years out-of-date, the official figure might be a serious underestimate, because (i) it is based on data collected from villages where primary health centres are located which are thus ideally placed in terms of access to health care, and (ii) as the data on cause of death are gathered through a retrospective,

---

[1] During the period 1970–72, a total of 649 maternal deaths and 164,936 live births were recorded in the survey villages, implying thereby a maternal mortality of 393 for 100,000 live births.

[2] However, the expert committee on health for all by 2000 AD in its report quoted a figure of 4.8 maternal deaths per 1000 live births for 1976, indicating its source as the cause of death survey in rural areas (India, Ministry of Health and Family Welfare 1981). The annual report of the survey, however, does not carry this information.

lay-reporting technique, a large number of deaths from indirect obstetric causes might be missed by the source.

In recent years, a study sponsored by the World Health Organization in Anantapur district of Andhra Pradesh has received much attention (Bhatia 1988). From a field investigation of deaths among women of reproductive ages, this study estimated a maternal mortality of 830 per 100,000 live births in rural areas, and 545 in urban areas during 1984–85. Though the study results have received wide publicity, one should be cautious in generalizing the estimates derived from a mere 391 maternal deaths from a backward region of Andhra Pradesh to the whole of India. It is also worth pointing out that a bias in favour of maternal deaths might have crept in while gathering data on deaths, or in classifying deaths from ill-defined causes, as the study was exclusively devoted to the estimation of maternal mortality levels, and had employed non-medically-trained personnel for the collection of data. Another important limitation of this study is that data on births needed for the computation of maternal mortality ratios were not collected along with the survey, but were estimated by assuming the fertility rates observed in another study (Bhatia 1988).

II. Building a Model for Estimation

In countries with deficient vital registration, a direct field investigation of the type undertaken in the Anantapur district would seem the best alternative to assess the level of maternal mortality of a community. However, even in countries where it is more common, maternal mortality is a rare event, and thus a large sample of women is required to estimate its level with a fair degree of accuracy. For example, in a country with a general fertility rate of 150 per thousand women in the reproductive age group, and a maternal mortality ratio of 5 per thousand births, over two million women of reproductive ages would have to be followed for a year to estimate maternal mortality and have a margin of error within five per cent.

Because of the requirement of a large sample in such investigations, alternative approaches are being explored to estimate maternal mortality. One of these is the so-called 'Sisterhood Method', wherein women are asked to recall the number of sisters who died during pregnancy, delivery and puerperium among those who were ever-married and not surviving at the time of the survey (Graham, Brass and Snow 1989). While this method cuts the sample size requirement drastically, it relies heavily on the women recalling events which occurred some time ago. The estimates derived from this procedure might not be for a period as recent as one might wish, and also could be sensitive to the assumed level of fertility. The method is more suitable in countries where fertility and mortality levels have been relatively stationary in the recent past.

Another method suggested is to estimate maternal mortality indirectly from age- and sex-specific death rates, without having data on cause of death. This approach does not necessarily cut down on the sample size requirement, but it makes use of information routinely collected on a large scale in censuses, surveys and registration systems. Recently, Blum and Fargues (1990) have proposed two methods utilizing this information. In the first method they assume that in the absence of maternal deaths, the ratio of women's to men's mortality would change linearly between ages 10 and 45, and deviations of the observed ratios from this norm could be attributed to maternal mortality. In the second method, they assume that in the absence of maternal mortality, the age schedule of female mortality would follow the well-known Gompertz law. They claim that while estimates from the first method give good approximations to maternal mortality from direct obstetric causes, estimates from the latter method are closer to the overall maternal mortality, including indirect obstetric causes.

Blum and Fargues appear to underestimate the significance of mortality from accidents and violence among adults in developing countries. As our studies on India and China indicate, mortality from accidental fire and suicide is a major cause of fatality among women of reproductive ages in Asia (Bhat 1991). Although there are fewer vehicles on the roads of developing countries, because of poor road conditions, lack of safety regulations, overcrowding, etc., a substantial number of passengers and pedestrians (more men than women) succumb to motor-vehicle accidents. It is therefore incorrect to assume, as Blum and Fargues do, that once the maternal mortality is removed, the age profile of female mortality or the sex-ratio mortality would have a more regular pattern. Indeed, it is very likely that their two methods give different estimates of maternal mortality because of the varying sensitivity of the methods to the disturbances from accidents and violence, and not because of the inclusion or exclusion of indirect obstetric causes, as they claim. The estimates from the two methods are also not influenced to the same degree by the under-enumeration of deaths.

We have proposed below a new method of estimating the level of maternal mortality by relating sex differentials in mortality in reproductive ages to the age-schedule of fertility.[3] Even though our method needs information on age-specific fertility rates in addition to the data that Blum and Fargues have used, this is essential to be able to separate the influence of maternal mortality on the sex differentials of mortality from that of external causes. Further, unlike Blum and Fargues, we do not make an attempt to estimate age-specific maternal mortality ratios; instead we aim at computing its overall level in the age group 15–49, by employing a standard age pattern of maternal mortality. Such an approach helps in suggesting a parametric method for estimating the level of maternal mortality in place of the non-parametric methods adopted by Blum and Fargues. Although it is possible to suggest a method of estimation similar to the second procedure outlined by Blum and Fargues (i.e., using only mortality rates of females), in our judgement it holds less promise because of greater sensitivity to mortality from accident or violence and inadequacies in death registration.

The Model

Notations

$\mu_f(x)$ = Instantaneous death rate of females at age x from all causes.

$\mu_m(x)$ = Instantaneous death rate of males at age x from all causes.

$R(x)$ = The ratio of female to male mortality risk at age x.

$m(x)$ = Ratio of maternal deaths to live births at age x.

$f(x)$ = Instantaneous fertility rate of women aged x.

$\mu^o(x)$ = Instantaneous death rate at age x from obstetric causes.

---

[3]In a paper under preparation, the method is more fully developed and its validity tested using data for populations having reliable, direct information on maternal mortality (Bhat, forthcoming).

$\mu^{-o}(x)$ = Instantaneous death rate of females at age x from causes other than maternity.

$N(x)$ = Number of women at age x in the population.

MMR = Average maternal mortality ratio for the interval 15–49.

Since in an instantaneous time interval mortality risks from maternal and non-maternal causes can be assumed as independent risks, we have

$$\mu_f(x) = \mu^o(x) + \mu^{-o}(x).$$

Further, the risk of mortality at age x from obstetric causes is the product of the risk of giving birth at that age, and the risk of dying after having given birth. That is

$$\mu^o(x) = m(x) \, f(x)$$

By substitution, we get

$$\mu_f(x) = \mu^{-o}(x) + m(x) \, f(x) \tag{1}$$

Let the maternal mortality ratio for women aged 20–24 be equal to m. We may then define the relative maternal mortality ratio as

$$w(x) = m(x)/m.$$

Equation (1) can now be rewritten as

$$\mu_f(x) = \mu^{-o}(x) + m \, w(x) \, f(x). \tag{2}$$

By dividing equation (2) by the force of mortality among males at age x, we get

$$\frac{\mu_f(x)}{\mu_m(x)} = \frac{\mu^{-o}(x)}{\mu_m(x)} + m \, \frac{w(x) \, f(x)}{\mu_m(x)},$$

or

$$R(x) = \varphi(x) + m \, \frac{w(x) \, f(x)}{\mu_m(x)} \tag{3}$$

where $\varphi(x) = \mu^{-o}(x)/\mu_m(x)$.

What we propose is to estimate m from equation (3) by the method of least-squares. Since instantaneous death rates are not observable, we employ the annual rates instead. This results only in a minor violation of the assumption of independency of risks. However, to implement the method, it is necessary (i) to find a suitable closed-form expression for $\varphi(x)$ whose parameters are to be estimated along with m, and (ii) to assume a standard age-pattern of maternal mortality (i.e., $w(x)$'s). While the latter is not a difficult task, our experience with the method suggests that it is not easy to find a single expression for $\varphi(x)$ that is applicable to all countries (Bhat, forthcoming). Nonetheless, a simple straight line fits the data well in many cases, and if excessive male mortality from accidents and violence is a problem (which is often indicated by a kink in the sex ratio of mortality at the age interval 20–24), inclusion of a dummy for that interval is found sufficient to capture its impact.

There is another econometric problem that we ought to address. While estimating the parameter m from equation (3) through the method of least-squares, one may either choose to implement

$$\frac{\mu_f(x)}{\mu_m(x)} = \varphi(x) + m \frac{w(x) f(x)}{\mu_m(x)} + e(x), \quad (3a)$$

or

$$\mu_f(x) = \varphi(x) \mu_m(x) + m\, w(x)\, f(x) + u(x) \quad (3b)$$

where the errors $e(x)$ and $u(x)$ are assumed to be random. The two may not necessarily give the same estimate of m. In theory, if equation (3a) is correct, the residuals of equation (3b) would be heteroscedastic with variance proportional to the square of $\mu_m(x)$. If equation (3b) is correct, the reverse would be true with the residuals of the former being inversely proportional to the square of $\mu_m(x)$. But in practice, the heteroscedasticity test may not be able to conclusively show which form is correct. Since equation (3b) gives more weight to the observed rate at older ages than equation (3a), the difference in the two estimates is often a reflection of how well the model fits the data at the beginning and end of the reproductive span. Therefore using an alternative form for $\varphi(x)$, or changing the values used for $w(x)$, might help in narrowing the difference.

After estimating m, the average maternal mortality ratio for the age group 15–49 can be computed using the identity

$$\text{MMR} = \frac{m\, \Sigma\, w(x)\, f(x)\, N(x)}{\Sigma\, f(x)\, N(x)} \quad (4)$$

One of the main advantages of the above method is that the estimated level of maternal mortality is robust to the incompleteness of vital registration. Indeed, if fertility rates and male and female mortality rates were affected to the same degree by the under-enumeration, the maternal mortality estimate remains free of error. However, if female deaths were more under-counted compared to male deaths, or if under-enumeration was greater in the case of deaths than in the case of births, the maternal mortality would be underestimated. The main disadvantage of the method is that the estimate is sensitive to the assumed mathematical expression for $\varphi(x)$. Therefore we suggest estimating the form of $\varphi(x)$ from the data themselves. This is possible if age-specific fertility and mortality rates are available for a large number of subnational populations having varying levels of maternal mortality.

The key assumption made here is that in the absence of maternal mortality, female-male mortality ratios in the reproductive ages would have the same slope in all subnational units, but might be uniformly higher or lower at all ages (i.e., have different intercepts) depending on region-specific factors. Then the ratio $\mu^{-o}/\mu_m(x)$ for the jth subnational population can be written as

$$\varphi(x, j) = B(x) + C(j)$$

where the $B(x)$'s are the age-specific effects on the sex ratio of mortality, and the $C(j)$'s are the region-specific effects on the same. We may now write equation (3) for the subnational population as

$$R(x, j) = B(x) + C(j) + m(j)\frac{w(x)\,f(x,\,j)}{\mu_m(x,\,j)} \qquad (5)$$

The parameters $B(x)$, $C(j)$ and $m(j)$ of equation (5) can be estimated by dummy-variable regression, or by the analysis of the covariance, of pooled cross-sectional data. A priori specification of the functional form for the $B(x)$'s is not necessary here because the pooled cross-sectional data contain invaluable information on how sex ratios of mortality change when the level of maternal mortality varies. However, as with equation (3), in actual estimation, the stochastic errors could be specified in two different ways which might not give the same result:

$$R(x, j) = B(x) + C(j) + m(j)\frac{w(x,\,j)\,f(x,\,j)}{\mu_m(x,\,j)} + e(x,\,j), \qquad (5a)$$

or

$$\mu_f(x, j) = B(x) \mu_m(x) + C(j) \mu_m(x)$$
$$+ m(j) w(x, j) f(x, j) + u(x, j) \tag{5b}$$

It may also be noted that once $B(x)$'s are estimated for a country, they may be reused in another application to estimate maternal mortality as follows:

$$R(x) - \hat{B}(x) = C + m \frac{w(x) f(x)}{\mu_m(x)} + e(x), \tag{6a}$$

or

$$\mu_f(x) - \hat{B}(x) \mu_m(x) = C \mu_m(x) + m w(x) f(x) + u(x). \tag{6b}$$

It may be noted that equation (6b) is a regression model without the intercept term.

III. Application to Indian Data

The data on age- and sex-specific death rates and age-specific fertility rates are available for India and its major states from the Sample Registration System and National Sample Surveys. They provide a good testing ground for demonstrating the usefulness of the above procedure. We begin by discussing the age pattern of maternal mortality (i.e., $w(x)$'s) employed in the estimation.

Standard age pattern of maternal mortality

Table 1 provides data on age-specific maternal mortality ratios from four different sources for South Asia. Among these, the information from Sri Lanka is perhaps the most reliable as it is based on a large number of maternal deaths from the civil registration system between 1954 and 1972. It indicates a sharp rise in maternal mortality after age 35. However, the Sri Lankan data do not show the higher risk of maternal mortality among mothers of under age 20, perhaps because the majority of those who gave birth in the age interval 15–19 did so when they were nearing 20 years of age, the age at marriage being higher in that country. On the other hand, the survey data from Matlab, Bangladesh, do indicate that teenage mothers have a higher risk of maternal mortality than those giving birth at ages 20–24.

Surprisingly, the maternal mortality study done in Anantapur district of Andhra Pradesh does not show the expected U-shaped age pattern of maternal mortality. In fact, the maternal mortality ratio

Table 1: Maternal Mortality Ratio for 1000 Live Births by Mother's Age from Vital Registration of Special Surveys in South Asia

Age interval	MMR for 1000 live births				Ratio to MMR of 20-24				Assumed $w(x)$
	Sri Lanka 1954-72	Matlab 1968-72	Matlab 1976-85	Anantapur dist. A.P. 1984-85	Sri Lanka 1954-72	Matlab 1968-72	Matlab 1976-85	Anantapur dist. A.P. 1984-85	
10-14	–	17.7	–	–	–	4.7	–	–	2.0
15-19	2.3	7.4	7.4	5.4	1.1	1.9	1.8	0.7	1.0
20-24	2.1	3.8	4.1	7.9	1.0	1.0	1.0	1.0	1.1
25-29	2.4	5.2	4.5	6.0	1.1	1.4	1.1	0.8	1.3
30-34	2.8	6.2	4.6	10.9	1.3	1.6	1.1	1.4	1.3
35-39	4.4	4.8	9.9	12.9	2.1	1.3	2.4	1.6	2.0
40-44	5.9	8.0	7.9	4.4	2.8	2.1	1.9	0.5	3.0
45-49	11.3	–	–	2.2	5.4	–	–	0.3	5.0
All ages	–	5.7	5.5	8.0					
No. of maternal deaths	–	119	387	391					

Source: ESCAP (1976), Chen et al. (1974), Koenig et al. (1988), Bhatia (1988).

was significantly lower among mothers under age 20, and those giving birth after age 40! Extreme caution is therefore necessary in interpreting the results of this survey.

Therefore, in choosing the standard age pattern of maternal mortality, we have accepted the pattern shown by the Sri Lankan data for ages above 20. For the age interval 15–19, we assumed the MMR to be twice that of the age interval 20–24, as suggested by the Matlab studies.

Age pattern of sex ratios of mortality

In the procedure described above, we have to either choose a functional form for the sex ratios of mortality in the absence of maternal mortality (i.e., $\varphi(x)$'s), or we have to estimate their age pattern (i.e. $B(x)$'s) from the regression of cross-sectional data. Since we had the requisite data for the Indian states, we adopted the second strategy.

The data on the age-specific fertility and mortality rates were taken from the Sample Registration System (SRS), which is considered to be very nearly complete with respect to the coverage of vital events. To reduce the sampling errors in the age-specific rates, we have used the average rates for 1982 to 1986. Although data were available for the 15 major states, information for Kerala, Punjab, Orissa and Rajasthan were not used in the pooled regressions as they appear to possess distinct age patterns of sex ratios.[4] Instead, to improve the information content on how the age pattern of sex ratios responds to the change in maternal mortality level, data on rural and urban areas of India were included in the analysis. The dummy-variable regression method was used in estimating the parameters of the model contained in equation 5. Two regressions were performed, one with the sex ratio of mortality as the 'dependent' variable (equation 5a), and the other with female mortality as the dependent variable (equation 5b). In all cases, data for the quinquennial age intervals, 10–14 to 50–54, were considered for the analysis.

Table 2 gives the results of this step. It is evident from the table that the regression with sex ratio of mortality as the dependent

---

[4] These states either had sex ratios of mortality substantially different from others at the age intervals 10–14 and 50–54, or values for some age intervals were extreme outliers.

Table 2: Estimates of Model Parameters from Regressions of Pooled Cross-Sectional Data for 1982–86 from Sample Registration System

Region/ age interval	D.V.: Female-Male Mortality Ratios		D.V.: Female Age-Specific Death Rates	
	Estimate of MMR of 20-24 age interval[+]	Standard error of MMR estimate	Coefficient of dummy variable	Estimate of MMR of 20-24 age interval[+]	Standard error of MMR estimate	Coefficient of dummy variable

Region/age interval	Estimate of MMR of 20-24 age interval[+]	Standard error of MMR estimate	Coefficient of dummy variable	Estimate of MMR of 20-24 age interval[+]	Standard error of MMR estimate	Coefficient of dummy variable
Andhra Pradesh	276	106	1.125	96	135	1.112
Assam	734	143	1.212	659	142	1.201
Bihar	534	144	1.176	270	114	1.216
Gujarat	274	133	1.079	104	136	1.055
Haryana	324	102	1.116	290	109	1.042
Karnataka	293	119	1.113	317	139	1.008
Madhya Pradesh	366	114	1.105	198	115	1.114
Maharashtra	288	97	1.037	215	124	0.965
Tamil Nadu	226	196	1.090	14	197	1.046
Uttar Pradesh	625	129	1.134	548	105	1.063
West Bengal	388	120	1.175	272	130	1.140
India, Rural	426	136	1.124	316	128	1.091
India, Urban	276	116	1.052	152	141	1.007
Age Intervals:						
10–14			0.000			0.000
15–19			-0.039			0.106
20–24			-0.108			0.047
25–29			-0.171			-0.037
30–34			-0.286			-0.176
35–39			-0.360			-0.287
40–44			-0.393			-0.333
45–49			-0.455			-0.414
50–54			-0.394			-0.358
R^2*			0.995			0.997
N			117			117

* R^2 of a regression model through the origin.   + For 100,000 live births.

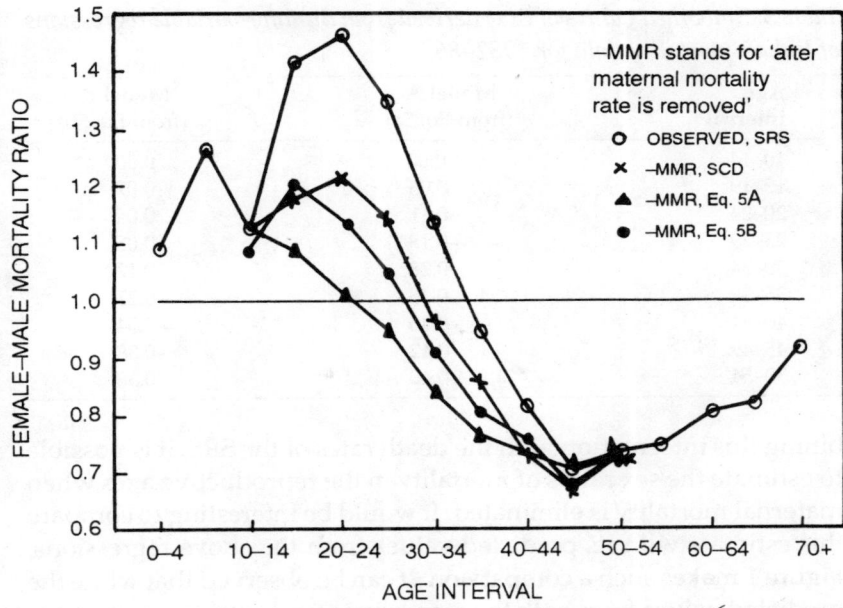

Fig 1: Observed and Predicted Sex Ratio of Mortality by Age, Rural India, 1982–86

variable gives significantly higher maternal mortality than the regression with female mortality in the reproductive ages. There is, however, a good agreement between the two sets of estimates on the regional variation in maternal mortality ($r = 0.90$). The coefficients of the regional dummies give the estimated sex ratio of mortality for the age interval 10–14 for each region (i.e. intercept). The coefficients of the age dummies provide, for each age interval, the sex ratio of mortality in the absence of maternal mortality, relative to that of the age interval 10–14. It ought to be evident now that the regression employing female death rates as the dependent variable gives significantly lower estimates of maternal mortality because it understates the fall in the sex ratio of mortality in the reproductive ages when maternal mortality is controlled. The heteroscedasticity test reported above failed to identify which specification is correct in this case, as residuals from both the equations did not exhibit significant correlation with the male death rate.

As reported in the introduction, the Registrar General's annual surveys of cause of death provide some useful information on the proportion of deaths from maternal causes in rural areas. By com-

Table 3: Smoothed values of $B(x)$ derived from dummy-variable regressions of Indian mortality data for 1982–86

Age interval	Model A (from Eq. 5a)	Model B (from Eq. 5b)
10–14	0.00	0.00
15–19	–0.05	0.07
20–24	–0.11	0.04
25–29	–0.18	–0.05
30–34	–0.28	–0.17
35–39	–0.35	–0.27
40–44	–0.40	–0.34
45–49	–0.42	–0.38
50–54	–0.40	–0.38

bining this information with the death rates of the SRS, it is possible to estimate the sex ratios of mortality in the reproductive ages when maternal mortality is eliminated. It would be interesting to compare this estimate with its predicted values from the above regressions. Figure 1 makes such a comparison. It can be observed that while the predicted values from both the regressions tend to be lower than the estimates derived using the survey of cause of death (SCD) data, those of the regression using the female death rates are closer to the survey-based estimates. Could we then conclude that the results based on this regression should be accepted? The answer, of course, is no, because it could very well be the case that the SCD had significantly underestimated the proportion of deaths from obstetric causes. Therefore, we ought to examine the state-level estimates before passing judgement on the validity of the two estimates.

The pooled regressions have, of course, provided the estimates of maternal mortality for the age interval 20–24. But we have omitted a number of states from this analysis, in the apprehension that their inclusion might unduly influence the estimates of sex ratios of mortality when maternal mortality is eliminated from the population. Now, with the estimated sex ratios of mortality in the absence of maternal mortality (i.e., $B(x)$'s), we can use equation (6a) or (6b) to compute maternal mortality for all the states by performing separate regressions for each of them. However, we have slightly smoothed the estimated $B(x)$'s before using them. The smoothed values are given in Table 3.

The model-A pattern was employed with equation (6a), and the model-B pattern was used in equation (6b).

Estimates of maternal mortality

Table 4 shows the results of the regressions done for each state in the above manner. It can be seen that for the states which also figured in the pooled regressions, the estimates of MMR for the age interval 20–24 differ only marginally from those reported in Table 2. In fact they would have been the same had we used the unsmoothed values of $B(x)$'s in the second step. However, the standard errors of maternal mortality estimates shown in Table 4 are significantly lower than those reported earlier because they were not adjusted for the fact that $B(x)$'s were estimated from an earlier regression.

In the case of states not included in the earlier step, the estimate of MMR is less than zero for Punjab under both the specifications. Either there is a problem in the mortality data from the SRS for Punjab, or the sex differentials in mortality there are somewhat unique. For Kerala, Orissa and Rajasthan, estimates using the model-A pattern seem acceptable; whereas for Kerala, and perhaps for Rajasthan too, the estimate using the model-B pattern appears to be too low. The model-B pattern, of course, gives exceptionally low values of maternal mortality even for states included in the earlier step, such as Tamil Nadu, Gujarat, Andhra Pradesh, Bihar and Madhya Pradesh—and this appears to be the main problem with this pattern.

By employing the weights, $w(x)$'s, the estimates of m can easily be converted into maternal mortality estimates for the age interval 15–49. Table 5 presents these estimates from both the versions of the model. For India as a whole, the MMR is estimated as 555 and 364 per 100,000 births during 1982–86 under the model-A and model-B patterns, respectively. The percentage of female deaths from maternal causes is estimated as 20 and 13 per cent under the two versions of the model. For the rural areas, the two versions give 619 and 414 as estimates of MMR and 22 and 15 per cent as the share of maternal deaths among all deaths. As expected, the estimates from the model-B pattern compare favourably with the estimates from the cause-of-death surveys in rural areas. For 1982–86 these surveys reported 14 per cent of all female deaths in the age interval 15–44 as maternal deaths. But estimates from this model pattern for a number of states are unbelievably low, thus forcing us to reject the entire set of estimates based on this pattern. Although on the basis of the all-India estimates it could be claimed that the model-B pattern gives the level

Table 4: *Maternal Mortality Estimates from State-Specific Regressions of Mortality Data for 1982–86 from Sample Registration System*

Region	D.V.: Female–Male Mortality Ratios			D.V.: Female Age-Specific Death Rates		
	Estimate of MMR of 20–24 age interval[a]	Standard error of MMR estimate[b]	Model R^2	Estimate of MMR of 20–24 age interval[a]	Standard error of MMR estimate[b]	Model R^{2*}
Andhra Pradesh	289	64	0.744	86	104	0.993
Assam	751	128	0.831	645	128	0.995
Bihar	543	79	0.871	236	88	0.993
Gujarat	285	108	0.498	90	120	0.991
Haryana	334	77	0.726	278	65	0.993
Karnataka	306	49	0.846	300	65	0.997
Kerala	188	72	0.492	5	92	0.993
Madhya Pradesh	379	47	0.903	183	64	0.995
Maharashtra	299	44	0.868	211	50	0.997
Orissa	574	197	0.548	508	148	0.986
Punjab	–128	98	0.196	–340	174	0.962
Rajasthan	662	121	0.810	343	95	0.985
Tamil Nadu	248	94	0.497	11	101	0.995
Uttar Pradesh	635	116	0.811	518	95	0.990
West Bengal	401	41	0.933	254	38	0.999
India, Rural	439	30	0.968	294	46	0.998
India, Urban	288	58	0.781	137	47	0.999
India, Total	400	22	0.980	262	35	0.999

* R^2 of regression model through the origin.   [a] Per 100,000 live births.   [b] Per 100,000 women in the age interval 15–49.

Table 5: Indirect Estimates of Maternal Mortality for 1982–86, and Direct Estimates from Survey of Cause of Death in Rural Areas for 1970–72

Region	D.V.: Female–Male Mortality Ratios			D.V.: Female Age-Specific Death Rates			Maternal mortality ratio from SCD, 1970–72
	Maternal Mortality		% of maternal deaths[c]	Maternal Mortality		% of maternal deaths[c]	
	Ratio[a]	Rate[b]		Ratio[a]	Rate[b]		
Andhra Pradesh	402	51	13.7	120	15	4.1	417
Assam	1028	140	25.8	883	120	22.2	1438
Bihar	813	139	26.6	353	61	11.6	229
Gujarat	355	49	14.5	112	15	4.6	245
Haryana	435	69	22.3	362	58	18.6	189
Karnataka	415	50	15.7	407	49	15.4	498
Kerala	234	20	14.2	6	1	0.4	196
Madhya Pradesh	535	89	22.1	258	43	10.7	416
Maharashtra	393	48	16.8	278	34	11.9	403
Orissa	778	105	21.9	688	92	19.4	415
Punjab	–	–	–	–	–	–	177
Rajasthan	938	164	44.1	486	85	22.9	957
Tamil Nadu	319	32	8.6	14	1	0.4	329
Uttar Pradesh	931	162	32.3	759	132	26.4	292
West Bengal	551	71	19.9	349	45	12.6	138
India, Rural	619	93	21.8	414	62	14.6	393
India, Urban	373	43	16.0	178	20	7.6	–
India, Total	555	78	20.2	364	51	13.2	–

[a] Per 100,000 live births.
[b] Per 100,000 women in the age interval 15–49.
[c] Among all female deaths in the age interval 15–49.

Table 6: Indirect Estimates of Maternal Mortality for India since the 1960s

Source	Year	Regression results with model-A pattern			Estimates for 15–49 age interval		
		MMR for 20–24 age interval	Standard error of MMR estimate	Model R-square	Maternal Mortality		% of maternal deaths[c]
					Rate[a]	Ratio[b]	
NSS, 14th and 16th rounds[d]	1957–60	919	199	0.914	1306	212	39.2
NSS, 19th round	1963–64	849	105	0.903	1211	195	44.0
SRS	1972–76	622	68	0.923	898	136	26.2
SRS	1977–81	602	61	0.933	855	119	27.0
SRS	1982–86	400	22	0.980	555	78	20.2

[a] Per 100,000 live births.
[b] Per 100,000 women in the age interval 15–49.
[c] Among all female deaths in the age interval 15–49.
[d] Information from the 14th round for rural areas and from the 16th round for urban areas were combined. Also, because of the broad age groups utilized in the tabulation, we could use data for the age intervals 15–24, 25–34, 35–44 and 44–55 only.

of maternal mortality from direct obstetric causes while the model-A pattern gives an estimate that includes deaths from both direct and indirect obstetric causes, such an assumption is untenable in the case of several state-specific estimates where the difference between the two estimates is too large to be accounted for by indirect obstetric causes alone. Moreover, there is nothing intrinsic to the technique to suggest that one version ought to give mortality from direct obstetric causes only, and the other should include deaths from indirect obstetric causes also. In principle, both estimates should include deaths from direct and indirect obstetric causes since they are derived by relating the excess female mortality in reproductive ages with fertility rates.

The estimates of maternal mortality can also be derived for the periods before 1982–86 using the equation (6a) or (6b). Table 6 presents such estimates derived from NSS and SRS all-India data. Since it seems to provide more reliable estimates, we have quoted only results derived using the model-A pattern of $B(x)$'s in equation (6a).[5] It is evident from the table that maternal mortality has declined rapidly in India from its 1960 level of 1300 per 100,000 live births. Even though the estimates of fertility and mortality from the NSS are considered to be too low, the high level of maternal mortality they imply shows the robustness of the present technique to under-enumeration of vital events. However, the estimated share of maternal deaths in all female deaths for the early 1960s (estimated at around 40 per cent) is probably too high because of the underestimation of deaths from all causes in the NSS.

IV. Discussion

In this section we will use the estimates derived using the model-A pattern to discuss a few important issues. The first issue that needs some attention is the overall level of maternal mortality in India. Blum and Fargues (1990), using the sex ratios of mortality as we do, but with different methodology, have estimated the maternal mortality in India during 1971–76 to be 584 per 100,000 live births, while our estimate for the corresponding period is 898 (see Table 6). However, using another method they arrive at levels closer to our es-

---

[5] Although the estimates derived from the model-B pattern are not shown here, they confirm the rapid decline in MMR indicated by the figures presented in Table 6.

timate. As we reported in the introduction, a community survey in Anantapur district of Andhra Pradesh has indicated a figure as high as 798 per 100,000 live births in 1985 while our estimate for the state as a whole is only 402 in 1982–86 (see Table 5). What is then the true level of maternal mortality in India?

Although it has received inadequate attention, in our judgement the best available information on cause-of-death data in India comes from the surveys of cause of death in rural areas gathered through the lay-reporting technique. The source is especially valuable in analysing deaths from such easily identifiable causes as accidents and violence, maternal mortality, etc. In Table 7 we have presented some data from this source for 1982–86 for the purpose of identifying causes that might have been over-emphasized due to the mis-classification of maternal deaths using this source. It can be seen that, compared to males, more females in the reproductive ages die from burns, anaemia, tetanus and 'fever'. The higher exposure of females to the risk of death from fire is probably genuine in Indian conditions (see Bhat 1991), and should not be attributed to mis-classification of maternal deaths. However, a good case can be made for attributing the excess female mortality from anaemia, tetanus and fevers (especially malaria) to obstetric causes. But even if we treat all the excess female mortality from these causes as maternal deaths, the percentage of deaths attributed to maternal mortality would only increase from 14 per cent to 20 per cent in the age interval 15–44. It may be recalled that our estimate based on the model-A pattern was 22 per cent for the age interval 15–49 in rural India (see Table 5). Studies done in Matlab, Bangladesh, have also suggested a level around the value we have estimated for India (Chen et al. 1974; Koenig et al. 1988). Viewed against this background, the estimate of 38 per cent recorded by the survey in Anantapur district appears to be too high.

The second issue that deserves some attention is the regional pattern in maternal mortality implied by our estimates. Our estimates disclose wide variation in maternal mortality among Indian states. Maternal mortality is the highest in Assam, where it is over 1000 per 100,000 live births, and the lowest in Kerala where it is around 200. Other states having high maternal mortality are Rajasthan, Uttar Pradesh, Bihar and Orissa. Generally, states in the southern and western parts of the country have relatively low

Table 7: Sex Differentials in Mortality from Selected Causes in Reproductive Ages (Survey of Cause of Death, Rural India, 1982–86)

Cause of death	Female deaths for 100 male deaths by age interval				% deaths from each cause in ages 15-44	
	15–24	25–34	35–44	15–44	Males	Females
Burns	493	291	146	316	1.2	4.3
Suicide	94	68	48	75	3.8	3.1
Other external causes	47	34	29	37	19.7	8.1
Maternal	–	–	–	–	–	14.2
Fevers[a]	122	127	76	107	11.3	13.4
Respiratory T.B.	102	76	45	64	17.4	12.3
Other coughs[b]	95	107	64	82	7.8	7.0
Anaemia	171	158	138	154	2.4	4.0
Jaundice	96	130	64	93	2.1	2.1
Tetanus	107	293	92	153	0.8	1.4
Rest	92	93	68	81	33.5	30.1
All causes	112	103	67	91	100.0	100.0

[a] Mainly malaria, influenza and typhoid.   [b] Mainly bronchitis and pneumonia.

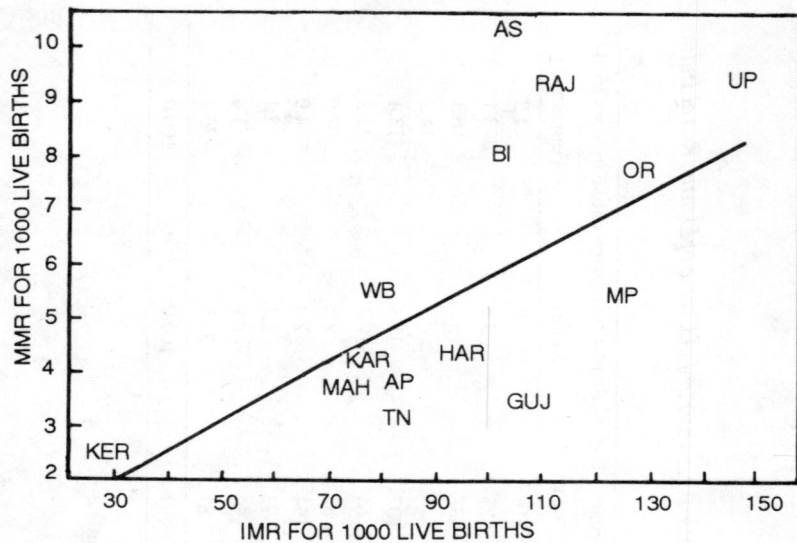

Figure 2: Relationship Between Maternal Mortality Ratios and Infant Mortality Rates for Indian States, 1982–86.

maternal mortality levels. In the urban areas of India, maternal mortality is only 60 per cent of the level observed in the rural areas.

Is there independent evidence in support of these estimates? For the major states of India, data on maternal mortality ratios are available from the survey of cause of death for 1970, 1971 and 1972. Since, for the country as a whole, only 649 maternal deaths were recorded for the three years, the state-specific estimates have large sampling errors. The average estimates of MMR from this source for 1970–72 are shown in Table 5. They confirm the presence of extremely high levels of maternal mortality in Assam and Rajasthan, and low levels in Kerala and Punjab. However, the estimates of MMR from this source for Uttar Pradesh, Bihar and West Bengal are unbelievably low, and this could be responsible for the underestimation of maternal mortality at the all-India level.

We may also check the accuracy of the regional variation in maternal mortality by comparing it with infant mortality levels, as both are influenced by the same factors. Figure 2 shows the relationship between the state-level estimates of maternal mortality and infant mortality rates for 1982–86. Again, our estimates appear to pass muster as they show a strong relationship with infant mortality rates ($r = 0.69$). However, the relation is far from perfect. Assam,

Table 8: *Percentage of maternal deaths in total deaths in reproductive ages*

Period	SCD, Rural (for 15–54)	Table 5 (for 15–49)
1972–76	11.5	26.2
1977–81	10.8	27.0
1982–86	10.8	20.2
1987–89	8.9	--

Rajasthan, Bihar and Uttar Pradesh have higher maternal mortality relative to their infant mortality levels. On the other hand, Tamil Nadu, Gujarat and Madhya Pradesh have relatively low maternal mortality. The following equation fits the data reasonably well:

$$\ln \text{MMR} = -2.33 + 0.89 \ln \text{IMR} \qquad R^2 = 0.55$$
$$(0.23)$$

The elasticity estimate of 0.89 indicates that a one per cent decline in the IMR is associated with a nearly one per cent decline in the MMR.

Another issue we would like to comment on is the rapid decline in maternal mortality that our estimates imply. Like our estimates, data from the survey of cause of death also suggest a fall in maternal mortality in recent years (Table 8).

The actual decline in maternal mortality is larger than the figures in Table 8 indicate because, as the data from the SRS suggest, there was a general fall in mortality from all causes in the last two decades. The figures indicate that the decline in maternal mortality was larger than the decline in general mortality in the reproductive ages. It may be noted that though there is broad conformity between the two sets of estimates regarding the trend, there is some variation in the detail. The data from the SCD suggest a relatively larger decline between 1972–76 and 1977–81 than between 1977–81 and 1982–86. The reverse is true in the case of our estimates. The stagnation in the maternal mortality level during the 1970s indicated by our estimates could be defended as due to the resurgence of malaria in India. However, the evidence is only circumstantial in nature.

It should be pointed out that the downward trend in maternal mortality in India is not a new phenomenon. As stated in the introduction, Visaria has presented evidence suggesting the fall in maternal mortality even before the 1960s. He attributes it mainly to the eradication of malaria. The decline since the 1960s could be attributed to the extension of health services to rural areas and improvements in transportation and communication. The data from the SRS suggest that the percentage of births at medical institutions and by trained birth attendants has gone up from around 25 per cent in the early 1970s to 40 per cent in the mid-1980s.

However, what is puzzling is the deterioration in the sex ratio of the population at a time when maternal mortality was declining. There could be two reasons for this. First, the evidence of declining sex ratios (F/M) might be erroneous, at least for the period after 1961. It is possible to argue that in both the 1971 and 1991 censuses—which registered a fall in the sex ratios—under-enumeration was more in the case of females than in the case of males. Second, inter-censal analyses suggest that while the decline in adult mortality was more for females than for males, the opposite was true in the case of child mortality (see Bhat 1987). While female children have probably been discriminated against in the provision of heath care since the days of Manu, this probably had little impact on the sex differentials in mortality until effective treatment for infectious diseases became available.

Finally, for policy purposes, it is important to know how much of the decline in maternal mortality is due to the decline in fertility. A simple decomposition of the decline in maternal mortality between 1972–76 and 1982–86 showed that 20 per cent of the decline in the maternal mortality rate (i.e. per woman) could be attributed to the decline in fertility, and 8 per cent of the decline in the maternal mortality ratio (i.e. per birth) is explained by the change in the age schedule of fertility (i.e. from the fall in the fertility rates at early and late ages of childbearing).

V. Summary

In this paper we have outlined a new technique for the estimation of maternal mortality by relating the sex differentials in mortality in reproductive ages to the age schedule of fertility. The method is well suited to the data circumstances in India. The application of this method to the SRS data for 1982–86 indicated a level of maternal mortality of 555 per 100,000 births for India as a whole. Maternal mortality appears to be relatively high in the eastern and northern parts of the country. Our estimates also suggest a substantial decline of maternal mortality in India since the 1960s. According to our estimates 20 per cent of the decline in the maternal mortality rate, and 8 per cent of the decline in the maternal mortality ratio, between 1972–76 and 1982–86 could be attributed to the decline in fertility.

References

Bhat, M. (1987), 'Mortality in India: Levels, trends and patterns'. Unpublished Ph. D. Dissertation, University of Pennsylvania, Philadelphia, U.S.A.
———(1991). 'Mortality from accidents and violence in India and China'. Research Report 91-06-1, Centre for Population Analysis and Policy, University of Minnesota, U.S.A.
———(forthcoming), 'An econometric approach to the estimation of maternal mortality from incomplete data'. Paper under preparation.
Bhatia, J.C. (1988). *A Study of Maternal Mortality in Anantapur District, Andhra Pradesh, India*. Bangalore: Indian Institute of Management.
Blum, A. and P. Farguès (1990). 'Rapid estimation of maternal mortality in countries with defective data: An application to Bamako (1974–85) and other developing countries'. *Population Studies* 44:155–71.
Chen, L. C. et al. (1974). 'Maternal mortality in rural Bangladesh'. *Studies in Family Planning* 5(11):334–41.
ESCAP (1976). *Population of Sri Lanka*. Country monograph series No. 4. Bangkok: United Nations.
Graham, W., W. Brass and R. W. Snow, (1989). 'Estimating maternal mortality: The sisterhood method'. *Studies in Family Planning* 20(3): 125–35.
India, Ministry of Health and Family Welfare (1981). *The Report of the Working Group on Health for All By 2000 A.D.* New Delhi: National Institute of Health and Family Welfare (reprinted 1983).
Koenig, M.A. et al., (1988). 'Maternal mortality in Matlab, Bangladesh, 1976–85'. *Studies in Family Planning* 19(2):69–80.
Visaria, P. 1971. *The Sex Ratio of the Population of India*. Monograph No. 10, Census of India, 1961, Volume 1. New Delhi: Manager of Publications.

5

Unsafe Motherhood:
A Review of Reproductive Health

SHIREEN J. JEJEEBHOY and SAUMYA RAMA RAO*

In recent years, levels of mortality in India have been declining and gender differentials in mortality narrowing. This however should not be interpreted to mean that reproductive *health* does not continue to be a matter of critical importance. This review of India's reproductive health situation underscores this note of caution. The review focuses on the fertility-related aspects of reproductive health in India, its levels, determinants and interventions designed to improve it; it touches on such issues as sterility and sexually transmitted diseases. Recognizing that reproductive health goes beyond the medical, we attempt here to synthesize the evidence available from a variety of sources: social science, public health and medical.

There is a tendency to equate reproductive health with maternal mortality, so at the outset we must note that reproductive health encompasses both mortality *and* health (WHO 1991; Sai and Nassim 1989). Such measures as maternal, foetal, perinatal and neonatal mortality are undoubtedly the most critical manifestations of poor reproductive health, but this should not detract from other important quality-of-life concerns such as anaemia, morbidity, obstetric conditions, birth weight, abortion and related complications, closely-spaced pregnancies, unmet need for contraception, infertility and incidence of STDs. Together, these mortality and morbidity in-

---

*We are grateful to Shantha Rajgopal for research assistance and to Sumati Kulkarni, Jyoti Moodbidri, K. Srinivasan and Yoshiteru Uramoto for comments and suggestions.

dicators are a true reflection of reproductive health. Equally important are factors underlying reproductive health. Reproductive health in India is largely influenced by poverty-related and socio-cultural factors on the one hand, and programme interventions on the other. Socio-cultural factors which impinge on reproductive health include women's lack of awareness of health practices, strong seclusion norms which inhibit health-seeking, adolescent marriage, large family size norms which encourage frequent and closely spaced pregnancies, and a general devaluation of women which makes them the last to obtain food or health care and which requires of them long periods of physical activity. Interventions directed towards reproductive health include the Maternal and Child Health, Integrated Child Development Services and Family Planning Programmes. This review considers each of these underlying sets of factors and the ways in which they affect reproductive health at various stages of the life-cycle.

1. Levels of Maternal, Perinatal and Neonatal Mortality

Currently the main indicator of women's health, maternal mortality, is recognized as the tip of the iceberg of the problems caused by sexuality and reproduction (Sai and Nassim 1989). Unfortunately, maternal deaths are notoriously under-reported even in the more developed world, since often when the cause of death is a non-obstetric condition, precipitated by an obstetric condition, the latter is not reported; underestimates in the range of 33–50 per cent have thus been observed even in the U.S.A. (Royston and Armstrong 1989). In India, mis-classification is compounded by sparse and unreliable civil registration data, and few community level studies. Results from hospital studies are more numerous and point to high rates but are mis-leading since they are not representative of the population at large.

India's maternal mortality ratio[1] is estimated at 400–500 per 100,000 live births—about fifty times higher than that of many

---

[1] Maternal mortality is measured in two ways: a *rate* and a *ratio*. The maternal mortality rate refers to deaths resulting from pregnancy-related causes per 100,000 women in the reproductive ages. The maternal mortality ratio is based on a different denominator, 100,000 live births; the number of live births is used as a proxy for the number of pregnancies, which, though more appropriate, is generally unavailable and difficult to obtain. There is considerable confusion on this issue in the literature, in which the term *rate* is frequently used in reference to a *ratio*.

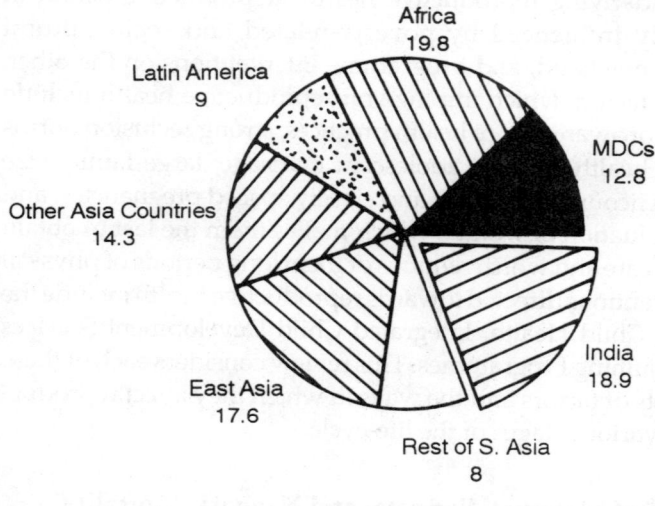

FERTILITY

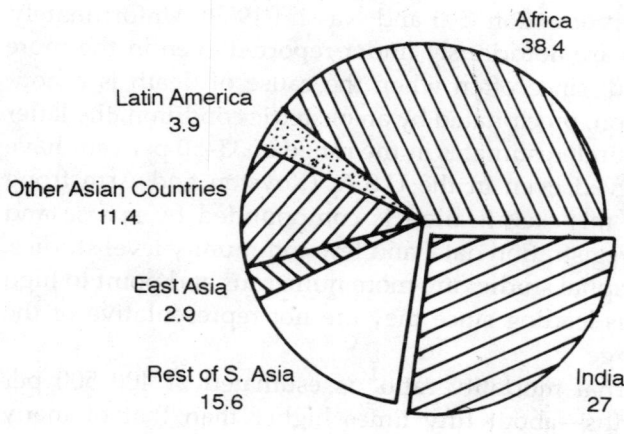

MATERNAL MORTALITY RATIOS

Fig. 1: Estimates of Live Births and Maternal Deaths (Average Annual Figures for 1985–1990)

Source: Acsadi and Johnson-Acsadi, 1990

industrialized nations and six times as high as that of neighbouring Sri Lanka (UNICEF 1991; Acsadi and Johnson-Acsadi 1990). This appears to be an underestimate and a more realistic estimate is probably 555 as estimated by Mari Bhat et al. (1992), though higher estimates in the range of 700–900 (Mathai 1989) have also been made. Even so, using the estimated MMR of 400–500, in the global perspective, it is estimated that India accounted for 19% of all live births worldwide, and for as much as 27 per cent of all deaths (Figure 1).

Not only is the risk of dying from maternal causes high, but also, women in India are repeatedly exposed to these risks as a result of high and closely-spaced fertility stretching from adolescence to menopause. Maternal deaths in India account for about one per cent of all deaths and two per cent of all female deaths annually—but this translates into over ten per cent of all deaths among women in the reproductive ages and 13.2 per cent among rural women in 1987 (UNICEF 1991). The lifetime risk of dying from pregnancy-related causes in India—with a total fertility rate of 4–5 and a maternal mortality ratio of around 500 per 100,000 live births—is as high as one in 27 (Royston and Armstrong 1989).

More intensive investigations of maternal mortality come from small field studies. There are few community or household level studies of maternal mortality. Notable among these is a 1985–86 village level study in Anantapur, Andhra Pradesh, which found a ratio of 830 and 545 in rural and urban areas respectively (Bhatia 1988). Maternal deaths accounted for 38 per cent of all deaths to women in the reproductive ages in rural areas and 28 per cent in urban. Maternal mortality ranges from 2166 per 100,000 live births in the least developed villages (as measured by location, communication and transport facilities, educational and other amenities), to 1523 and 803 respectively among somewhat and adequately developed villages, to 516 in highly developed villages. As many as 66 per cent of maternal deaths had not been recorded by health workers; reasons could range from inability in attributing cause of death to simply a vested interest in minimizing reported maternal deaths.

Hospital based studies of maternal mortality are more widely available. Ratios observed among these are expected to be higher than those for the community in general because given that no more than 20 per cent of all deliveries occur in hospitals, it is the high risk cases who are more likely to be observed. A look at hospital based

Table 1: Estimates of the maternal mortality ratio in India: various sources

Area	Year	MMR Survey	MMR Hospital	Sources, notes
India	1980–87	500		UNICEF, 1990
India	1982–86	555		Mari Bhat et al., 1992
India—rural	1982–86	619		
India—urban	1982–86	373		
India	1978–79		703	Bhasker Rao, 1980

State specific findings

1. Andhra Pradesh
Anantapur: Rural	1984–85	830		Bhatia, 1988
Anantapur: Urban	1984–85	545		

2. Bihar: Patna
	1976–80		553	Sinha, 1986

3. Haryana: Rohtak
	1978–88		1606	Tewari and Gulati, 1990
	1978–83		2243	
	1984–88		1071	

4. Madhya Pradesh: Rewa
	1975–80		1315	Agarwal et al., 1982

5. Maharashtra
	1983	333		Chandrakapure and Ranganathan, 1985
Bombay	1974–83		994	Lopez et al., 1986
Pune	1980–85		315	Panat and Mehendale, 1987

6. Tamil Nadu: Madras
	1981–85		224	Nafeesa Beebi, 1987

7. West Bengal: Calcutta
	1975–79			Roy Chowdhury et al., 1982
	1975		997	
	1976		1047	
	1977		677	
	1978		1157	
	1979		2000	
Calcutta	1974–1980		1053	Mitra and Khara, 1983

8. Uttar Pradesh: Kanpur
	1975–79		1025	Mathur and Rohatgi, 1981

9. Delhi
	1983–84		650	Sen Gupta and Gode, 1988
	1975–83		705	
	1979–87		638	Raichowdhuri et al., 1990
	1979		825	
	1987		484	

studies indicates wide variation in maternal mortality ratios—ranging from 224 in a study in Madras to over 2000 in certain years in studies in Haryana and West Bengal (Table 1), with the majority reporting ratios around 1000–1500.

Data on maternal mortality from vital registration systems, health service statistics and the few sample surveys that exist are unreliable, incomplete and of limited coverage. Indirect techniques to estimate maternal mortality seem promising in these circumstances; one example is the 'sisterhood' method (Graham et al. 1989), which derives estimates of maternal mortality from faulty data.[2]

Aside from maternal mortality, high rates of miscarriage and stillbirth as well as of perinatal and neonatal mortality are a direct consequence of poor reproductive health and antenatal, natal and neonatal care. For example 1.5 million perinatal deaths occur annually; the perinatal mortality rate is 66 per 1000 live births as compared to 10–20 in many developed countries. In limited prospective studies, perinatal mortality rates ranging from 46–80 in rural areas, and 39 to 47 in urban, have been observed (Singh and Paul 1988).

Table 2 presents the infant mortality rate and its components for India over the years 1976–87. Over this eleven-year period, there has been a modest decline of roughly 25 per cent, that is, about 2.2 per cent annually in each measure of mortality: infant mortality fell from 129 to 94, post-neonatal mortality from 52 to 38; neonatal and perinatal mortality from 77 to 58 and from 67 to 50 respectively; and stillbirths from 18 to 13. Over the 1980–85 period, it has been post-neonatal rather than neonatal or perinatal mortality which has recorded major declines, suggesting that the exogenous causes of death have been more effectively controlled than the endogenous: while the infant mortality rate fell by 17 per cent, post-neonatal mortality recorded an 18 per cent decline compared to a decline of 13 per cent in neonatal and 14.2 per cent in perinatal mortality, and 10 per cent in the stillbirth rate. On the whole, neonatal deaths account for about 60 per cent of all infant deaths and 50 per cent of neonatal deaths occur in the first week of life; nearly 25 per cent of all neonatal deaths (i.e. 15 per cent of all infant deaths) occur in the

---

[2]This method uses the proportion of elder sisters dying during pregnancy, childbirth or the puerperium reported by adults during a census or survey to derive a variety of indicators of maternal mortality, and may be appropriate for application in the Indian context. However, as Trussell and Rodriguez (1990) point out, this method has two drawbacks: that of double counting when the mother has many siblings and under-counting if she has none; and problems of the validity of the cause of death. More research on these lines on the development of indirect techniques is necessary to combat the paucity of data.

Table 2: Mortality indicators, 1976–1987

	1976	1977	1978	1979	1980	1981	1982	1983	1984	1985	1987
A. Rural											
1. Crude death rate	16.3	16.0	15.3	13.9	13.5	13.7	13.1	13.1	13.8	13.0	12.0
2. Infant mortality rate	139.0	140.0	137.0	129.7	123.8	119.1	113.7	113.8	113.8	107.0	104.0
3. Neonatal mortality rate	83.0	88.0	85.2	77.7	75.5	75.6	72.9	73.6	72.2	66.6	63.6
4. Postneonatal mortality rate	56.0	52.0	51.8	52.0	48.3	43.5	40.8	40.2	41.1	39.9	40.5
5. Perinatal mortality rate	76.6	69.5	67.9	63.1	59.8	58.8	57.7	57.7	58.3	52.4	54.4
6. Stillbirth rate	18.7	16.8	16.0	13.3	12.0	11.4	9.8	9.4	11.0	10.8	13.6
B. Urban											
1. Crude death rate	9.5	9.4	9.4	8.4	8.0	7.8	7.4	7.9	8.6	7.8	7.4
2. Infant mortality rate	80.0	81.0	74.0	72.2	65.2	62.5	65.2	65.8	66.1	59.0	61.0
3. Neonatal mortality rate	49.0	42.0	38.0	42.4	39.1	38.5	38.8	39.3	39.7	38.3	33.3
4. Postneonatal mortality rate	31.0	39.0	36.0	29.8	26.1	24.0	26.4	26.5	26.4	25.6	27.3
5. Perinatal mortality rate	43.7	35.4	33.5	38.7	35.3	31.5	33.1	35.4	35.7	30.4	32.4
6. Stillbirth rate	11.1	8.7	10.3	9.1	7.9	6.2	5.2	8.4	7.9	8.9	9.8
C. Combined											
1. Crude death rate	15.0	14.7	14.2	12.8	12.4	12.5	11.9	11.9	12.6	11.8	10.9
2. Infant mortality rate	129.0	130.0	127.0	120.0	113.9	110.4	104.8	104.9	104.0	97.0	95.0
3. Neonatal mortality rate	77.0	80.2	77.4	71.7	69.3	69.9	66.7	67.2	65.8	60.1	57.7
4. Postneonatal mortality rate	52.0	49.8	49.6	48.3	44.6	40.5	38.1	37.7	38.2	37.1	37.7
5. Perinatal mortality rate	66.8	63.7	62.2	59.0	55.7	54.6	53.2	53.6	53.8	48.1	50.1
6. Still birth rate	17.5	15.5	15.0	12.6	11.3	10.6	8.9	9.3	10.4	10.4	12.9

Source: Registrar General, 1987.

first 24 hours of life (Holla 1985). In short, the evidence reiterates the importance of endogenous factors which are a reflection of poor reproductive health.

2. Causes of Maternal, Perinatal and Neonatal Deaths

2.1 Maternal deaths

India is typical of a high mortality setting as seen in Table 3. Sepsis, abortions, haemorrhage, toxaemia and anaemia account for the large majority of all maternal deaths over the decade of the 1980s (Registrar General 1987; Bhatia 1988). In 1981, for example, these five conditions accounted for three-quarters (75 per cent) of all maternal deaths, and 72 per cent in 1986. Anaemia accounts for 17–25 per cent of all deaths; haemorrhage for 16–22 per cent; sepsis for 8–13 per cent of all deaths; and, despite legislation, roughly 10 per cent of all maternal deaths are attributed to abortion. Toxaemia accounts for another 10–12 per cent. That infective diseases become exacerbated and life-threatening in pregnancy is evident from both hospital and local level sample surveys (Bhatia 1988); Bhatia in fact observes that 10 per cent of all maternal deaths resulted from infective hepatitis and 7 per cent from gastro-enteric diseases.

This cause of death distribution suggests that a large number of maternal deaths are preventable, if attention is paid to three principal underlying conditions among women in India: poor health care, poor nutrition and high and closely spaced fertility stretching from adolescence to menopause. A number of medical studies report on preventable maternal deaths: by and large, well over two-thirds of all maternal deaths are held to be preventable (Agarwal et al. 1982; Bhaskar Rao 1980; Panat and Mehendale 1987; Roy Chowdhury and Sikdar 1982; Mitra and Khara 1983; Sinha 1986). A multicentric study from some eleven states and union territories in the late 1970s suggests that 70 per cent of all deaths were preventable; a more recent study of deaths in New Delhi suggests that about 90 per cent were (Raichowdhuri et al. 1990). The Anantapur study of maternal mortality suggests that 41 per cent of the deaths could have definitely been prevented and 37 per cent could have possibly been prevented (Bhatia 1988).

Table 3: *Percentage distribution of deaths (maternal) by causes related to childbirth and pregnancy 1978–1986 All India (rural)*

Specific causes	1978	1979	1980	1981	1982	1983	1984	1985	1986
Abortion	11.0	11.7	12.5	13.7	10.1	10.7	10.8	11.5	8.0
Toxaemia	21.2	16.1	12.4	8.0	12.5	12.1	10.8	6.7	11.9
Anaemia	14.6	15.0	15.8	17.7	24.4	18.9	23.3	23.1	17.0
Bleeding of pregnancy and puerperium	18.2	20.0	15.8	23.4	26.2	23.8	18.8	15.9	21.6
Malposition of child leading to death of mother	9.5	10.5	13.4	9.2	7.2	8.3	6.2	7.7	6.2
Puerperal sepsis	12.4	11.7	12.4	13.1	8.3	11.6	10.8	13.9	13.1
Not classifiable symptoms	13.1	15.0	17.7	14.9	11.3	14.6	19.3	21.2	22.2

Source: Registrar General, 1987.

2.2 Perinatal and neonatal deaths

Table 4 shows that between 1980 and 1986, diseases peculiar to infancy accounted for a steady three-fifths or more of all infant deaths. More specifically, over one-quarter of all infant deaths in 1986 were attributed to prematurity (27 per cent), almost one-tenth to respiratory infection (9 per cent), and 7 per cent to diarrhoea of the newborn. Another 8 per cent resulted from other causes including cord infection.

Local level studies reiterate that perinatal and neonatal mortality are overwhelmingly due to maternal factors, notably poor nutrition and inadequate ante- and intra-natal care. Various studies report that prematurity and low birth weight are directly responsible for about one-quarter of all infant deaths and are associated factors in about 50 per cent of all neonatal deaths (Roy Choudhary and Jayaswal 1989; Agarwal and Agarwal 1987; Singh and Paul 1988). Bacterial infection (mostly tetanus) is responsible for about one-tenth of all early infant deaths (Singh and Paul 1988).

Study after study reports the links between maternal education, age and parity and early infant mortality (Roy Choudhary and Jayaswal 1989; Agarwal and Agarwal 1987). A multicentric hospital study (Mehta 1983) reports a perinatal mortality rate of 58 per 1000 live births among uneducated women, compared to 41 among women with any education. A study in Bihar and Uttar Pradesh (Agarwal and Agarwal 1987) observes that neonatal mortality is even more sensitive to maternal factors than is infant mortality. Neonatal mortality was about three times as high among illiterate women (99 in Bihar and 78 in Uttar Pradesh) as among women with more than a primary school education (36 and 29 respectively); corresponding disparities in infant and in post-neonatal mortality are less dramatic.

3. Childhood and Adolescence

This pattern of high maternal and early infant mortality in India is a reflection of a series of social, cultural and economic circumstances which can be traced to the low status women occupy relative to men, and its seeds are sown long before the occurrence of pregnancy. Here we examine childhood and adolescence factors which impinge subsequently on reproductive health.

Table 4: Percentage distribution of all infant deaths by causes: India (rural) 1979–1986

Major cause groups	1979	1980	1981	1982	1983	1984	1985	1986
1. Digestive disorders	3.3	2.2	3.4	2.3	2.6	3.0	3.7	4.0
2. Coughs (disorders of respiratory system)	11.9	11.7	15.0	14.8	15.1	15.2	16.9	16.8
3. Fevers	4.8	2.8	4.5	5.0	7.3	6.2	6.9	6.4
4. Diseases peculiar to infancy	69.1	73.1	66.3	67.3	65.6	67.0	62.9	64.6
Pre-maturity	31.4	33.5	36.2	37.3	43.6	45.3	41.4	41.0
Respiratory infection of newborn	16.3	17.5	15.5	12.1	13.7	15.5	13.5	14.5
Malnutrition	13.1	11.3	11.7	10.3	1.8	–	–	–
Diarrhoea of newborn	10.8	9.4	10.0	10.4	9.5	8.9	11.3	10.2
Convulsions	8.3	6.1	7.0	7.0	0.7	–	–	–
Other causes	20.1	22.3	19.6	22.9	30.7	30.3	33.8	34.3
5. Others	10.9	10.2	10.8	10.6	9.4	8.6	9.6	8.2

Note: 'Malnutrition' and 'Convulsions' have been dropped from 1984.
Source: Registrar General, 1987.

3.1 Nutrition and health care

The poor nutritional and growth status of the mother is a reflection of her own growth as a foetus, newborn, child and adolescent. Nutritional status is recognized as a major risk factor for maternal and peri/neonatal mortality as well as the incidence of low birth weight and pre-term infants. Follow-ups of cohorts of girls (Ramachandran 1989) confirm that growth levels in childhood are an important determinant of age at menarche, nutritional status and weight in adulthood.

Under conditions of wide gender disparities which exist in India, malnourishment and limited access to health care are considerably more evident among females than among males from birth onwards (Das Gupta 1987; Acsadi and Johnson-Acsadi 1990). Boys are fed better (Das Gupta 1987; Khan et al. 1988) and are much more likely to receive early access to health care in case of illness. Studies which have monitored growth and nutritional status among children (Srikantia 1989; Government of Maharashtra and UNICEF-WIO 1991) confirm gender disparities in growth and severe malnutrition from an early age. One consequence of this is poor adolescent weight and height: it is estimated (Gopalan 1989) that 47 per cent of 15-year-olds in India have body weights less than 38 kg and 39 per cent have heights less than 145 cm. Another consequence is high levels of anaemia (Chatterjee 1989).

3.2 Early marriage and adolescent childbearing

The early onset of childbearing has disturbing consequences for reproductive health. As many as 6.2 per cent and 43.4 per cent of girls aged 10–14 and 15–19 respectively are already married. In some northern states in fact a number of household surveys suggest that between 20 and 40 per cent of all girls are married by age 15. Following marriage, there are socio-cultural pressures on the young woman to conceive as soon as possible—this is one means whereby she can attain both prestige and security in her new home. Hence, adolescent marriage is synonymous with adolescent childbearing. And while most adolescent fertility occurs within marriage, there is some evidence of sexual activity among unmarried girls, not only in urban but also in rural areas.[3]

---

[3] A rather extreme example of this comes from a village level study in rural Maharashtra (Bang et al. 1989), which reveals, on the basis of physical examinations, that nearly half of all unmarried girls had experienced sexual activity.

It is estimated that as many as 10–15 per cent of all births annually occur to women in their early teens, before they are physically fully developed (Mathai 1989; Kapil 1990). The extra nutritional demands of pregnancy come at the heels of the adolescent growth spurt, which itself requires additional nutritional inputs, and results in the poor nutritional status of the pregnant adolescent (Ramachandran 1989). As a result of the combined effects of shorter average maternal height, competition for nutrients between the mother's growth needs and the growth needs of her foetus, and also due to poorer placental functions of adolescent mothers, the risks of maternal mortality and peri- and neonatal mortality are exceptionally high among adolescents (Leslie 1991).

Hence it is not surprising to note that maternal deaths are concentrated in the youngest ages: 1986 data from rural India suggest that as many as 45 per cent of all maternal deaths took place among women aged under 24 (Registrar General 1987; rates for adolescents are not separately available). Evidence of differentials in age-specific maternal mortality levels come from both small-scale surveys and hospital studies. Estimates derived from Bhatia's village level study in Andhra Pradesh (Acsadi and Johnson-Acsadi 1990) suggest that adolescent maternal mortality ratios are almost twice as high as those reported for women aged 25–39: 1484 per 100,000 live births among women aged 15–19 compared to 735, 708 and 736 for women aged 25–29, 30–34 and 35–39 respectively. A hospital study in a relatively low mortality setting in Bombay (Pachauri and Jamshedji 1983) indicates that compared to women aged 20–29, adolescents experienced (a) a higher mortality rate (206 and 138 respectively); (b) higher spontaneous abortion (158 and 77) and stillbirth (35 and 29) rates; and (c) more difficulties in the ante- (29 and 28 per cent) and intra- (12 and 9 per cent) natal periods.

Not only are adolescent mothers more likely to die or suffer from morbidity, but the children they bear are also exposed to considerable risk. Neonatal mortality rates among adolescents are reported to be six times those of older women in a high mortality setting in rural Bihar and Uttar Pradesh (203 and 34 respectively; Agarwal and Agarwal 1987) and 1.4 times that of older women in a low mortality hospital setting in Bombay (Pachauri and Jamshedji 1983). Adolescent mothers are also more likely to give birth to low-birth-weight and pre-term babies and experience other pregnancy-related complications (Aras et al. 1990; Pachauri and Jamshedji 1983), even when exposed to identical levels of antenatal care and immunization and despite virtually identical levels of weight and haemoglobin at 20 weeks of pregnancy (Aras et al. 1989).[4]

4. Pregnancy and Antenatal Factors

The concept of special care during the antenatal period is not unknown traditionally in India. Pregnancy is associated with a number of cultural practices, ranging from those concerning diet to special rites. By and large however, existing traditional practices concerning diet, combined with traditional omissions, notably the reluctance to seek antenatal care, do little to enhance reproductive health.

4.1 Antenatal care (ANC): registration, visits

Traditionally, little attention has been paid to women in the antenatal period, even traditional dais coming into the picture only at delivery. The maternal and child health programme seeks to address this period of neglect. Under this programme, all pregnant women are to be routinely followed up either in the health centre or at home, and provided immunization, iron supplementation and regular check-ups to monitor the pregnancy. The available evidence on this programme however suggests that while antenatal care undoubtedly improves maternal and infant well-being, this service reaches few pregnant women. Few women are even aware of these services. On the national level, it is estimated that no more than 40–50 per cent of all pregnant women in India receive any antenatal care at all (Singh and Paul 1988; Starrs and Measham 1990; Acsadi and Johnson-Acsadi 1990). And fewer women are actually registered for antenatal care: only 21 per cent of all pregnant women in the rural sector and 47 per cent in the urban (UNICEF 1991 quoting NSS 1986–87).

Local level sample surveys give a more disturbing picture of ANC service utilization and programme awareness (see also Gopalan 1989; Mathai 1989). A study of antenatal care services in Bihar,

---

[4] Among women under twenty, birth weights of as many as 83 per cent were under 2500 grams and 64 per cent were under 2000 grams; corresponding percentages among women aged 25–34 were 70 and 49 per cent (Aras et al. 1990). Adolescents are also more likely to deliver pre-term infants (11 per cent compared to 7 per cent among older women (Pachauri and Jamshedji 1983).

Rajasthan, Orissa, Maharashtra and Gujarat finds that MCH services hardly reached pregnant women: only between 5 and 22 per cent of all pregnant women in rural areas and between 20 and 50 per cent in urban areas (Kanitkar and Sinha 1989). These findings are reiterated by other studies in these and other states, including Uttar Pradesh, Bihar, Rajasthan (Khan and Prasad 1983; Mehta et al. 1983; Khan et al. 1988) and Punjab (Bhatinda district, Singh et al. 1988). It is only in Kerala where antenatal services are reported to have reached a large proportion of women (Khan and Prasad 1983; Mehta et al. 1983).

Where visits do occur, they occur infrequently and their content is unclear (Jain and Agarwal 1986; Murthy et al. 1990). Whereas at least five antenatal check-ups are considered ideal, pregnant women who received antenatal care have rarely had more than one or two contacts and that, too, only when halfway through the pregnancy (Gopalan 1989).

The reasons for this poor utilization of services are cultural and socio-economic on the one hand but also a result of poor quality of services on the other. Kanitkar and Sinha (1989) observe that the large majority of women who did not utilize antenatal services considered it unnecessary. This could reflect the traditional notion that childbearing is not an event worthy of medical attention. It could also reflect dissatisfaction with the accessibility, quality and effect of services; a disturbing minority cited such reasons as lack of knowledge and economic and transportation problems. All these factors underscore the need for concentrated mass education efforts, a stepped-up domiciliary visit schedule and a general improvement in the quality of services.

Women who have received antenatal care experience lower maternal and early infant mortality, fewer complications and higher birth weight. As far as maternal mortality is concerned, the study in Anantapur, Andhra Pradesh, observes significant differences in visits for antenatal care between women who had died and those who had survived childbearing. Of women who had died, only 16 per cent had at least one antenatal visit to the health centre, compared to 27 per cent among women who survived (Bhatia 1988). As far as perinatal mortality is concerned, a multicentric hospital study (Mehta and Jayant 1981) found that two-thirds of all women who suffered a perinatal death had not received a single antenatal check up; 30 per cent of all perinatal deaths (and half of all identifiable causes) are attributed to insufficient antenatal attention (Mehta 1983). Antenatal care also affects birth weight: a study in Bombay (Aras et al. 1990) reports that 59 per cent and 69 per cent of women whose infants weighed less than 2.0 and 2.5 kilograms respectively had received antenatal care, compared to 86 per cent of those whose infants weighed 2.5 kilograms or more.

4.2 Identification and referral of high-risk cases

As a result of limited antenatal contacts, high-risk cases escape identification. In Anantapur for example, 49 per cent of the women who had died suffered anaemia, hepatitis and hypertension, which should have been identified as high-risk factors. Other risk factors which are to be identified by grassroots workers include age, weight, height, birth interval, parity (one, or more than 4), previous history of difficult pregnancy or infant loss, evidence of antenatal haemorrhage, poor weight gain (under 5 kilograms), excessive weight gain (to detect toxaemia), diarrhoea, dysentery or fever during pregnancy (Singh and Paul 1988). However, frequently this is not done. And even if a high-risk case is identified, mothers frequently do not get satisfactory treatment at referral institutions (the PHC for example) because of lack of competent staff, equipment and even facilities for transporting the woman to the referral facility (Kapil 1990).

4.3 Immunization

Service statistics suggest that 16.18 million pregnant women were immunized against tetanus during 1988–89 (Ministry of Health and Family Welfare 1990). We estimate (from 1988 population figures and 1986–89 crude birth rates) that this represents no more than 62.4 per cent of all pregnant women, with wide statewise variation. Community and survey based assessments of antenatal immunization suggest that the situation may be far worse. In contrast to estimates from service statistics, surveys in rural Bihar, Gujarat and Orissa report rates under 15 per cent; and in rural Maharashtra, about 28 per cent (Kanitkar and Sinha 1989). A village level study in Uttar Pradesh (Khan and Prasad 1983) observed that of the 1800 women who were pregnant in the year preceding the survey, only ten per cent received tetanus immunization (compared to an estimated 46 per cent from service statistics).

As a result of poor antenatal immunization, neonatal tetanus persists. Tetanus is estimated to account for some 230,000 to 280,000 infant deaths each year, well over half of which occur in Bihar and Uttar Pradesh (Sokhey 1988; Singh and Paul, 1988; UNICEF 1991). Tetanus is held to account for anywhere between one- and two-thirds of all neonatal deaths (Sokhey 1988; Singh and Paul 1988; UNICEF 1984; Kapil 1980; Agarwal and Agarwal 1987).

4.4 Nutrition in the antenatal period

There exists in India a wide range of cultural practices regarding diet during pregnancy, both on how much and on what to eat. Unfortunately these are unlikely to foster improvements in antenatal nutrition since they tend to discourage increases in women's already meagre average daily food intake (Ramachandran 1989) and in such nutritional items as leafy vegetables during pregnancy. A village level study in Uttar Pradesh (Khan et al. 1988) suggests that even when women are aware of the importance of diet during pregnancy, cultural and economic priorities deny them access to better nutrition: one pregnant woman's daily food intake was four chapatis, two dishes of vegetables and two cups of tea only. Another study in rural Uttar Pradesh (Tripathi et al. 1987) observes that weight gain during pregnancy was of the order of only 6.0–6.5 kg among poorly nourished women and 8.1–8.3 kg among better nourished women.

As a result, anaemia is widespread among pregnant women (haemoglobin levels below 11 grams/dl); it is estimated to range from 40–50 per cent in urban areas to 50–70 per cent in rural areas (UNICEF 1991; Kapil 1990; Bhardwaj et al. 1990; Mathai 1989), higher in such states as Bihar and Uttar Pradesh (Agarwal and Agarwal 1987) and almost 90 per cent in rural areas where hookworm infestation is endemic (Ramachandran 1989). Haemoglobin levels tend to deteriorate in the course of pregnancy; compared to a mean level of 10.8 g/dl among non-pregnant women, haemoglobin levels fell steadily to 10.4 g/dl, 9.7 g/dl and 9.4 g/dl respectively in the first, second and third trimesters of pregnancy (Srikantia 1989a). Parity also affects haemoglobin levels: while 24 per cent of women with two or fewer pregnancies had haemoglobin levels below 9 g/dl, the corresponding proportion among women with three or more pregnancies was over 42 per cent.

Thus, not only is anaemia a leading direct cause of maternal deaths, but it also contributes indirectly by aggravating other complications of pregnancy such as eclampsia, antepartum haemorrhage, sepsis and genito-urinary tract infections. And not only does it affect mortality, but it impairs the health of many more women; puerperal morbidity tends to be 3–4 times higher in women with haemoglobin levels below 6.5 g/dl compared to normal women (Kapil 1990). Consequences of maternal anaemia for infants are equally acute. For example, three-fifths of all infants born to women with haemoglobin levels less than 5.0 g/dl were low birth weight, compared to one-quarter of those born to women with normal haemoglobin levels (Ramachandran 1989); perinatal mortality rates are ten times higher among severely anaemic women compared to normal women. A study in Uttar Pradesh shows that 62 per cent of infants born to women who gained less than 5 kg during pregnancy were low birth weight compared to 38 per cent among women who gained 7–9 kg (Mathai 1989). Links between low birth weight and early infant death are well known: low-birth-weight infants account for over 70 per cent of all perinatal deaths, 90 per cent of all early neonatal deaths and half of all infant deaths (Ramalingaswami 1985; Singh 1986).

4.5 Food and iron supplementation

Food and iron supplementation have been found to improve such maternal health attributes as weight gain, incidence of anaemia, complications during pregnancy and childbirth and birth weight (Dawn and Mitra 1990; Iyengar 1975). These findings have prompted a variety of strategies for supplementing the diets of pregnant women. The most ambitious of these is the Integrated Child Development Services (ICDS) programme, in which pregnant and lactating women are provided supplementary nutrition (500 kilocalories and 25 grams of protein) daily. Unfortunately, though this programme has been implemented for over a decade now, there is little information available on changes in reproductive health indicators in areas served by the programme. The little that is available from service statistics suggests that little more than half (51 per cent) of all pregnant and lactating women eligible for this supplementary nutrition actually receive it (Ministry of Welfare, Department of Women and Child Development 1991). In some states, the situation is worse: for example, both ICDS reports and an assessment of the utilization of ICDS services in Rajasthan (Jain and Agarwal 1986) put this figure at 40 per cent.

The national anaemia prophylaxis programme of iron and folic acid distribution, in which pregnant women are provided with 100 iron and folic acid tablets during pregnancy, was initiated as early as the 1950s. However, both service statistics and sample surveys confirm that this programme has not been very successful. From service statistics, we find that no more than an estimated one-third of all pregnant and lactating women (as estimated from population and birth rate figures for 1988–89) have received iron and folic acid supplementation. Even more discouraging are the results of the few sample surveys on antenatal care, particularly in the four large northern states. A village level study in Uttar Pradesh (Khan et al. 1988) observed that only seven per cent of all pregnant women received iron and folic acid supplementation (compared to 26 per cent for the state as a whole as estimated from service statistics). A micro-level evaluation by the Indian Council of Medical Research has shown that the programme has had little effect on the prevalence of anaemia among pregnant women (UNICEF 1991); worse, there was little difference in the prevalence of anaemia between those who were supplied the tablets (88.1 per cent) and those who were not (87.6 per cent). Reasons underlying this range from inadequate supplementation to low acceptance, to poor quality of tablets.

4.6 Work in the antenatal period

In India, the average rural woman neither increases her nutritional intake nor reduces her physical activity through her pregnancy (Ramachandran 1989). The combination of poor pre-existing nutritional levels, inadequate diet during pregnancy, heavy physical activity and frequent childbearing results in further deterioration of maternal nutritional status and poor growth of the foetus (Tripathi et al. 1987). A village level study in Uttar Pradesh (Khan et al. 1988) observed that pregnant women work for as long as 13–14 hours a day, and throughout the pregnancy; time use data of five pregnant women suggests an average of 13 hours of physical labour, including both wage and domestic work and no more than 6–7 hours of rest. Reports of similarly long average work days among pregnant women come from Andhra Pradesh, too (Mathai 1989). Walking long distances to collect fuel and water results in high calorie expenditure, which is rarely offset by additional food intake. Even when pregnant women are aware of the need for additional rest during pregnancy, economic and domestic demands on their time take precedence and few women can afford to reduce physical labour during pregnancy (Khan et al. 1986).

5. During the Birth

Contact with the health care network at the intranatal stage is even poorer than at the antenatal stage. At the time of delivery, no more than twenty per cent of all women have some contact with medical or paramedical personnel. Deliveries are largely conducted by untrained personnel and in unhygienic conditions, both of which contribute significantly to poor maternal health.

5.1 Attendance at birth

A decade ago, in 1984, no more than 15 per cent of all rural births were performed in an institution and as many as two-thirds were delivered by untrained workers and others. And in such states as Bihar, Jammu and Kashmir, Madhya Pradesh, Orissa, Rajasthan and Uttar Pradesh, more than three out of four births are delivered by an untrained attendant. And what is disturbing is the evidence that over the 1971 to 1987 period, the picture has hardly changed. The proportion of births conducted institutionally increased from 8 to 15 per cent in rural areas and from 32 to 47 per cent in urban. The proportion of births delivered by untrained attendants fell from 81 per cent in 1971 to 68 per cent in 1987 in rural areas and from 43 per cent to 39 per cent in urban areas. Even so, there are rural areas of the country where nine out of ten births are delivered by an untrained attendant (Khan et al. 1986 for Uttar Pradesh; Kanitkar and Sinha 1989 for Bihar, Rajasthan and Gujarat).

In these circumstances, the role of the estimated 500,000 traditional birth attendants in India—about one per 1000 population—becomes especially important (Singh and Paul 1988; Planning Commission 1985). Collaboration between the health sector and the traditional birth attendant is an important way of bridging two very different cultures concerning reproductive health but this link has not yet been effectively exploited. And the little evidence which is available (for example, Kumar and Walia 1983) suggests that trained attendants do in fact have significantly better health care knowledge and can better recognize high-risk conditions, suggesting the importance of training of traditional birth attendants. But we have little evidence on reproductive health outcomes in areas served by trained dais, and this is a topic worthy of further investigation.

5.2 Birth hygiene

For the most part, delivery continues to be conducted under unhygienic conditions. A 1984–85 study of traditional birth attendants (Sharma and Bali 1989) in slums in Delhi reveals that, among intranatal practices, as many as 80 per cent did not wash their hands before delivery (119/141) and two-thirds used an unsterilized (but fresh) blade to cut the cord. This is quite consistent with a hospital based study of neonates with tetanus which reports that in all cases, unsterilized blades, knives or broken glass were used to cut the cord (Kumar et al. 1988). We would do well to be reminded that China's success in reducing the number of deaths from sepsis and neonatal tetanus is attributed largely to the teaching of simple hygienic principles of clean hands, clean perineum and clean cord care.

6. Other Factors Affecting Reproductive Health

Other factors concerning reproductive health range from conditions in the immediate postnatal period (morbidity, breast-feeding and nutrition, and birth spacing) to more general concerns such as contraception and abortion on the one hand, and infertility and exposure to sexually transmitted diseases on the other.

6.1 Morbidity

For every maternal death in India, there are at least 20 mothers suffering from impaired health (Kapil 1990), suggesting an additional 2.4 million mothers with impaired health and efficiency as a result of pregnancy-related causes. Complications in pregnancy and childbirth can result in poor maternal health: incontinence, uterine prolapse and infertility are commonly associated with pregnancy-related complications. Pelvic inflammatory disease is commonly associated with unclean hands or instruments during delivery and can lead to infertility. Infectious diseases are more common and more serious in pregnancy.

Despite the fact that most maternal and neonatal deaths occur in the immediate postnatal period, few women are visited by health workers during this period. In Anantpur, for example, as many as 60 per cent of maternal deaths took place within five days of delivery (Bhatia 1988) and yet we have evidence that no more than one-third of all who have just given birth are visited by health workers in the first week after delivery (Mathai 1989). Given the cultural setting in which neither mother nor child is allowed out of the house in the first 40 days, this lack of contact during the early postnatal period could have serious implications for reproductive health.

Maternal morbidity has serious implications in terms of the chronic suffering and poor quality of life it brings. Yet universally, indicators of maternal morbidity remain undeveloped and no systematic attempt at classifying them has been made. The little evidence available from India suggests a high incidence of gynaecological diseases. A village level investigation of rural women in Maharashtra (Bang et al. 1989) observed on physical examination that some 92 per cent were found to have one or more gynaecological diseases; infections of the genital tract, including pelvic inflammatory disease, vaginitis and cervicitis, contributed half of this morbidity. Despite this high prevalence, only 8 per cent had undergone gynaecological examination and treatment in the past.

6.2 Breast-feeding and lactational amenorrhoea

Breast-feeding continues to be fairly universal and prolonged in India, up to about 24 months in rural areas. During lactation, women continue to subsist on average on 1200–1600 kilocalories daily—out of which 450–500 are required to meet the demands of milk production (Ramachandran 1989a), leaving 800 calories to meet the woman's requirements; this ratio is suggestive of considerable daily weight loss and maternal depletion. At the same time however, prolonged breast-feeding has tremendous advantages for the infant. Even so, unhealthy traditional breast-feeding practices continue which have a negative effect on early infant survival: even in the metropolis of Bombay (UNICEF-WIO 1991), colostrum is discarded, prelacteal feeds are given and the introduction of supplementary foods is delayed to well beyond six months. As a result of this, compounded by poor hygiene and sanitation, growth faltering is commonly observed after six months among low income households (Ramachandran 1989a).

6.3 Frequent childbearing

Women in South Asia have more pregnancies than in any other region of the world other than sub-Saharan Africa. Women in India remain largely valued for their reproductive performance, and large numbers of children and sons in particular (at least two) are widely desired. With a total fertility rate of 4.3, the average woman spends a large proportion—about one-third—of her reproductive years in pregnancy and lactation. Early, frequent and rapid childbearing is then the norm, reinforcing, in turn, women's already poor reproductive health and enhancing their chances of pregnancy-related complications. Unfortunately there are few studies in India on the relationship between birth intervals and maternal depletion, health or mortality. An analysis of all maternal deaths occurring in three hospitals in Bangkok, however, confirms that women with a previous birth interval of less than two years had a 250 per cent higher risk of dying than women with a longer birth interval (Royston and Armstrong 1989). Studies in India (Ramachandran 1989) indicate that morbidity among women who conceive during lactation is considerably higher than in other women; the mean birth weight of infants born within a twelve-month interval from a previous birth was significantly lower than those born after a twelve-month interval.

Finally, there is the familiar link between the length of the birth interval and infant mortality: a study in Punjab in the 1970s reports infant mortality rates of 206 for those born after an interval of less than one year, compared to 132 and 108 for births occurring after intervals of 2–3 and more than 4 years respectively (Sadik 1980). Another study (Chatterjee 1989) indicates that births occurring within 12 months of a previous one are exposed to a mortality rate of 200 compared to 100 in cases where the birth interval exceeds 12 months. Apart from higher mortality, short birth intervals are associated with growth faltering of the immediately older sibling.

6.4 Contraception

Though contraceptive prevalence rates have been increasing, more births in India continue to be averted by the practice of prolonged breast-feeding than by contraception. Where contraception is practised, it is usually for limiting rather than spacing fertility and, indeed, knowledge of non-terminal methods is poor. While 42 per cent of all currently married women in the reproductive ages practise some form of contraception, few (only 12 per cent) use a non-terminal method, reflecting the unbalanced focus of the family planning programme on terminal rather than reversible methods. As a result, the current pattern of contraception offers women little relief from closely spaced pregnancies. Rather, it compresses childbearing into fewer years, usually terminating childbearing by the early thirties, by which time over three children have already been born.

Morbidity (and even mortality) arising from contraception is not unknown. In particular, the camp approach to sterilization and the increasing focus on IUDs have been associated with a variety of side-effects and more serious conditions ranging from excessive bleeding to pelvic inflammatory disease—pointing once more to a need for more hygienic service delivery conditions in general.

There continues to be considerable unmet need for family planning (currently married women who want no more children but are not using a method of contraception). Estimates of unmet need for India are of the order of 20 per cent: if women who wanted no more children were able to avoid another pregnancy, it is estimated that maternal mortality ratios would fall by up to 40 per cent (see Acsadi and Johnson-Acsadi 1990).

6.5 Induced abortion

A sad reflection of the extent of unmet need is the fact that roughly five million abortions are performed annually in India, most of them illegally. In 1987–88, only about half a million abortions were performed under the health services network, while another estimated 4.5 million abortions occurred illegally (UNICEF 1991). About two out of five legal abortions occur because of contraceptive failure (Ministry of Health and Family Welfare 1989). There has also been a tendency in India to misuse amniocentesis to detect the sex of the foetus, and resort to abortion (usually of the female foetus) to arrive at the desired sex composition of children; this suggests the disturbing possibility of increased abortions and repeat abortions. Women resort to illegal abortions in large numbers for many reasons. Registered practitioners are unavailable: in 1984 for example, only about 1000 physicians of a total of roughly 15,000 trained to perform abortions were in rural areas. Abortion can involve a cost to the patient, for saline and drugs, and this can be prohibitive for the average rural woman. Information about legal termination services is inadequate; there is limited publicity about the law and there is a widely held perception that abortion is illegal. And abortion services at approved centres tend to be impersonal and unattractive.

Mortality and morbidity arising from abortion continue to be high. We have seen that about 10 per cent of all maternal deaths are due to abortions: largely from sepsis and haemorrhage (84 per cent from sepsis and 10 per cent from haemorrhage in one study (Kamalajayaram and Parameswari 1988)). Even so, the actual number of deaths due to abortion may be as high as 15–25 per cent (Starrs and Measham 1990) since the majority of deaths from abortion are unreported as such and most illegal abortions are conducted by untrained practitioners under unhygienic conditions. This is corroborated by evidence from hospital based studies (Bansal and Sharma 1985; Mathur and Rohatgi 1981; Kamalajayaram and Parameswari 1988) suggesting a high incidence of abortion-related mortality and morbidity.

6.6 Infertility and sexually transmitted diseases

Far less evidence is available on the levels and patterns of infertility. Evidence from the 1981 Census (Ministry of Health and Family Welfare 1989) and a village level study in Maharashtra (Bang et al. 1989) puts the level of infertility at 6–7 per cent, compared to 2–3 per cent in other developing countries (Sai and Nassim 1989). Infertility poses a serious threat to female well-being in a culture which prizes reproduction—preventing her from achieving the family size which she desires and exposing her to various kinds of emotional harassment or marital disharmony. Factors underlying infertility include, among other things, women's poor health and nutrition status which can lead to repeated miscarriages and foetal waste, unhygienic obstetric and abortion procedures and even such debilitating diseases as tuberculosis.

Even less is known of the levels and patterns of sexually transmitted diseases which have severe implications for the reproductive health of both women and men. The available evidence suggests a relatively high prevalence of STDs. For example, an intensive village level investigation of 650 women in Maharashtra (Bang et al. 1989) suggests that a disturbingly large proportion of women were suffering from syphilis (10.5 per cent) and gonorrhoea (0.3 per cent). Finally, about a million men and women are estimated to be suffering from HIV/AIDS with dangerous potential for its wider spread.

7. Prospects for Improvements in Reproductive Health

Reproductive health features prominently in the government's stated goals for Health For All by 2000. Targets have been set for a variety of reproductive health components ranging from mortality rates to such health-related measures as levels of antenatal care, trained attendance at delivery, immunization and birth weight. Unfortunately, despite these programmes and these goals, the situation today remains discouraging: the chances of achieving these goals seem remote.

Rather than simply a medical problem, poor reproductive health is, of course, ultimately a reflection of the series of social, cultural and economic circumstances, which are not responsive to short-term strategies and go beyond the health sector. The most basic long-term solutions are of course poverty- and gender-related and here changes in female status in general are the key, and the expansion of educational and economic opportunities for women, improvement in nutrition and prevention of adolescent marriage are of particular importance.

Short-term benefits to reproductive health can accrue through well-implemented interventions which reduce not only mortality but also morbidity. Such interventions do of course exist but the thrust of their services has been so skewed that health benefits have been limited. While an impressive array of programmes exist in India to improve reproductive health, in practice the focus has been on sterilization, so that maternal and child health care, health and nutrition education, birth spacing and safe abortion have been relatively neglected. Programmes suffer from poor outreach, quality of services and care, and an inability to adapt services and messages to the cultural milieu of their beneficiaries. First, improvements in the quality of services and care are an important means by which to encourage service utilization and dispel the cynicism with which services are currently viewed. Second, in a culture where few women seek health services and seclusion practices inhibit health centre visits, outreach is critical; domiciliary visits by health personnel have to be not only frequent but of good quality and must cover a range of services, from antenatal care to nutrition, immunization, birth spacing and health education. Third, and equally important in a society in which the large majority of women are uneducated and unexposed to new ideas, information needs of rural women must be satisfied through culturally acceptable messages.

The assessment of reproductive health levels is handicapped by a scarcity of good data on most reproductive health outcomes, including both mortality and especially quality of life indicators. Most of the work currently available is clinic based and medically oriented but this is inadequate when it comes to assessing reproductive health and its underlying causes. Rigorous indirect estimates of maternal mortality, at the state and district levels are essential. Micro-level analyses of the links between reproductive health outcomes and their socio-economic and cultural antecedents in different settings would go a long way in tailoring services in a locally relevant way. So would studies on the impact of interventions designed to redress reproductive health deficiencies.

Finally a word of caution. It is tempting to infer from the fact that mortality levels have declined and gender differentials narrowed that the *reproductive health* of women is not a matter of serious concern. Evidence presented in this review offer strong support countering this inference. There is no denying that reproductive health in India continues to be unacceptably poor, and that national commitment to and investment in its improvement have been inadequate.

References

Acsadi, George T.F., and Gwendolyn Johnson-Acsadi. 1990. 'Safe motherhood in South Asia: socio-cultural and demographic aspects of maternal health', Background Paper, Safe Motherhood South Asia Conference, Lahore.

Agarwal, D. K. and K. N. Agarwal. 1987. 'Early childhood mortality in Bihar and Uttar Pradesh', *Indian Pediatrics* 24, no. 8 (August): 627–32.

Agarwal, V., S. Patil and S. Khanijo. 1982. 'Study of maternal mortality', *Journal of Obstetrics and Gynaecology* 32, no. 5 (October): 688–92.

Aras, R., N. Pai, and A. Purandare. 1990. 'Perinatal mortality—a retrospective hospital study', *Journal of Obstetrics and Gynaecology* 40, no. 3 (June): 365–69.

Aras, R., N. Pai, A. Baliga, S. Jain and Naimuddin. 1989. 'Pregnancy at teenage—risk factor for lower birth weight', *Indian Pediatrics* 26, no. 8 (August): 823–25.

Bang, R. A. et al. 1989. 'High prevalence of gynaecological diseases in rural Indian women', *The Lancet*, 14 January.

Bansal, M. C. and Usha Sharma. 1985. 'Comparative study of septic abortions and medical termination of pregnancy', *Journal of Obstetrics and Gynaecology* 35: 705–12.

Bhardwaj, N. et al. 1990. 'Socio-economic factors affecting weight gain in pregnancy', *Journal of Obstetrics and Gynaecology* 40, no. 3 (June): 327–30.

Bhasker Rao, K. 1980. 'Maternal mortality in India—a cooperative study', *Journal of Obstetrics and Gynaecology* 30, No. 6 (December): 859–64.

Bhatia, J. C. 1988. *A Study of Maternal Mortality in Anantapur District, Andhra Pradesh, India*. Bangalore: Indian Institute of Management.

Chandrakapure and Ranganathan. 1985. 'Maternal mortality in rural Maharashtra', Paper presented at the Obstetrics and Gynaecology Conference, Aurangabad.

Chatterjee, Meera. 1989. 'Socio-economic and socio-cultural influences on women's nutritional status and roles' in C. Gopalan and Suminder Kaur (eds.), *Women and Nutrition in India*. New Delhi: Nutrition Foundation of India.

Das Gupta, Monica. 1987. 'Selective discrimination against female children in rural Punjab, India', *Population and Development Review* 13, no. 1 (March).

Dawn, C. S. and Bani Kumar Mitra. 1990. 'Effect of food supplementation on maternal weight gain, low birth weight incidence, infant weight gain and breast feed performance', *Journal of Obstetrics and Gynaecology* 40, no. 3 (June): 313–18.

Gopalan, C. 1989. 'Women and nutrition in India—general consideration' in C. Gopalan and Suminder Kaur (eds.), *Women and Nutrition in India*. New Delhi: Nutrition Foundation of India.

Government of Maharashtra and UNICEF-WIO. 1991. *Women and Children in Dharni: a Case Study after Fifteen Years of ICDS*. Bombay: UNICEF, Western India Office.

Graham, W., W. Brass, and R. W. Snow. 1989. 'Estimating maternal mortality: The sisterhood method', *Studies in Family Planning* 20, no. 3 (May/June).

Holla, M. 1985. 'Vital statistics system—a major source of information on infant and child mortality', *Indian Pediatrics* 52: 115–26.

Iyengar, L. 1975. 'Influence of the diet on the outcome of pregnancy in Indian women', in *Proceedings of the 9th International Congress of Nutrition*, Mexico, 1972, vol. 2, Karger, Nutrition, pp. 48–53.

Jain, M. L. and Dinesh Agarwal. 1986. 'Utilization of maternal services in an I.C.D.S. block', *Journal of Obstetrics and Gynaecology* 36, no. 5 (October): 842–44.

Kamalajayaram, V. and T. Parameswari. 1988. 'A study of septic abortion cases in the last 6 years', *Journal of Obstetrics and Gynaecology* 38, no. 4 (August): 389–92.

Kanitkar, Tara and R. K. Sinha. 1989. 'Antenatal care services in five states of India', in S. N. Singh, M.K. Premi, P.S. Bhatia and Ashish Bose (eds.), *Population Transition in India*, vol. 2, pp. 201–11. Delhi: B. R. Publishing Corporation.

Kapil, U. 1990. 'Promotion of safe motherhood in India', *Indian Pediatrics* 27, no. 3 (March): 232–38.

Khan, M. E., Richard Anker, S. K. Ghosh Dastidar and Sashi Bairathi. 1988. 'Inequalities between men and women in nutrition and family welfare services: an in-depth enquiry in an Indian village', *Social Action* 38 (October–December).

Khan, M. E. and C. V. S. Prasad. 1983. *Under-utilization of Health Services in Rural India: A Comparative Study of Bihar, Gujarat and Kerala*. Baroda: Operations Research Group.

Khan, M. E., S. K. Ghosh Dastidar and R. Singh. 1986. 'Nutrition and health practices among rural women—a case study of Uttar Pradesh, India', *Journal of Family Welfare* 33, no. 1 (September).

Kumar, Harish, S. Aneja, V. K. Prasad, S. K. Arora and D. N. Mullick. 1988. 'Tetanus neonatorum: clinico-epidemiological profile', *Indian Pediatrics* 25, no. 11 (November): 1054–57.

Kumar, Vijay and Inderjit Walia. 1983. 'Beliefs and practices of birth attendants during antenatal period in a rural area', *Journal of Obstetrics and Gynaecology* 33, no. 4 (August): 460–65.

Leslie, Joanne. 1991. 'Women's nutrition: the key to improving health in developing countries?' *Health Policy and Planning* 6, no. 1: 1–19.

Lopez, J. A., K. K. Deshmukh and K. S. Iyer. 1986. 'Maternal mortality due to sepsis', *Journal of Obstetrics and Gynaecology* 36, no. 3 (June): 411–13.

Mari Bhat, P. N., K. Navaneetham and S. Irudaya Rajan. 1992. 'Maternal mortality in India: estimates from an econometric model', *Population Research Centre, Dharwad: Working Paper* 24 (January).

Mathai, Saramma T. 1989. 'Women and the health system' in C. Gopalan and Suminder Kaur (eds.), *Women and Nutrition in India*. New Delhi: Nutrition Foundation of India.

Mathur, V. and P. Rohatgi. 1981. 'Maternal mortality in septic abortion', *Journal of Obstetrics and Gynaecology* 31, no. 2 (April): 272–75.

Mehta, A. and K. Jayant. 1981. 'Perinatal mortality survey in India (1977–79) Part I, identification of health intervention needs', *Journal of Obstetrics and Gynaecology* 32, no. 2 (April): 183–215.

Mehta, A. 1983. 'Strategies for reduction of perinatal mortality in India', *Journal of Obstetrics and Gynaecology* 33, No. 6 (December): 721–33.

Mehta, S., M. E. Khan, R. B. Gupta, M. M. Gandotra and O. S. Ojha. 1983. *Role of Health Service Delivery on Acceptance of Family Planning*. New Delhi: ICMR, mimeo.

Ministry of Health and Family Welfare, Central Bureau of Health Intelligence, Directorate General of Health Services. 1987. *Health Information of India*. New Delhi: Government of India Press.

Ministry of Health and Family Welfare. 1989. *Family Welfare Programme in India: Yearbook 1987–88*. New Delhi: Ministry of Health and Family Welfare.

Ministry of Health and Family Welfare. 1990. *Family Welfare Programme in India: Yearbook 1988–89*. New Delhi: Ministry of Health and Family Welfare.

Ministry of Welfare, Department of Women and Child Development. 1991. *15 Years of ICDS, an Overview*. New Delhi: Government of India.

Mitra, J. and B. N. Khara 1983. 'Maternal Mortality (a review of the current status in a teaching institution)', *Journal of Obstetrics and Gynaecology* 33, no. 2 (April): 209–13.

Murthy, G. V., Anil Goswami and Saroja Narayanan. 1990. 'Utilization patterns of antenatal services in an urban slum', *Journal of Obstetrics and Gynaecology* 40, no. 1 (February): 42-46.

Nafisa Beebi. 1987. 'Five year study of maternal mortality at the Institute of Obstetrics and Gynaecology, Madras (1981–85)', *Journal of Obstetrics and Gynaecology* 37, no. 6: 820–22.
Pachauri, S. and A. Jamshedji. 1983. 'Risks of teenage pregnancy', *Journal of Obstetrics and Gynaecology* 33, no. 3 (June): 477–82.
Panat, S. P. and S. S. Mehendale. 1987. 'Maternal Mortality—review of 6 years', *Journal of Obstetrics and Gynaecology* 37, no. 3 (June): 527–29.
Planning Commission, Government of India. 1985. 'Steering Group Report Part III. Rural and Urban Health Services in the Seventh Plan', *Indian Journal of Pediatrics* 52: 217–22.
Raichowdhuri, G., Veena Ganju and Rupali Dewan. 1990. 'Review of maternal mortality over nine year period at Safdarjang hospital, New Delhi', *Journal of Obstetrics and Gynaecology* 40, no. 1 (February): 84–88.
Ramachandran, Prema. 1989. 'Nutrition in pregnancy' in C. Gopalan and Suminder Kaur (eds.), *Women and Nutrition in India*. New Delhi: Nutrition Foundation of India.
Ramachandran, Prema. 1989a. 'Lactation-nutrition-fertility interaction' in C. Gopalan and Suminder Kaur (eds.), *Women and Nutrition In India*. New Delhi: Nutrition Foundation of India.
Ramalingaswami, V. 1985. *The state of life: Report of the National Seminar on reducing incidence of low birth weight babies in India*. New Delhi: National Institute of Public Cooperation and Child Development.
Registrar General. 1987. *Survey of causes of death (Rural): annual report 1984 and 1986*. A Report, Series 3, No. 17 and 19. New Delhi: Office of the Registrar General.
Roy Chowdhury, N. N. and K. Sikdar. 1982. 'Factors influencing maternal mortality', *Journal of Obstetrics and Gynaecology* 32, no. 4 (August): 507–10.
Roy Choudhary, S. and O. N. Jayaswal. 1989. 'Infant and early childhood mortality in urban slums under ICDS scheme—a prospective study', *Indian Pediatrics* 26, no. 6 (June): 544–49.
Royston, Eric and Sue Armstrong (eds). 1989. *Preventing Maternal Deaths*. Geneva: World Health Organization.
Sadik, Nafis. 1980. 'Family planning: improving the health of women', *Draper Fund Report*: 9 (October)
Sai, Fred T. and Janet Nassim. 1989. 'The need for a reproductive health approach'. *International Journal of Gynaecology and Obstetrics*, Supplement 3: 103–13.
Sen Gupta, Amit and A. G. Gode. 1988. 'A comparative study of maternal mortality and morbidity in a teaching hospital of Northern India'. *Journal of Obstetrics and Gynaecology* 38, no. 2: 177–81.
Sharma, N. and P. Bali. 1989. 'Care of the newborn by traditional birth attendants', *Indian Pediatrics* 26, no. 7 (July): 649–53.
Singh, Meharban. 1986. 'Hospital based data on perinatal and neonatal mortality in India', *Indian Pediatrics* 23, no. 8 (August): 579–84.
Singh, Meharban and V. K. Paul. 1988. 'Strategies to reduce perinatal and neonatal mortality', *Indian Pediatrics* 25, no. 6 (June): 499–509.
Singh, Surinder, Jagjeet Singh, Sushila Mittal, R. K. D. Goel, Tejbir Singh and S. K. Oberoi. 1988. 'A study of antenatal services in rural area of district Bathinda of Punjab', *Journal of Obstetrics and Gynaecology* 38, no. 1 (February): 22–26.

Sinha, Jyoti. 1986. 'A 5 year study of maternal mortality: analysis of its causative factors (1976–1980)', *Journal of Obstetrics and Gynaecology* 36, no. 3 (June): 404–406.
Sokhey, J. 1988. 'Magnitude of problem in India', in Ministry of Health and Family Welfare, *The Control of Neonatal Tetanus in India*, pp. 16–23. New Delhi: Government of India, quoted in Singh and Paul, 1988.
Srikantia, S. G. 1989. 'Pattern of growth and development of Indian girls and body size of adult Indian women' in C. Gopalan and Suminder Kaur (eds.), *Women and Nutrition in India*. New Delhi: Nutrition Foundation of India.
Srikantia, S. G. 1989a. 'Nutritional deficiency diseases' in C. Gopalan and Suminder Kaur (eds.), *Women and Nutrition in India*. New Delhi: Nutrition Foundation of India.
Starrs, Ann and Diane Measham. 1990. *Challenge for the Nineties: Safe Motherhood in South Asia*. New York and Washington: The World Bank and Family Care International.
Tewari, S. and N. Gulati. 1990. 'Maternal mortality: a study of 11 years at Medical College Hospital, Rohtak (Haryana)', *Journal of Obstetrics and Gynaecology* 40, no. 2 (March): 703–12.
Tripathi, A. M., D. K. Agarwal, K. N. Agarwal, R. R. Devi and S. Cherian. 1987. 'Nutritional status of rural pregnant women and foetal outcome', *Indian Pediatrics* 24, no. 9 (September): 703–12.
Trussell, James and Rodriguez, G. 1990. 'A note on the sisterhood estimator of maternal mortality', *Studies in Family Planning* 21, no. 6 (Nov./Dec.).
UNICEF, India. 1984. *An Analysis of the Situation of Children in India*. New Delhi: UNICEF, Regional Office for South Central Asia.
UNICEF, India. 1991. *Children and Women in India: a situation analysis*. New Delhi: UNICEF.
UNICEF-WIO. 1991. *Infant feeding practices in Bombay*. Bombay: UNICEF, Western India Office.
WHO. 1991. *The Special Programme of Research, Development and Research Training in Human Reproduction*. Geneva: World Health Organization.

6

Women's Roles and the Gender Gap in Health and Survival

ALAKA MALWADE BASU

I. Introduction

No other 'high-risk' population group has received as much academic and lay attention and interest in recent years as the female sex. The above average risks of this group have been especially highlighted for health and survival, at least partly because these risks are easier to observe and measure than are sex differences in other indicators of welfare such as employment opportunities, wage rates and control over resources. However, we have now passed the stage of establishing that gender differences in health and mortality do exist, especially in the South Asian region, and may even have widened over time in some areas (although the overall trend is probably towards a closing of the gap; see for example, Dyson 1984). The more interesting question now is how these sex differentials come about, that is, to use the language of Mosley and Chen (1984), what are the 'proximate determinants' of health and mortality responsible for the sex differential and, in turn, what aspects of the female situation lead to such sex differences in these proximate determinants?

But this paper begins with a more neutral objective. It examines some of the ways in which women's roles lead to gender differences in health and survival in either direction. While it is true that I will end up having many more examples of gender differences adverse to females, the complementary situation too does exist and deserves comment. The final aggregate outcome is therefore a balance of these two kinds of effects and in this sense, if overall differentials are unfavourable to females, their underlying disadvantage is in fact greater than that suggested by these overall differentials.

There is also the problem of devising independent measures to rank the position of women in order to relate these to health and survival differences by sex. This is because, while worse female health may reflect an anti-female socio-economic situation in general, the absence of a gender differential in health need not imply the absence of a gender differential in socio-economic status. The pattern of disease occurrence and control may be such that discriminatory practices against women in some spheres of life are less easily translated into excess female mortality or worse health. This is likely to be the picture in the developed world today (see, for example, Harris 1989). For example, a sharp fall in the incidence of or fatality from infectious diseases would reduce sex differentials in mortality without changing underlying social mores.

By the same token, worse health and survival prospects for women need not necessarily reflect only an inferior status of women, except tautologically if health is the measure of status. Indeed, as highlighted in a later section, the inferior position of women on one count, such as their freedom to smoke or to drive fast cars, can result in a male disadvantage on the other count of health and survival.

Then, there is biology (or what we often call biology in our inability to locate environmental explanations) as a determinant of sex differences in health. The higher male neonatal mortality observed in a large number of diverse populations is a classic example of the supposed greater 'biological hardiness' of the female. I will not touch upon such inherently produced sex differences here; the accent will be on ways in which differences in women's roles in different populations lead to differences in the sex differential in health and mortality, or more correctly, in the proximate determinants of health and mortality.

For the sake of convenience, these proximate determinants will be divided into two broad categories—those affecting exposure to an episode of ill-health and those affecting the outcome of such an episode, either in terms of survival or general debility. Women's roles are hypothesized to act somewhat differently on these two sets of determinants. But several of the arguments made about the effects of women's position do apply to both categories of determinants—where they appear in the paper is therefore somewhat arbitrary.

To anticipate an important conclusion, we will need to distinguish between two kinds of discriminatory effects when the female is at a disadvantage: (1) those effects which are due to behaviour which is consciously or directly discriminatory and part of some larger 'strategy' and (2) those effects which are due to behaviour conditioned by calculations not directly related to affecting a sex differential in welfare, except in some kind of long-term historical or institutional sense. This distinction is important, because the intervention points suggested to narrow the gender gap in health are different in the two cases. In particular, the second set of behaviours is more amenable to immediate short-term policy interventions.

II. Women's Roles Relevant to the Gender Gap in Health

There are several possible categorizations of women's roles depending on one's inclinations as much as on one's reasons for the categorization. One of the most general and exhaustive is that of Oppong and Abu (1985) who identify seven roles that women play during their lives—maternal, occupational, conjugal, domestic, kin, community and individual. Several of these roles are interrelated, so that by knowing the nature of one of the roles we are able to successfully predict the nature of one or more of the remaining roles.

For this reason and because several of these roles do not have an independent bearing on gender differences in physical welfare, the present paper restricts itself to three roles in a woman's adult life—the productive, the domestic and the reproductive. In turn, these three are also of course interrelated but I treat them separately here because their relations to sex differentials in health and survival are not merely through one another; each one of these also exerts an independent effect on the gender gap in the proximate determinants of health. This will became clearer in the next three sections.

Not only does this categorization leave out four of Oppong's roles, it also does not consider separately the effect of other women's status-related factors such as inheritance laws, kinship systems, property rights and the existence of dowry—all of which are believed to contribute to the disadvantaged position of women in survival in some groups. This is because such factors tend to be often related to female employment (for example, dowry is a lesser burden in areas where female employment is high) and because their effects are broadly those of economic dependency in general, which are captured by female employment. On the other hand female economic activity exerts several effects (especially the indirect ones) which are not captured by any of these factors.

In any case, what is needed now is some simple definition of these three roles. To begin with female employment, an attempt to define it certainly stirs up a hornet's nest. The literature abounds with examples of how conventional (that is, male-inspired) definitions of economic activity lead to a heavy undercounting of female productivity. This is especially the case for work categories in which women are disproportionately represented—such as unpaid farm work, home-based production and the service sector. What gets most easily measured is male oriented productive work—generally for wages, outside the home and with some regular schedule. All these accusations are certainly justified; however, we do not address them here and continue to measure women's productive roles by these conventional methods. This is not because the other kinds of work that women engage in are not directly productive, it is because the gender gap in health is even more affected by perceptions about female economic roles than by the reality. The NSS or census investigator is often doing no more than reflecting society's bias when he records low female labour force participation rates and our hypothesis is that such perceptions about women's economic potential (perceptions being shaped either by knowledge or by women's involvement in conventionally defined activities) determine the value attached to their very existence.

The second point to note is that as important as the individual women's economic role is the extent of female economic activity in her larger community in general (Basu 1993). It is suggested that in a situation of relatively high female labour force participation rates, even non-working women will experience some of the effects of female employment on gender differences in health and mortality. This is particularly the case for those effects which are related to the changed ideas and values associated with economic independence.

The control category here is therefore the non-working woman as defined by the conventional census or survey, and the following sections examine how economic activity works to increase or decrease the gender gap in health and survival that this non-working woman faces. Moreover, in addition to economic inactivity, the analysis includes a cultural variable which is strongly associated with and often determines the kind and level of female economic activity. This is the variable of female seclusion norms and refers not just to the literal veiling of women (or purdah) but also to the restrictions on their movements in and interactions with the extra-domestic world.

Next, there is the female domestic role. This is defined as the extent to which women's activities are confined to the domestic domain and the extent of their responsibility for the different chores needed for household maintenance. This is not merely the converse of the economic independence variable (in fact, it is more directly connected to the seclusion variable)—a woman can be economically inactive but nevertheless have a wider area of operations than her immediate home and may not take on full responsibility for all the mechanical tasks that keep this home going. The control here is the woman with no expected or actual extra-domestic role with the major responsibility for performing (though not necessarily, or even usually, deciding on the performance of) household maintenance tasks.

Finally, we have the woman's reproductive role. This refers to the extent to which the woman's position is defined by her reproductive behaviour and is therefore to some extent the converse of her importance in extra-domestic affairs. The control is the woman with high fertility whose social and domestic value diminishes if she has few children.

All these roles are usually defined culturally rather than purely by contemporary socio-economic circumstances. It is true that the cultural norms and institutions defining these roles may have their roots in material factors historically, but they tend to persist long after the rationale for their original emergence has expired and to today exist in economically diverse settings. However, this does not mean that the scope does not exist to tamper with them—it only means that the intervention points will often have to be non-economic and, even if economic, culture-sensitive.

The next three sections discuss some of the ways in which these three roles of women influence the proximate determinants of their health and life chances relative to males. Effects at different stages of the life-cycle are considered and an attempt made to identify, even if only qualitatively, conflicting effects.

III. Women's Roles and the Male Disadvantage

We already know that in the developed countries as well as in several parts of the developing world, life expectancies for females are well above those for males. Perhaps this is the natural order of things; what is interesting is that even in regions where there is an overall female disadvantage in health and survival, with this disadvantage being distressingly sharp for certain groups and at certain ages, there are other groups and other ages where the direction of the gender gap is reversed and it is the male that fares worse. Intrinsically determined male disadvantage (as for example in neonatal survival as already mentioned) is one thing; it appears that there is also a certain amount of male disadvantage (or, more correctly, female advantage) conferred by our present independent variable of interest—women's roles.

In the Indian context, the most striking example of excess male mortality is at the ages above thirty-five (Dyson 1984); life expectancy at this age is significantly shorter for males. Nor can this be attributed to the reduced risks of death faced by women past their active childbearing years. It is more likely to be due to the fact that the rise in age-specific death rates for men after this age is about twice that for women after thirty-five (Caldwell and Caldwell 1990). This may of course be partly because only the fitter women have survived the assault on their survival in childhood and young adulthood.

But what else could account for this reversal of fortunes? Dyson (1984) speculates that it may be linked to high levels of adult male tuberculosis mortality, on the basis of similar findings for some East Asian populations, (Goldman 1980) and on the basis of cause-of-death statistics for India. If this is indeed the case, even if partly, one needs a better understanding of the reasons for this gender gap in tuberculosis deaths. Is it due to a greater exposure to the disease? In that case, there is probably a link with sex differences in life-styles: through occupational differences by gender and through gender differences in other aggravating behaviours such as smoking—according to WHO estimates about 52 per cent of adult males in India are smokers compared to 3 per cent of adult females (United Nations 1991). Relatedly, heart attacks too seem to be the cause of death in a disproportionately large number of males (Registrar General of India 1987). Similar remarks can be made about alcohol-related deaths, primarily cirrhosis of the liver, which are unduly partial to older males.

How do all these behaviours result from different male-female roles? They certainly have a connection with the relatively limited extra-domestic role of women. Hand-in-hand with the restrictions on female movement and economic activity go the social restrictions on 'male' activities such as smoking and drinking. However, just as a convergence in roles and life-styles may be leading to a reduction in the gap between male and female health by improving the latter relative to the former in the case of excess female mortality, it is plausible that modernization can also reduce the gap by worsening female health to bring it more in line with male health. According to one estimate, the prevalence of lung cancer among women has increased 400 per cent in the last 30 years (United Nations 1991).

In the same way, male death rates are disproportionately high from some kinds of 'accidents and violence'. And nor is this confined to adulthood, (Chen et al. 1980; Gordon, Singh and Wyon 1965). The Registrar General's Cause of Death Survey (1987) recorded twice as many male as female deaths from drowning, falls and vehicular accidents in the 5–14 year age group. The relative restrictions on the free movement of even young girls in South Asian society has this benefit, even if it is more than compensated in the next age group by the female predominance in deaths due to 'burns'—a mysterious category which should be redistributed between accidental burns and homicide (see also Karkal 1985).

Then there is the male disadvantage in mortality during periods of famine or acute food shortages in general (see Dyson 1991). Contrary to expectation and earlier predictions (e.g. Chen and Chowdhury 1977; Caldwell and Caldwell 1987) it now appears that adult males are the worst sufferers at such times. While there is the possibility that their relatively good nutritional status at other times has made them less well adapted to nutritional stress, Dyson speculates on some other explanations related to male-female roles. Perhaps male and female propensities to migrate at such times differ; more importantly, perhaps rises in female mortality are attenuated by post-famine falls in fertility; in the absence of such falls, the effects of pregnancy and lactation would be compounded by the nutritional deficits of famine.

Finally there is the historical and (though less acute thanks to new technology) contemporary male excess mortality due to wars and feuds. Whether through socialization or through inherent skills, the traditional division of labour, whereby to women fall all domestic responsibilities and to men the task of protecting their property at whatever level of aggregation, has meant a preponderance of male deaths during war and, during periods when war-related deaths accounted for a large proportion of all deaths, a preponderance of male deaths among all deaths.

In the Indian context, these male disadvantages together with their biological inferiority at some ages have resulted in expectations of life after age five being greater for females since the late 1970s and perhaps even earlier in some parts of the country.

IV. Sex Differentials in the Outcome of Illness

This section should logically follow the next section—after all one has to first become ill before one does or does not do something about the illness episode and this influences the outcome. However, I place it here because in the course of discussing 'personal illness control' behaviour (Mosley and Chen 1984) I make several general remarks about the effects of women's roles on this behaviour, which apply equally to the effects of women's roles on the incidence of illness. At the same time these remarks on the whole fit better into this section than they do in the more restricted section on exposure to illness which follows. And finally, as a determinant of differentials in health and mortality, illness outcome is more important than the exposure to illness, so on that count at least it bears earlier discussion.

As already mentioned more than once, the motivations underlying apparently discriminatory behaviour are not easy to deduce. This is especially so because the most common situation is probably for a mixture of conscious and unintentional discrimination to be involved and the best one can do is demonstrate the existence of each type without trying to attribute relative values. Connections between women's roles and these two kinds of discriminatory behaviour are easy to draw intuitively, but there is increasingly also a fair (but scattered) amount of empirical support for much of this intuition.

For example, one would expect that in a sufficiently rational or practical set-up, women's economic roles will have a bearing on the value attached to their survival and, given our ability to manipulate events of life and death, on the sex differential in health and survival. There certainly seems to be some evidence that such calculations are important, however subconscious or institutionalized. Viewed in this way, it is hardly surprising that Rosenzweig and Schultz (1982) found a negative correlation (in a district-level analysis) between female employment rates and the male-female differential in survival. Similar conclusions have been drawn by several others (for example, Miller 1981; Bardhan 1974) with cross-sectional as well as longitudinal data. Wadley and Derr (1987) for example, speculate that declining opportunities for female employment have led to increases in sex differentials in mortality in poor households in their study area in Uttar Pradesh.

But why should this connection be an outcome of 'planned' discriminatory behaviour? I do not enter here into a discussion of what constitutes 'planned' or 'deliberate' behaviour beyond defining it as behaviour which leads to an outcome that is not unwelcome.

Table 1: State-wise differentials in female employment, the sex ratio of child mortality and son preference

Region/State	% women aged 30–34 employed (1981—rural)	Sex ratio (m/f) of child mortality (1981—rural)	Index of son preference*
India	27.8	0.93	20.2
North			
Punjab	4.1	0.87	29.0
Haryana	9.1	0.81	20.7
Uttar Pradesh	10.4	0.83	25.0
Rajasthan	18.0	0.90	31.3
Madhya Pradesh	44.5	0.96	21.9
South			
Andhra Pradesh	52.5	1.05	9.0
Karnataka	39.4	1.01	11.2
Tamil Nadu	44.3	1.13	11.5
Kerala	27.3	1.01	17.2

Sources: 1. Census of India, 1981
         2. Bhatia, 1978

*Index of son preference = $100 \times E/C$, where E is the excess of the number of sons over daughters considered ideal and C is the ideal family size. The index varies between –100 and 100. *Source:* Bhatia, 1978.

Table 1 illustrates the answer to this question quite plausibly. The first part of the table does not contradict the hypothesis that high female labour force participation rates are associated with greater gender equality in child survival (Basu and Basu 1991). The last column also finds an association between female labour force participation rates and the sex ratio of ideal family size, the direction of the association being able to correctly predict the relative sex ratio of child mortality if one assumes that child survival is open to behavioural influences. That is, where the economic productivity of women is low, this is matched by a smaller demand for daughters and apparently some success in translating this demand into reality.

Even stronger support for the existence of such family building strategies is available from Das Gupta's (1987) Punjab data which demonstrate a wider sex differential in survival for second and higher order daughters; that is, there is a clear element of conscious neglect of certain children. Not surprisingly, Das Gupta's study area is also known for its social aversion to female economic activity. However, it may be mentioned that Pebley and Amin's (1991) data analysis for the same region finds a similar birth order effect for sons, confirming the existence of a family building strategy but suggesting that boys do not necessarily lie on a bed of roses either.

1981 census data (see Table 2) bring out another hopeful side of women's employment—the sex ratio of child survival relationship (Basu and Basu 1991). Not only do areas with high female labour force participation rates exhibit greater gender equality; even in areas of low labour force participation by women, working women (as conventionally defined), experience less sex-biased child loss. This suggests that it does not take long for the value of women's productive work to be perceived as a reason to rear daughters that live, cultural compulsions in favour of mistreating daughters notwithstanding.

As to how the handling of an illness contributes to this differential survival of boys and girls, there is now a fairly large body of evidence on the role of prompt and efficient (meaning, usually, modern and often paid for) health care in determining child mortality differentials in general and differentials by sex in particular (see among others, Basu 1989; Singh, Gordon and Wyon 1962; Aziz 1977, Beals 1976; Das Gupta 1987; Kielmann et al. 1983; Khan et al. 1988, Chen et al. 1981).

Table 2: Sex Ratio of Child Mortality according to maternal work status

Region/State	Sex ratio (m/f) of child mortality for non-working women	Sex ratio (m/f) of child mortality for working women
India	0.90	0.99
North		
Punjab	0.87	0.92
Haryana	0.82	0.91
Uttar Pradesh	0.82	0.91
Rajasthan	0.88	0.92
Madhya Pradesh	0.91	1.00
South		
Andhra Pradesh	1.07	1.04
Karnataka	1.02	1.01
Tamil Nadu	1.01	1.02
Kerala	1.12	1.15

Source: Registrar General of India, 1988.

Differential investment in children's welfare according to their perceived potential contributions to household welfare thus seems a distinct possibility. What about women's economic roles and the investment in their own well-being? That is, does women's economic activity lead to a narrowing of the gender gap in health and mortality among adults in this direct sense? Increased investment in economically active women is certainly rational from the household's point of view. In addition Drèze and Sen (1990) have proposed that more equal investment in such women is likely because of the increase in their bargaining position in the situation of 'cooperative conflict' that characterizes relationships such as the marital one. That is, one reason for women's acquiescence in the continued relative under-investment in them is to do with the greater cost to them in the event of a 'breakdown' in cooperation. Presumably this cost is lower if the woman is economically independent or has access to other reliable family or community sources of support. But, as pointed out by Sen (1987), the 'perceptions' about women's bargaining position both among women and among men may be more important than the reality in determining welfare outcomes.

This brings us to some other possible connections between women's roles and differential health care for the two sexes. Can one really attribute the latter entirely to the materialistic calculations determined by women's economic roles? As discussed in an earlier section, low female labour force participation rates tend to be associated with high levels of female seclusion and norms about female interaction with extra-kin males. These norms take effect at an early age and must assume at least partial responsibility for sex differentials in health care and consequently in mortality for both young girls and (especially) young adult women. Salman Rushdie was not being wildly imaginative in his description of the medical examination of a young girl standing behind a sheet with the affected part of her anatomy visible to the doctor through a hole in this sheet (*Midnight's Children*). More usually, inhibitions about having girls and women seen and (especially) touched by non-related males are expressed in less exotic forms such as delaying treatment until it is seen to be essential (by when it might well be too late), making do with home treatment (Basu 1989), obtaining treatment through symptoms being described to the doctor by a male relative or seeking the services of a doctor in the next village who is less likely to recognize his patient on the street the next morning (for empirical evidence on the last two, see Khan et al. 1988). The irony is that these same factors of female seclusion and low female economic activity outside the home lead to a shortage of female medical and paramedical staff in the very areas where the need for them is the most desperate.

To summarize this section thus far, while women's economic potential is an important determinant of discriminatory behaviour, direct economic value is not everything. At least a part of the apparent bias against females must be attributed to something less calculative. This something is the intangible variable of culture and custom. While such cultural practices and inhibitions may have had their origins in economic factors, their persistence often implies little more than the observance of norms jelled over generations; so that, for example, if the women in a household eat last, it is not essential to take this to mean that a woman's welfare is considered unnecessary or irrelevant. It may just be that such an eating order has become established in that particular culture. Similarly, a disinclination to take a girl to a doctor (especially a male doctor) may be the result of an overprotective attitude towards daughters rather than one of callousness towards their health. While it is important to change such norms because of their adverse impact on one group, it may be self-defeating to assume a conscious ill-motive behind every action which results in a sex differential in welfare.

This kind of distinction is also important for practical policy reasons. That part of the sex differential in health and survival which is unintentional in its motives is the part least resistant to change from outside—both through education on these often unappreciated effects of discriminatory behaviour, and through the provision of services which lessen the need for such behaviour. The most obvious example of the latter is of course the provision of more domiciliary health services and the availability of more female staff in existing services.

In any case, to return to the effect of women's roles on the sex differential in ill-health outcomes, in addition to health care use, a neglected and probably significant determinant of such outcomes is food and rest during illness and convalescence. Unfortunately there is very little empirical information available on gender differences in this variable; intuitively it seems the advantages conferred by women's productive activities on health care use become disadvantages in this case. For instance, rest is likely to be shorter after an illness if rest means wages lost. More indirectly but perhaps more significantly, after a bout of illness, rest may also be shorter for the daughters of working mothers because of their household and sibling care responsibilities—once again, the longer the mother stands in for the daughter, the greater the wage loss. Both these possibilities are in the direction of an increased sex disparity in the intensity and duration of an illness in adulthood as well as late childhood in households where women have an important economic role. But this is a question which deserves more empirical investigation.

So far, we have discussed only the sex differential in mortality in childhood and early adulthood, because of the generally clear female advantage in health and survival at the later adult ages. But perhaps, as suggested by Caldwell and Caldwell (1990), we need to distinguish between the health and mortality of older women who are currently married and those who are widowed. The latter certainly seem to get the short end of the stick compared to both married women and widowed men. The adverse condition of widows as compared to widowers is also important for another reason—given the age difference between spouses and the higher level of widower remarriage, there are so many more widows than widowers.

How do women's roles impinge on the situation of widows? While direct economic activity may not be the determining factor at the older ages that characterize widowhood, the material underpinnings are nevertheless still strong. Widows with direct access to some material assets, be it land or money, stand a better life chance than those entirely dependent on their kin for support (the question of state support for security has not even appeared on the horizon as yet). Drèze (1990) has pointed out an interesting and illuminating contrast in the regional incidence of widowhood in India. There are far fewer widowed women in the states (predominantly in North India) with an overall population sex ratio adverse to females. A higher incidence of widow remarriage or a higher survival rate in their husbands offer inadequate explanations—what is more likely is that the same factors of economic and social dependency that lead to higher female death rates at younger ages operate among widows to negate the effects of the increasing authority and autonomy of women with age, and these factors account at least partly for the lower mortality of older women in general.

Finally, there is the effect of women's reproductive roles on the outcomes of ill-health according to gender. Given the association between women's economic, domestic and reproductive roles discussed earlier, one mechanism for the effect of high fertility on sex differentials in ill-health outcomes is naturally through the intermediate effect of economic dependency and domestic seclusion. But high fertility can also have direct independent effects on the sex ratio of health and mortality, effects which are accentuated by the simultaneous presence of socio-economic dependence.

It is of course well established that one of the consequences of several and (especially) closely spaced births is an increased risk to the health of women and children. In the case of maternal health, this means that high fertility is associated with an increased gender gap during the reproductive years. Higher fertility leads to a higher number of deaths due to causes related to pregnancy for two reasons—because it increases the number of times the woman is exposed to the risk of maternal mortality and because the risk of maternal death is higher for higher order pregnancies. A maternal mortality rate of around 300 per 100,000 live births is high by any reckoning.

The regional variations in maternal mortality and morbidity are the subject of another paper in this volume; here I would like to mention two aspects of women's roles which heighten the regional disparities. First there is the indirect effect of the inhibitions about seeking modern health care that characterize a culture where norms about female seclusion are strong. It is no surprise therefore to find in Basu (1990) that while in the south Indian study sample 30 per cent of live births had been in an institution, only 10 per cent of the north Indian births had occurred under similar medical supervision—this in a situation where the two groups faced identical access to health services. This kind of difference influences both our proximate determinants of maternal mortality—the exposure to complications associated with pregnancy as well as the outcome of any complications that arise.

But there is probably another cultural practice which contributes to this disadvantaged position of northern Indian women during pregnancy and delivery. This is the custom in much of South India of the woman going to her parental home at least for the first one or two deliveries—the attention and care she can demand and obtain in this location are qualitatively and quantitatively different as several fictional and real accounts testify. It is certainly not inconsistent that the use of and demand for professional services for delivery is the lowest in those areas where the woman remains in her husband's home through her pregnancy—however exaggerated our notions about the frictions between a young wife and her husband's family, there is certainly less personal interest in making things easier for the daughter-in-law than there is for the daughter.

So much for reproduction and its effect on the sex differential in adult mortality. What about the sex differential in child mortality, as distinct from overall child mortality? If the sex differential in child mortality is greater for higher order births (example, Das Gupta 1987), one can see high fertility being associated with a larger sex differential for 'strategic' reasons. But, given the evidence that higher order boys also face some (but smaller) disadvantages compared to their older living brothers (Pebley and Amin 1991; Beals 1976), this increased differential is still narrower than it might have been if the demand for sons had been endless.

V. Sex Differentials in the Exposure to Illness

'Exposure to illness' refers here to attributes and behaviours that predispose one to the risk of ill-health. This section will consider some of the aspects of women's roles, as defined by their involvement in production, reproduction and domestic duties, which increase their exposure to potentially debilitating or life-threatening conditions relative to males. Whether this potential to debilitate or kill is then differentially realized was the subject of the last section, reversing somewhat the order of things in real life.

First, there is the effect of women's real or potential economic independence. How does this differentially affect the exposure to illness in males and females? The evidence is mixed. Economic activity can improve things for women through indirect factors such as knowledge, autonomy and control over resources, but this has to be balanced against the hazards of employment (a) in a time schedule that is packed to begin with, (b) in activities which carry special risks and (c) under conditions where the host (that is, the woman) is already weakened by her other 'female' roles.

The good effects of women's access to and use of employment opportunities on sex differentials in exposure to illness are theoretically obvious. Economic independence should increase the woman's incentive to treat her male and female offspring equally and the extra resources she now commands should give her the means and the freedoms to exploit this incentive. Several studies have documented how income earned by women, even keeping total household income constant, is more likely to be used for household (and especially child) welfare (for example, Mencher 1988; Kumar 1977). At the same time, there is also ample evidence that female employment is not synonymous with female control over income (see, for example, some of the papers in Dwyer and Bruce 1988), indeed, it is not at all uncommon for the two to be divorced altogether.

What about the more direct effects of women's employment on sex differentials in the exposure to physical ill-health? Here, the disadvantages seem to outweigh the benefits. To consider the relative health status of women themselves, female employment carries with it all the physical burdens of a double shift of work. The Indian situation is no different from the one in the developed countries where even today women carry the responsibility for some 80–90 per cent of household chores (United Nations 1991). These chores are much more labour- and energy-intensive in the typical Indian (especially rural) setting and the additional demands of outside work cannot but add to the physical strain. It is not surprising therefore that Khan et al. (1988) recorded a higher level of nutritional stress among the working women in their field study in U.P.

In addition there are the occupational hazards of the jobs that women crowd into. For example, the concentration of women in the transplanting of paddy in South India is associated with a series of health risks specific to this occupation (Mencher and Sardamoni 1982). Similar arguments apply to the disproportionate representation of women workers in the construction industry in urban India.

One wonders how much the higher levels of female employment in South India contribute to the smaller difference in the male-female survival gap in the 20–24 year age-group between north and south India, as compared to large regional differences in the gender gap in childhood mortality. Caldwell and Caldwell (1990) point out this poorer southern advantage in survival by sex among young adults but do not speculate on the possible causes. It would be interesting to see if this southern advantage is again striking for non-working women.

However, when the access to employment is low for cultural reasons, the gain to women in terms of less exposure to ill-health may still be offset by other aspects of this same culture—the norms about female seclusion that tend to accompany norms about not working outside the home. The results of such domestic confinement and sole responsibility for a range of back-breaking domestic activities (fuel and water collection in particular) carry with them a number of different kinds of sex-selective exposure to illness. For example, Caldwell and Caldwell (1990) report how in their field work in Karnataka they found the long hours spent by women and young girls in dark, smoke-filled and secluded kitchens to appreciably increase the incidence of bronchitis and asthma in this group. Similarly Cohen (1987) attributes the higher incidence of trachoma in females to their role in nursing sick family members.

These increased risks of exposure to illness are aggravated by the nature of our development. Ecological policies for example have made little attempt to include in their calculations the special costs to women of declining and shifting sources of fuel (Agarwal 1988).

The increased time and energy required to collect fuel in many parts of the country today cannot but be detrimental to women's health. Similarly the relative absence of innovation in cooking technology for poor homes means that women's (and young girls') exposure to domestic pollutants continues to increase their exposure to serious or fatal diseases (Batliwala 1983). Indeed Batliwala (1982) suggests that the energy conserved (and consequently the health status protected) by developing alternative domestic technology for, say, fuel collection and use, may at least partly offset the need for more calories in the diets of poor women.

But several data sources suggest that sex differences in the incidence of illness are not a serious determinant of sex differences in health and mortality. However, exposure factors can still be important according to recent research by Aaby (1988) and others. To cite one example, which relates directly to the situation where women's value is defined primarily and perhaps even solely by their domestic and reproductive duties, in such a situation there is a hesitation in letting girls attend school or even move around freely outside the home. Caldwell and Caldwell (1990) have underscored the relation between sex differentials in schooling and sex differentials in child health in terms of the beneficial effects of school on the health behaviour of children—faster recognition of illness, insistence on treatment and rest, and so on.

However, it now appears that schooling or outdoor activity in general may also be an important determinant of the intensity of an infection—children who are primary cases, that is, infected from an outsider, receive a smaller dose of infection than secondary cases, that is, persons infected from another household member. Since girls are more likely to be secondary cases in situations where they are relatively more confined to the home, they are also likely to suffer a more severe infection than their brothers, leading to higher case fatality rates which are made worse by their poorer health care as discussed in the last section.

Finally, there is the effect of women's reproductive roles on exposure to the risk of ill-health. Much of this effect is similar to that of female employment and to do with energy loss and general nutritional stress. High fertility imposes what has been called the maternal depletion syndrome, whereby the rigours of pregnancy, delivery and breast-feeding are translated into protein-calorie malnutrition, anaemia and other complications (especially during delivery) to compound the protein-calorie malnutrition and anaemia which are in any case the lot of poor women in the region whatever their fertility.

As far as sex differentials in childhood exposure to illness go, high fertility cannot be clearly associated with these, although it certainly increases the exposure of children to ill-health regardless of their gender.

VI. Conclusion

If the last few pages have a message, it is that the relationship between women's economic, domestic and reproductive roles and the gender gap in health and survival is not clear-cut and unidirectional. To repeat just one example, while female employment may result in more equal treatment of sons and daughters, it may increase the gender gap in the exposure to and intensity of several diseases among adults. Nevertheless, the broad finding is that where women are economically active, not restricted to the domestic domain and not defined primarily by the number of children they bear, the gender gap in health and survival in smaller than it is for women who are cut off from economic independence, cut off from the extra-domestic world and dependent on their reproductive success for their status.

There is another question that has not been touched upon in this paper. This is the role of poverty. How does a constraint on resources mediate in these relations between women's roles and gender differences in health? While there is a tendency to assume that when resources are limited, things worsen for females much more than for males (for example, World Bank 1991), the empirical support for this assumption is rather weak. If anything, it appears that the poor believe in greater gender equality. This is evident for example in the smaller sex differentials in mortality typically found in the lowest socio-economic groups (as defined by factors such as caste, income and education) and suggests that women's roles are the intervening variable that determine the relationship between poverty and the sex differential in physical well-being. If women belong to high-risk categories in all socio-economic classes then certainly a further constraint on resources might increase their disadvantage. But women's roles themselves seem to be conditioned by socio-economic status.

That poverty cannot be the excuse for such gender inequalities is also suggested by inter-regional analyses. For example, as pointed out by Sen (1987a) and others, sub-Saharan Africa is a prime illustration of the fact that greater poverty and greater gender disparities in physical welfare need not go together.

This paper has also not considered the complementary issue of the effects of gender differences in health and survival on gender differences in productivity and welfare as well as on overall household productivity and the quality of life. One can think of several such effects and some of the more general (that is, not differentiated by sex) ones are discussed in Das Gupta et al. (1995).

Finally, the South Asian female disadvantage in health and survival risks is becoming the all-consuming passion of research on health differentials in this area. This attitude is not warranted for two reasons: (a) gender differences in health are narrowing down and may well be reversed in the near future and (b) gender differences in health are often small compared to differences by other kinds of categorizations such as caste, rural-urban residence and education.

At the same time, it is also true that even if sex differences in health and mortality are now less adverse to females, there is much of female ill-health and mortality that is still 'preventable'. That is, in a situation of no discrimination, conscious or otherwise, there would continue to be a marked sex differential in health and mortality but the direction of this differential would be reversed with males bearing the larger brunt. If this is the 'natural' situation, then, even with similar health and mortality levels in the two sexes, we are still not close enough to the ideal of gender equality in opportunities and treatment that a truly egalitarian system should aspire to.

References

Aaby, P. (1988), *Malnourished or Overinfected: An analysis of the determinants of acute measles mortality*, Copenhagen, Copenhagen University.

Agarwal, B. (1988), 'Neither Sustenance nor Sustainability' in B. Agarwal (ed.), *Structures of Patriarchy*, London, Zed books.

Aziz, K. M. A. (1977), 'Present trends in medical consultation prior to death in rural Bangladesh', *Bangladesh Medical Journal*, vol. 6.

Bardhan, P.K. (1974), 'Little girls and death in India', *Economic and Political Weekly*.

Basu, A.M. (1989), 'Is discrimination in food really necessary for explaining sex differentials in childhood mortality?', *Population Studies*.

Basu, A.M. (1990) 'Cultural influences on health care use when accessibility is held constant', *Studies in Family Planning*.

Basu, A.M. (1993), *Culture, the Status of Women and Demographic Behaviour*, Oxford, Oxford University Press.
Basu, A.M. and K. Basu (1991), 'Women's economic roles and child survival', *Health Transition Review*.
Batliwala, S. (1992), 'Rural energy scarcity and undernutrition', *Economic and Political Weekly*.
Batliwala, S. (1993), 'Women and cooking energy', *Economic and Political Weekly*.
Beals, A.R. (1976), 'Strategies of resort to curers in South India' in C. Leslie (ed.), *Asian Medical Systems: A Comparative Study*, Berkeley, University of California Press.
Bhatia, J. (1978), 'Ideal number and sex preference of children in India', *Journal of Family Welfare*.
Caldwell, J.C. and P. Caldwell (1987) 'Famine in Africa', paper presented to the IUSSP Seminar on Mortality and Society in Sub-Saharan Africa.
Caldwell, P. and J.C. Caldwell (1990), *Gender Implications for Survival in South Asia*, ANU, Health Transition Working Paper No. 7.
Chen, L.C. and A.K.M.A. Chowdhury (1977), 'The dynamics of contemporary famine', in IUSSP International Population Conference, Mexico,
Chen L.C., A. Rahman and J. Sardar (1980), 'Epidemiology and causes of death among children in a rural area of Bangladesh', *International Journal of Epidemiology*.
Chen, L.C., E. Huq and S. D'Souza (1981), 'Sex bias in the family allocation of food and health care in rural Bangladesh', *Population and Development Review*.
Cohen, N. (1987), 'Sex differences in blindness and mortality in the Indian subcontinent: Some paradoxes explored', Paper presented at the workshop on differential female mortality, Dhaka, January.
Das Gupta, M., T.N. Krishan and Lincoln C. Chen (eds.) (1995) *Health, Poverty and Development in India*, Bombay, Oxford University Press.
Das Gupta, M. (1987), 'Selective discrimination against female children in India', *Population and Development Review*.
Drèze, J. (1990), *Widows in Rural India*, Paper No. 26 of the Development Economics Research Programme, London School of Economics.
Drèze J. and A. Sen (1990), *The Political Economy of Hunger*, Oxford, Clarendon Press.
Dwyer, D. and J. Bruce (eds.) (1988), *A Home Divided: Women and Income in the Third World*, California, Stanford University Press.
Dyson, J. (1984), 'Excess female mortality in India: Uncertain evidence on a narrowing differential', in K. Srinivasan and S. Mukherji (eds.), *Dynamics of Population and Family Welfare*, Bombay, Himalaya Publishing House.
Dyson, T. (1991), 'On the demography of South Asian Famines', *Population Studies*.
Goldman, N. (1980), 'Far eastern patterns of mortality', *Population Studies*, vol. 34.
Gordon, J. E., S. Singh and J. B. Wyon (1965), 'Causes of death at different ages by sex and by season in a rural population of the Punjab, 1957–59: A field study', *Indian Journal of Medical Research*, vol. 53.
Harris, B. (1989), 'Differential female mortality and health care in South Asia', *The Journal of Social Studies*.
Karkal, M. (1985), 'How the other half dies', *Economic and Political Weekly*.
Khan, M.E., R. Anker, S.K. Ghosh Dastidar and S. Bharati (1988), 'Inequalities between men and women in nutrition and family welfare services', *Social Action*.

Kielmann, A.A. and associates (1983), *Child and Maternal Health Services in Rural India: The Narangwal Experiment*, Baltimore, Johns Hopkins University Press.

Kumar, S. (1977), 'Role of the household economy in determining child nutrition at low income levels: A case study of Kerala', Ithaca, Cornell University, Deptt. of Agricultural Economics, Occasional paper No. 5.

Mencher J. and K. Sardamoni (1982), 'Muddy feet and dirty hands: Rice production and female agricultural labour,' *Economic and Political Weekly*.

Mencher, J.P. (1988), 'Women's work and their poverty: women's contribution to household maintenance in South India', in Dwyer and Bruce (eds.).

Miller, B.D. (1981), *The Endangered Sex*, Ithaca, Cornell University Press.

Mosley, W.H. and L.C. Chen (1984), 'An analytical framework for the study of child mortality in developing countries', *Population and Development Review*.

Oppong, C. and K. Abu (1985), *A handbook for data collection and analysis of seven roles and statuses of women*, Geneva, ILO.

Pebley, A. and S. Amin (1991), 'The impact of a public health intervention on sex differentials in childhood mortality on rural Punjab, India', *Health Transition Review*.

Registrar General of India (1987), *Survey of Causes of Death (Rural)*, Annual Report 1987, New Delhi, Government of India.

Registrar General of India (1988), *Child Mortality Estimates for India*, New Delhi, Government of India.

Rosenzweig, M.R. and T.P. Schultz (1982), 'Market Opportunities, Genetic endowments and intrafamily resource distribution: Child survival in rural India', *American Economic Review*.

Sen, A. (1987), 'Women, well-being and agency'. Paper presented at the seminar on 'Women's Issues in Development Policy' at the International Centre for Research on Women, Washington, D.C.

Sen, A. (1987a), *Africa and India: What do we have to learn from each other?* Oxford, All Souls College, mimeo.

Singh, S., J. E. Gordon and J. B. Wyon (1962), 'Medical care in fatal illnesses in a rural Punjab population: Some social, biological and cultural factors and their ecological implications', *Indian Journal of Medical Research*, vol. 50.

United Nations (1991), *The World's Women 1970–1990, Trends and Statistics*, New York, United Nations.

Wadley, S. and B. Derr (1987), 'Child survival and economic status in a North Indian village', paper presented at the workshop on differential female mortality, Dhaka.

World Bank (1991), *Gender and Poverty in India*, Washington D.C., The World Bank.

7

Women's Health in a Rural Poor Population in Tamil Nadu

T. K. SUNDARI RAVINDRAN

1. Introduction

The health status of women in India is an area which so far has received inadequate scholarly attention. The limited evidences from the few studies available present a dismal picture.

India is one of the few countries where life expectancy of women has been less than that of men till very recently. For rural women this still holds good.[1] More girls than boys die in infancy and childhood. This higher female infant and child mortality is a rare phenomenon not found even in countries with far higher mortality rates than India, and is believed to be the consequence of the discriminatory treatment of the female child. It is seen that 'Deaths of young girls in India exceed those of young boys by at least one-third of a million every year. Every sixth infant death is specifically due to gender discrimination.' (1). What is more, the gap shows no signs of narrowing: the ratio of female to male mortality in childhood has remained

---

[1] Trends in life expectancy at birth by sex are as follows (Source: Registrar General of India, Sample Registration System, various years).

Years	Rural		Urban		Total	
	Male	Female	Male	Female	Male	Female
1972–76	47.85	46.82	57.60	58.02	49.47	48.62
1977–81	48.40	47.53	59.92	61.66	52.69	52.33
1982–86	48.64	47.82	61.08	63.68	54.89	55.35

at around 1.1 since 1970 (Registrar General of India, Sample Registration System, various years).

This trend of excess female mortality is pronounced till the age of 35. High rates of maternal mortality contribute to excess female mortality in the reproductive years, the mortality rate being more than 50 per cent higher for females than for males. Maternal mortality rates in India (at 500 per 100,000 live births) are among the highest in the world, and more than 50 times the average for industrialized countries. Even this may be an underestimate.[2] Frequent pregnancies compound a woman's lifetime risk of dying from maternity-related causes. The absence of trained attendance at birth for the majority of women contributes greatly to high rates of maternal mortality. As recently as 1988, 66 per cent of all births in the country took place without trained medical attendance, and only 22 per cent of births took place in medical units (3).

Pregnancy outcome—the probability that a pregnancy results in a full-term, healthy live birth—is an important indicator of women's health status. According to community studies from different parts of the country, there were above 139 unsuccessful pregnancies per 1000 (4). In comparison, the rates range from 71 per 1000 pregnancies in South Korea to 126 per 1000 in Costa Rica (5). The levels of pregnancy wastage for women from poorer communities is steeper, in some cases reaching even a high of 300 per 1000 pregnancies (6).[3]

Morbidity Data

Sources of information on women's morbidity and nutritional status are even fewer than those on mortality. According to National Sample Survey data for 1973–74, the incidence of morbidity in women was 12 per cent for India as a whole. A 1990 national survey reported prevalence rates of 47 per cent and 60 per cent for urban and rural women respectively. However, the prevalence rate in the latter case is restricted to 'treated' illness rather than all illnesses (7 and 8). According to macro-level studies conducted by the NNMB,

---

[2] A community-based study reported maternal mortality rates of 545 and 830 per 100,000 live births, respectively, in urban and rural Anantapur (2).
[3] Casterline's figures (5) are from World Fertility Survey results for 8 developing countries, and Gopalan and Naidu's figures (6) are based on a survey of 2537 rural and 2021 urban women from a low socio-economic group, subsisting on a daily calorie intake of less than 1850 kcals per day.

only 20 per cent of girls below 5 years of age are adequately nourished, 77 per cent suffer mild to moderate malnutrition, and 3 per cent are severely malnourished (9). Interestingly, all the above studies indicate better morbidity and nutritional status for women/girls as compared to men/boys.

Nevertheless, two large-scale rural morbidity surveys, one in Kerala (10) and the other covering two districts each from Madhya Pradesh, Uttar Pradesh and Rajasthan (11), find the contrary. Prevalence rates reported by these studies vary from only 6 per cent in Alwar, Rajasthan, to 21 per cent in Kerala.[4] The prevalence of anaemia in women is again very high, especially in the reproductive age-groups. A study covering four centres found more than 70 per cent of rural women between 25 and 44 years to be anaemic (12).

Intensive community-level micro-studies, not attempting comparison by gender but documenting women's reproductive health problems in detail, have found very high morbidity rates: more than 50 per cent in the 15–45 age-groups (13 and 14). It therefore seems likely that macro-studies underestimate women's morbidity for reasons such as: (a) non-inclusion of reproductive morbidity; (b) the definition of prevalence being restricted to treated illness—as a result, if women tend not to treat their illnesses they would be recorded as having lower morbidity; (c) not questioning the women concerned, but only the male heads of their households, and so on.

Any attempt to arrive at an understanding of the extent and causes of morbidity from these sources of data are further hampered by the use of widely varying reference periods, definitions and classifications of health problems. There is also a near absence of information on socio-economic differentials of morbidity levels and the nature of health problems experienced.

[4]The male and female prevalence rates for morbidity in the Kerala study (10), which has a two-week reference period, were 203.4 and 209.2 per 1000, respectively, while the prevalence rates over a one-month reference period in the NCAER study (11) are as follows:

	Madhya Pradesh		Uttar Pradesh		Rajasthan	
	Gwalior	Datia	Mathura	Hardoi	Alwar	Tonk
Male	158	184	209	154	68	143
Female	182	194	202	190	62	156

In short, serious lacunae exist in the information available on Indian women's health status. A number of crucial questions remain unanswered:

(1) What is the extent of illness burden experienced by women?
(2) What are the main causes of illnesses?
(3) How do socio-economic and demographic characteristics (such as age and parity) of the women concerned influence (a) their susceptibility to illnesses, and (b) their health-seeking behaviour?

The present study is an attempt at addressing some of these questions through a case study of women from a rural poor population. The focus is especially on women's reproductive health, about which far less is known as compared to their other health problems.

Framework, Indicators, Data sources and Limitations

We start from the basic premise that disease is a socially produced natural/biological reality, influenced by the economic environment at both macro- and micro-levels.

This approach is at variance with the biomedical paradigm which views disease in purely biological terms, as an impairment in the functioning of one or more components making up the body. Within this paradigm, it is usual to take into consideration only factors related to the natural environment which may increase risk of, or susceptibility to, certain illnesses.

Our framework also differs from approaches which recognize the influence of socio-economic factors on health status, but treat these factors in a social vacuum, as if individuals were just a mass of separate entities who 'happen to have' specific attributes such as a given level of income, education and so on.

The health status of an individual depends on two interrelated factors:

(a) the frequency with which he/she falls ill, and
(b) action taken in the event of illness, such as self-treatment and professional medical help.

It is inequitable resource distribution and the concentration of wealth and productive resources in a small section of the population which is at the root of mass poverty in many societies, including our own. Poverty increases a person's risk of disease due to chronic malnutrition, unhealthy living conditions, excessively strenuous work and so on. It often simultaneously makes people less able to take care of themselves or seek professional help in case of illness, because of lack of appropriate information, or limited access to health services owing to lack of time and money. Thus the same factors which make some sections of the population more vulnerable to disease through denial of basic resources also impedes their ability to deal with disease effectively. Differentials in health status across socio-economic groups, and across households and individuals varying in socio-economic characteristics are usually the result of these disadvantages resulting from inequitable distribution of/access to resources.

In societies where gender-based discrimination limits women's access to resources, one may expect to find gender differentials both in susceptibility to illnesses and in access to health care. The health status of women from poor communities suffers from the compounded disadvantages of being poor and female.

Within the specific context of a community with a given resources base and resource distribution, social stratification by class/caste/gender, and health culture (beliefs and practices affecting well-being), the following set of factors have been considered, as having a major influence on women's health at the household level:[5]

(1) Household resource base.
(2) Women's access to resources.
(3) Demographic characteristics of women, such as age and parity.

The resource base of the household sets the context for defining women's susceptibility to illness, mediated by women's access to resources and women's demographic characteristics. These factors also have a role to play in women's health-seeking behaviour: i.e. what women do when they have a health problem. The functioning of these factors becomes evident through their influence on women's self worth; women's awareness of illnesses and their causes; and the time, money and social support at their disposal.

The community's health culture and the accessibility, quality and range of health services provided are also major influences on whether women feel inclined to seek medical help.

---

[5] A more detailed discussion of the various background factors mentioned here is given in a recently published article by this author, entitled 'Research on Women's Health—Some Methodological Issues', in *Development in Practice*, vol. 2, no. 3, 1992.

Two indicators are used to express women's susceptibility to illness:
Prevalence M_p = Number of women ill/Target Population
Frequency M_p = Number of times illness reported/Target Population

Since high fertility considerably increases the risk of morbidity and mortality from pregnancy-related causes, the Marital Fertility Rate is also used as an indicator of women's health status. Pregnancy outcome is the other indicator used. Both these indicators were computed from data on women's' pregnancy histories collected during the baseline survey.

Contraceptive prevalence and place of delivery are the preventive health measures considered, while type of health care resorted to in case of illness, including self-care, constitute the indicators related to curative care.

Women's access to resources is expressed in terms of their educational status, and participation in the labour force.

The main indicators of household resource base are caste status and the extent of land owned. In addition, indicators such as quality of housing, access to safe water and sanitation have been considered. The extent and causes of women's morbidity and the nature of their health-seeking behaviour have been analysed with respect to these variables.

The prevalence of morbidity was computed from a household interview survey covering 1452 households, conducted during August–October 1989. The reference period was 24 hours, to minimize recall errors and false positive reporting. To compute frequency, a follow-up survey was carried out over a period of six months (January–June 1990) for a representative sub-sample of the reference population, and all episodes of illnesses and their causes were documented. Data on causes of illnesses were used to arrive at cause-specific prevalence and frequency rates.

The data were collected by a nongovernmental rural women's organization (NGO) committed to health promotion among Scheduled Caste women, in Chengalpattu district of Tamil Nadu, South India. The choice of households was not random, but consisted of all the 1452 households and 1017 women covered by the NGO's activities. The majority of them are illiterate and landless agricultural wage workers and belong to the Scheduled Castes. They live in abject poverty, and have limited access to basic amenities and services. Consequently, the morbidity profile and health-seeking behaviour found in this study is not representative of the general population, but perhaps more indicative of the worst possible scenario.

The data pertain only to married women in the reproductive age group of 15 to 40 years, who form the main clientele of the NGO. The numerous health problems of older women, single women or unmarried adolescents have therefore not been captured.

The baseline survey's concern with women's reproductive health problems, moreover, was prompted by the virtual absence of information on women's reproductive health even for the state as a whole, and the need for information on this area as a necessary basis for the NGO's programme directions. The follow-up data however, included both general and reproductive health problems. Data on general health problems suffered by women were thus available only for a sub-sample of 351 women, while data on reproductive health problems are for 1017 women covered by the baseline, and for the smaller sample of women observed over the six-month period.

Another limitation is that data on morbidity are based on health interviews and not on clinical examination. A number of steps were taken at the data collection stage to ensure reliability of data collected. These included limiting the reference period of illness reported to 24 hours; using a checklist of specific symptoms rather than asking general questions on prevalence of illness; talking to the women concerned on an individual basis; and carrying out clinical examinations on a small sub-sample of women to get a rough estimate of the probability of false positive or false negative reporting.[6]

---

[6]25 women underwent a follow-up with a clinical examination by a physician on the same day. It was found that symptoms reported coincided with those of physical examination in 20 out of 25 women, and that there were no false positives. However, vaginal infections went unreported—i.e. there were false negatives in 4 out of 10 women who actually had a problem. It was discovered that under-reporting of reproductive tract infections was largely due to women's inability to identify symptoms. A series of five one-day workshops were organized, each covering five hamlets/villages, and having a participation of five to six women from each settlement. A resurvey was done after these workshops in November–December 1989, to document gynaecological problems alone. The results of this resurvey are the ones considered for reproductive tract infections.

In the following section we have presented information on the extent and nature of the illness burden suffered by women belonging to the study population, and analysed their relationship to the socio-economic and demographic characteristics of the women. Section 3 looks at patterns of health seeking behaviour, while the fourth and concluding section highlights the major findings and discusses their implications for policy.

2. Health Status of Currently Married Women

2.1. Socio-economic Characteristics

The women covered by this study belong to a section of the rural population that suffers extreme social and economic deprivation. They live under harsh circumstances and bear a heavy work burden. 95 per cent of the women belong to the Scheduled Castes and the remaining 5 per cent to Backward Castes. About 60 per cent of them come from agricultural households that are totally landless. Most of these landless households (80 per cent) do not even own the sites on which their huts stand, while 60 per cent do not own any other productive assets, including livestock. This group is completely dependent on agricultural wage labour for its subsistence.

The vast majority of women (85 per cent) have not had even a single year of schooling. Given their lack of resources and education, the women have little option but to work and earn money for their families' subsistence. Only 13 per cent of the women are home-based (not working outside the home, and not participating in any regular remunerative activity). Further analysis shows that non-participation in paid work is related more to women's reproductive responsibilities, being higher among young mothers than among any other demographic or socio-economic category. Three-quarters of the women are wage labourers in agriculture, while the rest work on their own or leased farms. Only 2 per cent are engaged in salaried employment, usually in their own villages as teachers and helpers in the Balwadis and state-sponsored nutrition (feeding) centres. Wages in agricultural employment are very low, and do not exceed Rs 10 per day for women, hardly enough to buy one kilo of rice, the staple food.

Hours of work on the other hand, can extend from dawn to dusk, and in peak seasons are even longer.

Housing conditions are poor: 75 per cent live in mud huts with thatched roofs, with only one room inclusive of kitchen. There is little space around the houses. These are crowded together in a locality called the 'cheri', specifically allocated in every village under traditional land tenures for habitation by the 'untouchable' Scheduled Castes.

Public wells and taps (47 per cent each) are the main sources of water for all purposes, while about 6 per cent have to rely for water supply on irrigation pumpsets belonging to landed households. In most cases the source of water is at least five minutes away, and gathering water from public taps takes a couple of hours. Water supply in summer is unpredictable, with water levels in wells dipping and taps often running dry. Toilets are virtually non-existent. Only 5 women have a toilet in their homes, and the remaining 1012 use the fields.

2.2. Demographic Profile

The picture that generally emerges is one of women characterized by a low age at marriage trapped into high fertility and repeated pregnancies by high rates of child loss, which not only increases their risk of pregnancy wastage, but also seriously compromises their health and well-being.

(a) Age at marriage

Marriage is universal for women, and the vast majority marry and begin childbearing while still in their teens. The average age at marriage is 16.9 years, far below the average of 20.22 reported for Tamil Nadu (15).

59 per cent of currently married women in the 15–44 age-group were married before they were 18, 96 per cent before 20 and only 4 per cent were married after they were 20 years old. However, a shift in the age at marriage is indicated, on analysing age at marriage by current age of women. There is a jump from median age at marriage of 15 for women above 25 years of age, to 18 for women who are currently below 20 years old.

(b) Fertility

Fertility is high: the average number of children ever born to women in the 45–49 age-group is 5.12. The total marital fertility rate (TMFR), calculated on the basis of number of births to women over the last one year, is 5.75, higher even than the all-India figures for rural SC of 5.56 in 1978 (16). When computed on the basis of children ever born, the total marital fertility rate is 5.04. Even this is higher than

Table 1: Total Marital Fertility Rates by characteristics of women, rural India (1978) and Chengalpattu (1989)

Characteristics	Total Marital Fertility Rate	
	Chengalpattu[a]	Rural India
Caste		
SC	5.04	5.56
Non SC	4.86	5.40
Land ownership (of household)		
Landed	5.04	n.a.
Landless	4.95	n.a.
Literacy status		
Illiterate	5.18	5.48
Literate[b]	4.02	4.98
Occupation		
Agricultural		4.90
Wage labourer	5.03	4.91[c]
Home-based	4.94	5.61
All women	5.04	4.60

n.a. : not available.
[a]Calculated from field survey data.
[b]For rural India, figures for women with primary and secondary education are given.
[c]Includes all workers.
Source: India, Rural—Registrar General of India 1979 and 1988.
        Chengalpattu—Baseline Survey, 1989.

the corresponding rate for women of rural Tamil Nadu, which was 4.8 in 1988 (17).

Differences in total marital fertility rates exist according to caste, ownership of land, literacy status and participation in economic activity. The sharpest difference is seen between illiterate and literate women, the TMFR being 5.18 and 4.02 respectively.[7] It is marginally higher for Scheduled Caste women as compared to Backward Caste women, and for women from landed households as compared to those from landless households. While these differences are in the expected directions, the

---

[7]The TMFR for different sections of the study population have been computed from data on children ever born to currently married women, by age of women, using the MORTPAK software of the UN Population Division.

TMFR for agricultural wage workers is found to be higher not only as compared to those engaged in other occupations, but also compared to women who do not work outside the home (Table 1). This is contrary to all-India trends, where non-workers have higher marital fertility rates than all workers (16). The demand for children among female agricultural wage workers is likely to be related to their need for children to help in domestic work and participate in wage labour to supplement the household income, as well as to the higher probability of child loss.

The first five years of marriage result in less than 1 birth (0.7) on an average. The number of children added to the family is highest in the next five years of marriage (1.3), to make the total number of children ever born 1.98. The average number of children ever born increases to 2.94, 3.95 and 4.23 in subsequent five year periods, and reaches 4.9 only for women who have been married for 25 years and more (Table 2). Childbearing is thus spread over the women's whole reproductive span. This may be explained by the high rates of child loss

Table 2: *Mean number of children ever born and children surviving to currently married women, by age and duration of marriage, Scheduled Caste women (1989)*

	Mean number of children ever born	Mean number of children surviving	Proportion dead
Age groups			
15–19	0.37	0.31	0.162
20–24	1.21	1.10	0.091
25–29	2.50	2.22	0.112
30–34	3.51	2.98	0.151
35–39	4.16	3.51	0.157
40–44	4.66	3.84	0.176
45–49	4.93	4.01	0.187
Duration of marriage (yrs)			
0–4	0.67	0.63	0.060
5–9	1.98	1.76	0.112
10–14	2.94	2.58	0.123
15–19	3.95	3.38	0.144
20–24	4.23	3.49	0.175
25–29	4.85	4.00	0.175
30–34	4.92	4.01	0.185

Source: Field survey

and pregnancy wastage. In addition, it has a bearing on contraceptive prevalence and choices (see section 3.1).

(c) Child loss

A comparison of information on children ever born and children surviving to currently married women, indicates a high level of child loss. Six per cent of all children born during the first five years, and 11 per cent of children born during the second five years of marriage die (Table 2). For every 5 mothers in the study population, there have been two child deaths. 20 per cent have lost one child each, while 11 per cent have lost 2 or more children (Table 3). The under-five mortality rate works out to 184 per 1000 births, far higher than the estimated figure of 114 for the state in 1988 (17).

(d) Pregnancy wastage

Of every 1000 pregnancies, only 906 result in a live birth. 60 foetuses are lost due to miscarriage, 27 as a result of intra-uterine death, and 7 are terminated. The stillbirth rate is 29.8 per 1000 live births, more than twice that for rural India (13.9/1000 live births) and 1.5 times that of rural Tamil Nadu (17.8/1000 live births) in 1988 (17).

Socio-economic differences do not proportionately reflect the number of pregnancies ending in miscarriages or stillbirths (Table 4). Unlike in the present case, higher pregnancy wastage rates for higher caste groups is reported from a community study from rural Haryana. Here, the rate of pregnancy wastage is 8.1 per 1000 live births for the Scheduled Caste population, 12.33 for Rajputs and 9.32 for other Backward Castes. The rates of miscarriages and of stillbirths were higher for higher castes (18).

The rate of miscarriages is high for women in the younger age-groups of 15–19 and 20–24, and tapers off thereafter. The stillbirth

Table 3: *Distribution of mothers by number of children lost in childhood for children ever born to currently married women (1989)*

	Child deaths							
	0	1	2	3	4	5	6	Total
Number of mothers	609	176	64	30	4	3	1	887[a]
Per cent	68.7	19.8	7.2	3.4	0.5	0.3	0.1	100

[a]Women who have had at least one live birth
Source: Baseline Survey, 1989.

Table 4: Pregnancy wastage in currently married women (1989)

Age in years	Miscarriages/ 1000 pregnancies	Stillbirths/ 1000 live births	Pregnancy wastage/ 1000 pregnancies[a]
Current age			
15–19	71.5	0	71.5
20–29	80.0	27.8	104.9
30–34	41.9	39.4	81.0
35–39	49.1	26.0	72.3
Caste			
SC	61.0	28.2	86.5
BC	28.4	62.0	85.0
Land-ownership			
Landed	48.2	26.2	72.3
Landless	68.3	32.7	97.5
Education			
Illiterate	70.2	27.0	94.8
Literate	74.1	51.4	118.1
Occupation			
Wage labourer	61.2	31.1	89.3
Other occupations	51.1	23.1	72.6
Home-based	57.0	28.4	82.3
All women	59.6	29.8	94.0

[a] Includes pregnancies medically terminated.
Source: Baseline Survey, 1989.

rate, however, is highest for women between 30 and 35 years of age. There is no incidence of stillbirths among women below 19. The mean number of miscarriages as well as stillbirths increases significantly, in a step-wise fashion, with increasing parity. Women of parity 6 and above have, on an average, three times as many miscarriages and six times as many stillbirths as women of parity 2 and 3 (Table 5).

2.3. Morbidity Associated with Pregnancy and Childbirth

The complications and problems experienced by women in their most recent pregnancy are taken up here. Maternal morbidity would be best captured by a prospective study covering all pregnant women. The present study, being retrospective in nature, is likely to

Table 5: Mean number of miscarriages and stillbirths by parity of women (1989)

Parity	Miscarriages	Stillbirths
1	0.0211	0.0158
2 & 3	0.1532	0.0520
4 & 5	0.2570	0.0964
6+	0.4732	0.3036
All parities	0.1709	0.0776

Source: Base Line Survey, 1989.

be fraught with underestimations due to memory lapses in reporting, especially by women whose most recent pregnancy was several years ago. Further underestimations may also result because the information we have pertains only to complications directly related to pregnancy and childbirth as perceived by the respondent, instead of obstetric morbidity which includes also illnesses aggravated or complicated by pregnancy and childbirth, such as anaemia.

Extent and causes

Of the 887 women who have had at least one prior delivery, 42 per cent have suffered from one or more serious problems related to pregnancy and childbirth. 22 per cent of the women encountered problems during pregnancy or childbirth, while 32.9 per cent had complications in the postpartum period. This includes 119 women (11.7 per cent) who suffered complications in both periods.

Problems included here are antepartum haemorrhage, obstructed labour (at times, but not always, caused by breech presentation) often resulting in stillbirth, excessive bleeding during delivery; as well as perineal tear and other injuries of the birth passage, excessive bleeding, reproductive tract infection, and/or fever within the first week following childbirth. Details of the proportions of women affected by these problems are given in Table 6.

As expected, the incidence of problems increases with parity, but is significantly higher only for those whose parity is six or more, at 53 per cent. Teenage mothers have a significantly higher incidence of postpartum problems, which are mainly related to injuries resulting from difficult deliveries, while women above

Table 6: *Complications during pregnancy, childbirth and postpartum in the most recent pregnancy, currently married women (1989)*

Complications	Number of women[a]	Percent.
Pregnancy and delivery		
Antepartum bleeding	17	1.9
Prolonged labour (24 hrs)[b]	163	16.0
Obstructed labour due to breech presentation	16	1.6
Complicated labour/obstructed labour[c]	42	2.7
Eclamptic fits[d]	22	2.2
Excessive bleeding during delivery	106	10.4
Within a week following delivery		
Excessive bleeding	136	13.4
Fever	81	8.0
Perineal tear (unrepaired)	122	12.0
Reproductive tract infections	6	0.6

[a] Several women had more than one problem
[b] not included as part of obstetric morbidity
[c] 12 cases led to stillbirth
[d] 15 cases led to stillbirth
Source: Baseline Survey, 1989.

30 encounter a significantly higher rate of problems during pregnancy and childbirth.

Socio-economic factors seem to have an important influence on the incidence of complications related to pregnancy and childbirth. Complication rates are significantly higher for Scheduled Caste women and women from landless households. They are lower for women from the owner-farmer or tenant-farmer category when compared to all occupational categories. A puzzling finding is the higher complication rates for literate women (53 per cent) as compared to illiterate women (40 per cent). It is possibly because of higher reporting as a consequence of better awareness, or perhaps because of a medical diagnosis from hospital delivery. The lower prevalence rates for current reproductive health problems point in this direction (Table 7).

Out of the 351 women included in the follow-up, 32 were pregnant at the time of the initial survey. Only 12 of these pregnancies resulted in a normal and healthy birth, implying an even higher rate

Table 7: *Incidence of complications of pregnancy and childbirth in the most recent pregnancy (by characteristics of women and the household) (1989) (Figures in brackets give prevalence rates M_p)*

Characteristic	Had one or more problems			Had no problems	Total
	Pregnancy & delivery	After delivery	All		
Age in years					
15–19	5 (20.0)	11 (44.0)	11 (44.0)	14	25
20–29	94 (20.6)	163 (35.7)	198 (43.3)	259	457
30–34	53 (29.1)	50 (27.5)	77 (42.3)	105	182
35–39	43 (19.2)	68 (30.4)	82 (36.8)	141	223
All ages	195 (22.0)	292 (32.9)	368 (41.5)	519	887
Parity					
1			74 (39.8)	112	186
2–3			130 (38.2)	210	340
4–5			105 (42.2)	144	249
6+			59 (52.7)	53	112
Caste					
SC			355 (42.2)	487	842
BC			13 (29.5)	31	44
Others			0	1	1
Land-ownership					
Landed			108 (29.2)	260	368
Landless			260 (50.2)	258	519
Education					
Illiterate			303 (39.7)	461	764
Secondary education			40 (54.1)	34	74
Primary education			25 (51.0)	24	49
Occupation					
Owner farmer/Tenant			25 (26.0)	71	96
Wage labourer			282 (42.3)	384	666
Non-farm employment			10 (50.0)	10	20
Home-based			51 (48.6)	54	105
Total			368 (41.5)	519	887

Source: Baseline Survey, 1989.

of pregnancy-related complications (63 per cent) than captured by the baseline whence information was retrospective.[8]

Comparison with a number of studies from rural India show that pregnancy and childbirth-related morbidity among Scheduled Caste women in Chengalpattu is very high. According to a study conducted in rural Uttar Pradesh, only 4.6 per cent of Scheduled Caste women reported having had complications during delivery, as compared to around 18 per cent in Chengalpattu (19). A 1979 study from Rajasthan reports complication rates of only 6.8 per cent (20). In yet another study from Gujarat in 1983 (21), postnatal problems were found in only 2.25 per cent of the women, while another study in 1982 (22) gave a postnatal complication rate of 26.7 per cent.[9] Although differences in definitions and details probed by the questionnaire are likely to have caused some difference in reporting of complications, it seems unlikely that this is the only reason for the considerably higher rates of morbidity observed in the present study.

2.4. Women's Illness Burden

Compared with the baseline survey which is restricted to reproductive health problems, the follow-up survey gives a more comprehensive picture of the burden of illness borne by poor women. In all, 150 women out of 351 had a health problem during the six months of follow-up. The prevalence rate M_p for all health problems thus works out to 43 per cent, and the frequency M_f is a stupendous 68 per cent. More than two-fifths of the population reporting illness points to a prevalence rate far exceeding that normally reported, even making allowances for the fact that our period of coverage is six months.[10]

---

[8] One pregnancy ended in a miscarriage. In one case the childbirth was complicated by prolonged labour and foetal distress. It ended in a c-section, but the infant died soon after birth. Four women had premature deliveries, and one of the premature babies died within a week of birth. Two of these women had shown symptoms of hypertensive disorders of pregnancy with high blood pressure and fluid retention. In ten other cases, labour was prolonged, resulting in perineal tear, accompanied by severe blood loss in five of them.

[9] References 21 and 22 are as quoted in Saramma Mathai (reference 25).

[10] The highest prevalence rates for women over various seasons, in six rural districts in North India was only 20 per cent, according to a study conducted by NCAER (11). In the study of health status in rural Kerala (1987), prevalence of acute illnesses in women was only 21 per cent (10). Comparison with a number of community studies with reference periods of one to three months confirms this situation (ref. 25, p. 272, Table 6).

Table 8: Prevalence of health problems in women (January–June 1990)
(Figures in brackets give prevalence rates M_p)

Charac-teristic	Had one or more problems			Had no problems	Total
	All problems	Reproductive	General health		
Age in years					
15–19	6 (22.3)	1 (3.7)	5 (18.5)	21	27
20–24	23 (28.8)	10 (12.5)	16 (20.0)	57	80
25–29	60 (52.6)	33 (28.9)	44 (38.6)	54	114
30–34	36 (52.2)	19 (27.5)	30 (43.5)	33	69
35–39	25 (41.0)	10 (16.4)	19 (31.1)	36	61
Parity					
0	11 (28.2)	3 (7.7)	9 (23.0)	28	39
1	17 (28.3)	8 (13.3)	14 (23.4)	43	60
2–3	58 (43.9)	32 (24.2)	41 (31.1)	74	132
4–5	44 (51.7)	20 (23.5)	35 (41.2)	41	85
6+	20 (57.1)	10 (28.6)	15 (42.9)	15	35
Land-ownership					
Own ≤ 1.5 acres	139 (43.4)	70 (21.9)	105 (32.8)	181	320
Own > 1.5 acres	11 (35.4)	3 (9.7)	9 (29.0)	20	31
Education					
Illiterate	139 (44.6)	69 (22.1)	103 (33.0)	173	312
Literate	11 (28.2)	4 (10.2)	11 (28.2)	28	39
Occupation					
Owner-farmer/tenant	6 (54.5)	4 (36.4)	4 (36.4)	5	11
Wage labourer	125 (43.6)	65 (22.6)	93 (32.4)	162	287
Non-farm employment	3 (37.5)	2 (25.0)	2 (25.0)	5	8
Home-based	16 (35.6)	2 (2.3)	15 (33.0)	29	45
Total	150 (42.7)			201	351

Source: Follow-up Survey, January–June 1990.

Prevalence rates vary across socio-economic groups, with educated women from landed families who are home-based or in salaried employment being less affected. However, the differentials are far more significant by age and parity groups, being more than twice as high for older and high-parity women as compared with women below 25 years and those who have had less than two pregnancies (Table 8).

Table 9: Nature of health problems in women (January–June 1990)

Causes	Number of episodes	M_f (%)	Number of women affected*	M_p (%)
General Health Problems				
Total	122	34.8	114	32.5
Fevers	42	12.0	39	11.1
Aches and pains	30	8.5	28	8.0
Respiratory infections	23	6.6	22	6.3
Oral infections	11	3.1	9	2.6
Diarrhoea and dysentery	9	2.6	8	2.3
Acute anaemia	—	9.0	2.6	
Injuries	8	2.3	7	2.0
Eye infection (conjunctivitis and stye)	7	2.0	6	1.7
Jaundice	1	0.3	1	0.3
Chickenpox	2	0.6	2	0.6
Others	13	3.7	13	3.7
Reproductive Health Problems				
Total	118	33.6	73	20.8
Menstrual disorders	5	1.4	5	1.4
Reproductive Tract Disorders (RTDs)	73	20.8	44	12.5
Urinary Tract Infections	9	2.6	9	2.6
Urinary incontinence with urinary tract infection	2	0.6	2	0.6
Uterine prolapse with reproductive tract infection	14	4.0	7	2.0
Miscarriage	1	0.3	1	0.3
Postpartum infection	1	0.3	1	0.3
Infection following tubectomy	4	1.1	3	0.9
Hypertensive disorders of pregnancy	9	2.6	8	2.3

* The same woman may suffer from different causes at different times, and the same episode of illness may include more than one cause.
Source: Follow-up Survey, January–June 1990.

(a) General health problems

For general health problems the prevalence rate is 33 per cent, and the frequency is nearly equal at 34 per cent. In other words, general health problems were for the most part one-time occurrences.

The single most important cause of morbidity was non-specific fever, accounting for 27 per cent of all affected. Nineteen per cent of

Table 10: Prevalence of reproductive health problems in currently married women (1989)
(Figures in brackets give prevalence rates M_p)

	Had one or more problems	Had no problems	Total
Age in years			
15–19	8 (11.2)	63	71
20–29	136 (25.8)	390	526
30–34	72 (38.3)	116	188
35–39	99 (42.7)	133	232
Parity			
0	14 (11.7)	106	120
1	44 (22.6)	146	190
2–3	94 (28.6)	252	346
4–5	99 (39.7)	150	249
6+	64 (57.1)	48	112
Caste			
SC	302 (31.3)	660	962
BC	12 (22.2)	42	54
Others	1	0	1
Land-ownership			
Landed	124 (30.1)	288	412
Landless	191 (31.6)	414	605
Education			
Illiterate	275 (31.8)	586	861
Primary education	13 (22.8)	44	57
Secondary education	27 (27.3)	72	99
Occupation			
Owner farmer/Tenant	23 (20.9)	87	110
Wage labourer	247 (32.6)	510	757
Non-farm employment	8 (38.1)	13	21
Home-based	37 (28.6)	92	129
Total	315 (31.0)	702	1017

Source: Baseline Survey, 1989.

the women complained of severe backaches or joint pains that restricted them to bed, while respiratory infections accounted for a further 15 per cent. Other important problems reported include oral infections, diarrhoea, eye infections and injuries related to work and to domestic violence (Table 9). This cause pattern is similar to those reported by the various morbidity studies discussed above.

(b) Reproductive health problems

Direct gynaecologic morbidity such as menstrual disorders, reproductive tract disorders (RTD) (both sexually and otherwise transmitted), and sequelae of complicated deliveries such as uterovaginal prolapse constitute reproductive health problems. Urinary incontinence, and urinary tract infections (UTI) may also be included in this category. Although they cannot be strictly termed reproductive health problems, they have been included since they are more common in women than in men and are related to physiological differences by sex.

(i) Prevalence: Thirty-one per cent of women covered by the base-line survey reported having a reproductive health problem at the time of the survey. A third of those with problems, or 106 women, were suffering from more than one ailment. If morbidity reported as a sequela of sterilization for birth control is also considered, the prevalence rate rises to 39 per cent.

Gynaecologic morbidity, as in the case of complications related to pregnancy and childbirth, increases dramatically with age and parity. Only 11 per cent of the teenagers reported current reproductive health problems; the figure more than doubled for women between 20 and 29 (26 per cent), rising to as high as 43 per cent for women above 35. With parity, the prevalence of reproductive morbidity rises from 11 per cent for nulliparous women to a stupendous 57 per cent for women of parity above 6 (Table 10).

The prevalence of reproductive health problems is significantly higher among illiterate women, and lower for women who are from owner-farmer and tenant families (Table 10). This is perhaps a consequence of the resource base of women's households, as per evidence from the follow-up survey. In the latter, women from households owing less than 1.5 acres of land—i.e. households dependent primarily on wage labour—have twice the prevalence rate of women from households with more land (see Table 8).

A comparison of morbidity rates (reference period 24 hours) with those of Maharashtra and Gujarat in 1983 shows prevalence rates of 4.71 and 3.1 per 100 women respectively, for all illnesses (not only gynaecologic morbidity), and 6.6 per 100 women in Madhya Pradesh

(23, 21 and 24). Female morbidity figures over a reference period of one month also do not present rates higher than 17 per cent, almost half the rate for Chengalpattu women, despite our taking a restricted definition of morbidity (25).

However, the few health examination surveys on rural Indian women present a different picture, reporting higher gynaecologic morbidity. A WHO study conducted in Gandhigram, Tamil Nadu, in the mid-seventies found 59 per cent of all women to be suffering from gynaecological diseases (14). In rural Maharashtra it was found that 55 per cent of 650 women medically examined suffered from a gynaecological disease (13).

The six month follow-up of the baseline survey points to some interesting trends. A programme of health education and provision of basic health services at the door-step accompanied the follow-up. While this has made an impact on the proportion of women affected,[11] the frequency of episodes has not come down substantively. Among the 351 women covered, 118 episodes of reproductive health problems were reported, by only 73 women. Thus while prevalence is only about 21 per cent, frequency is 34 per cent. The high frequency is a consequence of the repetitive or chronic character of a number of reproductive health problems, with the same women being affected over and over again, by the same or a related health problem.

Another interesting finding from the follow-up is that differentials by socio-economic status are far more pronounced in the case of reproductive health problems than in the case of general health problems. Women from lower socio-economic groups had twice as high a prevalence of reproductive health problems as compared to their better-off counterparts (Table 8).

(ii) Nature of problems: Twenty per cent of all the women had problems associated with menstruation, such as excessive bleeding, extremely painful periods, and irregular periods, apart from those suffering from urinary tract infections (9 per cent), reproductive tract infections (10 per cent), and uterine prolapse (2 per cent). Irregular

---

[11]We believe that the significantly lower prevalence rates when compared to the baseline survey are a result of the health intervention programme. However, the different months of the year covered by the two surveys (January to June in the case of the follow-up and August to October in the case of the baseline) may also have had some influence on prevalence of morbidity in these periods.

Table 11: Causes of reproductive morbidity by characteristics of currently married women[a] (1989)
(Figures in brackets give prevalence rates M_P)

	Menstrual problems	RTD[b]	UTI[c]	Incontinence	UP[d]	All
Age in years						
15–19	8 (11.6)	1 (1.4)	0	0	0	71
20–29	94 (17.8)	42 (7.9)	8 (7.2)	4	9 (1.7)	526
30–34	39 (20.7)	24 (12.8)	26 (13.8)	1	5 (2.7)	188
35–39	61 (26.3)	32 (13.7)	28 (12.1)	1	5 (2.2)	232
Parity						
0	12 (10.0)	3 (2.5)	1 (0.8)	0	0	120
1	31 (16.3)	10 (5.2)	11 (5.7)	1	0	190
2–3	60 (17.3)	35 (10.0)	30 (8.7)	3	9 (2.6)	346
4–5	61 (24.5)	27 (10.8)	34 (13.7)	2	5 (2.0)	249
6+	38 (33.9)	24 (21.4)	16 (14.2)	0	5 (4.5)	112
Caste						
SC	190 (19.8)	98 (10.2)	91 (9.5)	6	19	962
BC	11 (20.4)	1 (1.9)	1 (1.9)	0	0	54
Land-ownership						
Landed	79 (19.2)	37 (8.9)	26 (6.3)	1	7 (1.7)	412
Landless	123 (20.3)	62 (10.2)	66 (10.4)	5	12 (2.0)	605
Education						
Illiterate	171 (19.9)	88 (10.2)	81 (9.4)	4	19	861
Literate	31 (19.8)	11 (7.1)	11 (7.1)	2	0	156
Occupation						
Owner farmer/ Tenant	11 (10.0)	9 (8.2)	5 (4.5)	0	1	110
Wage labourer	158 (20.9)	77 (10.2)	76 (10.0)	6	15	757
Non-farm employment	4 (19.0)	6 (28.5)	2 (9.5)	0	1	21
Home-based	29 (22.4)	7 (5.4)	9 (7.0)	0	2	129
Total	202 (20.0)	99 (9.7)	92 (9.1)	6 (0.6)	19 (1.9)	1017

[a]The same person may have more than one problem.
[b]Reproductive tract disorders.
[c]Urinary tract infections.
[d]Uterine prolapse.
Source: Baseline Survey, 1989.

periods were common not only in older women who were nearing menopause, but also in younger women who seemed to be in very poor general health. All women with uterine prolapse had associated genital infections and, sometimes, urinary tract infections as well. Incontinence was also similarly accompanied by urinary and reproductive tract infections (Table 11).

Some patterns in the nature of problems suffered by women of varying demographic and socio-economic characteristics were apparent. Menstrual problems were higher for older and higher parity women. This was also true of urinary tract infections. This trend is most pronounced in the case of reproductive tract disorders, which are 10 times more prevalent in women of parity six and more when compared to nulliparous women. There is not much difference by socio-economic class in the nature of reproductive health problems, save for the fact that Backward Caste women as well as home-based women have a significantly lower prevalence rate of reproductive tract infections.

The more problematic and serious conditions, namely incontinence, uterine prolapse and cancer, are all found in women between 20 and 29 years of age, of parity two and more, who are all from the Scheduled Castes, predominantly landless, and all illiterate wage workers in agriculture (Table 12). Early marriage, strenuous manual labour, coupled with early childbearing complicated by prolonged labour, and inadequate delivery care—predisposing factors for uterine prolapse, were all simultaneously present in women covered by the present study (26).

In addition to these problems, 91 of the 242 women who had undergone sterilization for birth control (38 per cent of family planning acceptors or 9 per cent of all women) complained of a variety of chronic health problems. These ranged from menstrual irregularities and recurring reproductive tract disorders, to backaches, extreme weight loss and non-specific lower abdominal pain.

In the follow-up survey, the most frequent problem reported was reproductive tract disorders, accounting for 73 out of the 118 episodes or 62 per cent, in 44 women, pointing to repeated episodes in the women affected. In 39 of the 44 women, the problem was not present during the baseline survey. The situation was similar for cases of uterine prolapse and urinary incontinence.[12] Over all, ten

---

[12] One new case of urinary incontinence and 7 new cases of uterine prolapse complicated with reproductive tract infections were reported during the follow-up period.

Table 12: Contraceptive prevalence by characteristics of women (1989)

Characteristics	Number of women	Rate of prevalence
Method		
Female sterilization	230	22.6
Other methods	12	1.2
Age		
Below 20	1	0.6
20–24	23	8.7
Above 25	218	25.4
Years of marriage		
0–4	2	1.0
5–9	49	17.4
10 and above	191	37.3
No. of live children		
0	0	0
1	7	3.0
2	28	14.7
3	96	42.5
4–5	97	49.5
6+	14	56.0
Caste		
SC	222	23.0
BC	20	37.0
Land-owing status		
Landless	124	20.5
0.1–5.0 acres	115	28.4
Above 5.1 acres	3	42.9
Occupation		
Owner farmer/tenant	47	31.8
Wage labourer	163	22.9
Home-based	24	18.6
Non-farm employment	6	28.5
Education		
(Below 25 yrs)		
Illiterate	21	6.5
Literate	3	3.1
(Above 25 years)		
Illiterate	189	34.9
Literate	29	54.7
Total	242	23.8

Source: Baseline Survey, 1989.

per cent had more than one reproductive health problem; 51 per cent, in addition, experienced other general health problems such as fevers and respiratory infections. Three of the 18 women who had undergone tubal ligation for birth control developed post-operative infections.

Effectively curing the above health problems, leave alone preventing their recurrence, would be a formidable task, as shown by the health intervention programme. Reproductive tract infections, for instance, were in a number of instances sexually transmitted. Treatment proved useless since both partners, not just the woman, were required to comply with it. The men did not want to be identified as the source of infection. More tragically, they repeatedly infected their wives. Other causes of RTDs, such as poor menstrual hygiene, were, once again, not a problem of awareness alone. They were related to affordability of better means of menstrual hygiene, water supply, waste disposal facilities, and women's strenuous working conditions in agriculture. Prevention of urinary incontinence and uterine prolapse also require a whole gamut of changes such as fewer births, better delivery care, avoidance of strenuous work during pregnancy and immediately following delivery, and of course, better general health and nutrition so that the muscles supporting the uterus and bladder do not give way.

3. Utilization of Health Care Services

Women's utilization of preventive care (such as the use of contraceptive services and choice of place of delivery) and of curative care is discussed in this section.

3.1. *Preventive care*

(a) Contraceptive prevalence

Only 24 per cent of the women (237) practised family planning, mainly sterilization (95 per cent).[13] This is exactly half the prevalence rate for Tamil Nadu which was 53 per cent in 1988 (15).

An overwhelming majority (90 per cent) of women who used a method of contraception were above 25 years of age. Contraceptive

---

[13] 5 women are protected against conception since their husbands have adopted a method of birth control, so that 242 women in all are covered by family planning methods.

Table 13: Proportion of institutional deliveries to all previous deliveries in currently married women (1989)

Characteristics of the woman	Total deliveries	Institutional deliveries	Percent.
Age in years			
15–19	26	18	69.2
20–29	1032	233	22.6
30–34	684	151	22.0
35–39	988	179	18.1
Parity			
1	208	92	44.2
2–3	897	274	30.5
4–5	1046	213	20.4
6+	579	101	17.5
Caste			
SC	2592	640	24.7
BC	137	43	31.4
Others	1	1	100.0
All deliveries	2730	684	25.1

Source: Baseline Survey, 1989.

prevalence was almost nil in women aged 20 or less, and was highest for women between 31 and 35 years of age, at 41 per cent (Table 13). Acceptance increased with number of surviving children: from 42 per cent for those with three surviving children to 60 per cent among women with 5 or more. But not until women were 30, perhaps married for fifteen years or more, did they have three surviving children.

Thus, practically none of the women who had been married for less than five years were practising contraception. After the fifth year of marriage, the proportion increased steeply, and was highest for women who had been married for 16 to 20 years. Significant differences by caste and land-ownership also existed in the extent of contraceptive prevalence: 37 per cent for Backward Castes and only 23 per cent for Scheduled Castes. Acceptance was lowest among women from landless households (20.5 per cent) as compared to those owning up to 5 acres (28.4 per cent).

Contrary to expectation, education did not influence family planning practice at all among young women below 25 years of age. The women's occupational status did not influence contraceptive prevalence as much as the land-owning status of her household. Both home-based women and wage labourers had a similar rate of lower contraceptive prevalence. A much higher proportion of women who worked in their own farms or in leased farms (32 per cent) had adopted family planning.

Thus, women's utilization of contraceptive services seems to be far less influenced by women's education or ability to earn an income than by the prevailing patterns of child survival and the asset base and social status of their households. In particular, because child survival is related to the household resource base, contraceptive prevalence also seems to be influenced by the latter.

(b) Place of delivery
Trained attendance at delivery is one of the most important health interventions necessary to bring down infant and maternal mortality, and considerably reduce obstetric morbidities. Kerala owes its remarkable achievement in lowering infant mortality rates in no small measure to the very high proportion of institutional deliveries in the state (90 per cent) (27). Even in rural Kerala, as shown recently (10), 76 per cent of all deliveries have taken place in hospitals.

Access to emergency obstetric care can reduce maternal mortality rates by 30 per cent. For every case of maternal death, there are estimated to be 16 women who suffer morbidities that can last a lifetime. These, again, can be avoided to a large extent with trained attendance and, where necessary, institutional care (26).

The contrast in the situation of the women under study is stark. Seventy-five per cent of all deliveries took place at home assisted by a traditional birth attendant. The remaining 25 per cent took place under the medical supervision of the auxiliary nurse midwife or, less often, of the doctor in the health centre or hospital. For rural Tamil Nadu, the proportion of untrained attendance at delivery was far lower (41 per cent), while even for rural India it was lower than the present case (67 per cent) (17).

A conscious choice of place of delivery was indicated, according to risk perceived in childbirth, and perhaps reflecting a tacit valuation of the woman by the family. Forty-four per cent of all first deliveries had taken place in a hospital, and the proportion of hospital births gradually declined with increasing parity, despite the higher rates of obstetric morbidites associated with

Table 14: Proportion of first deliveries in health unit (by socio-economic characteristics of currently married women) (1989)

Characteristic	Number of women of parity one	Proportion of institutional deliveries
Scheduled caste	197	43.1
Backward caste	10	60.0
Landed	77	49.3
Landless	131	41.2
Illiterate	173	40.8
Literate	35	62.9
Owner-farmer/Tenant	23	65.2
Wage labourer	153	37.9
Home-based	27	63.0
Total	208	44.2

Source: Baseline Survey, 1989.

high parities.[14] (Table 14). The increasing proportion of hospital deliveries with lower age-groups appears to be indicative, not of a gradual change in favour of medically supervised deliveries, but of the higher risk associated with first births and deliveries to very young women. Another reason seems to be the value placed on the birth of a first child (ideally a male child), which is seen as the raison d'etre of marriage, and in respect of which the family does not want to take unnecessary risks. The absence of a clear trend towards a gradual increase in institutional deliveries is underlined by the fact that the proportion of hospital deliveries at 26.6 years, the mean age at childbearing, was only about 22 per cent.[15]

Educational status and occupation significantly affect the proportion of first deliveries taking place in hospital. Sixty-three per cent of first deliveries to literate women were in institutions, as against only 41 per cent for illiterate women. Only 38 per cent of women wage labourers had their first deliveries in hospital, as compared to over 63 per cent of

---

[14] Another finding confirms this trend: 69 per cent of all births to teenage mothers took place in a health unit. The proportion declines dramatically to a mere 22 per cent for mothers in the age-group 20–29 years, and further to 18 per cent for those above 35.

[15] Mean age at childbearing has been computed from data on children ever born to women, by years of marriage, using the MORTPAK software of the UN Population Division.

Table 15: Type of health care sought by currently married women with a current reproductive health problem (1989)

Type of help	Number of women	Percent.
No help	187	59.4
Self-treatment at home	56	17.8
Traditional healer	7	2.2
Village health worker	17	5.4
Government facilities or personnel	36	11.4
Private facilities or personnel	12	3.8
Total	315	100.0

Source: Baseline Survey, 1989.

women engaged in all other occupations. Level of awareness and opportunity costs involved obviously play a determining role in choice of place of delivery even in the case of first births (Table 15).

3.2. Curative Care

Despite having an acknowledged reproductive health problem, inaction and self-neglect is pervasive among women. This situation contrasts strongly with these very women's utilization of health services for their children.[16]

Almost 60 per cent of the women affected ignored it, 19 per cent initiated self-treatment at home, and only 22 per cent sought external help[17] (Table 16).

An analysis of differentials in health care utilization reveals some unusual features (Table 16). Illiterate wage labourers, and women from lower socio-economic groups ignored their ailments far less frequently than their educated and economically better-placed counterparts. At the same time, unlike the latter, they also tended to resort at least as much to self-treatment, as to medical help.

---

[16] These same women had sought medical help for 51 per cent of their children who had a health problem. A further 6 per cent had been treated by a traditional healer, and 23 per cent treated at home. Only 20 per cent had received no help.

[17] Those who sought help from a medical facility were even lower, only 15 per cent. Five per cent sought help from the village health worker, and 2 per cent from a traditional healer.

Table 16: Utilization of health care services for reproductive health problems (by characteristics of women) (1989)

Characteristics of the women	No action	Self-treatment	Medical help	Total
Age in years				
15–19	8 (100.0)	0	0	8
20–29	80 (58.9)	23	33 (24.2)	136
30–34	32 (44.4)	18	22 (30.6)	72
35–39	67 (67.7)	15	17 (17.2)	99
Parity				
0	9 (64.3)	1	4 (28.6)	14
1	28 (63.6)	10	6 (13.6)	44
2–3	57 (60.6)	17	20 (21.3)	94
4–5	57 (57.6)	16	26 (26.3)	99
6+	36 (56.3)	12	16 (25.0)	64
Caste				
SC	178 (58.9)	56	68 (22.5)	302
BC	8 (66.7)	0	4 (33.3)	12
Others	1	0	0	1
Land-ownership				
Landed	83 (66.9)	15	26 (21.0)	124
Landless	104 (54.5)	41	46 (24.1)	191
Education				
Illiterate	161 (58.5)	49	65 (23.6)	275
Literate	26 (65.0)	7	7 (17.5)	40
Occupation				
Owner farmer/Tenant	16 (69.6)	3	4 (17.4)	23
Wage labourer	143 (57.9)	46	58 (23.5)	247
Non-farm employment	2 (25.0)	2	4 (50.0)	8
Home-based	26 (70.3)	5	6 (16.2)	37
Total	187 (59.4)	56 (19.0)	72 (21.6)	315
Nature of illness				
Menstrual problems	142 (70.3)	25	35 (17.2)	202
Reproductive tract diseases	44 (44.5)	13	42 (42.4)	99
Uterine tract infections	26 (28.3)	43	23 (25.0)	92
Incontinence	3 (50.0)	2	1	6
Uterine prolapse	10 (52.6)	0	9 (47.4)	19

Source: Baseline Survey, 1989.

In terms of demographic characteristics, the use of medical facilities increases progressively with parity. There is however, no difference in the extent of non-action by parity, being between 57 and 64 per cent for women of all parities. None of the teenagers sought any help; nor did they resort to self-treatment. The extent of utilization increased for women in their twenties, was the highest for those between 30 and 34, and tapered off thereafter. The extent of inaction followed an exactly inverse pattern: highest for teenagers, lower in the 20–29 age-group, lowest for 30–34-year-old women, and again higher for those above 35.

Health care utilization patterns suggest conscious selectivity in favour of those most at risk and who can least afford to be immobilized due to illness: wage workers, salaried workers, and mothers with one or more grown-up children to run the household or compensate for the loss of an adult's income.

Opinion has been expresed that female mortality has an inverse correlation with female labour force participation, and that this is because girls and women who are potential or current wage earners, are better valued and consequently better cared for (28, 29 and 30). Patterns of high morbidity among wage earners found in the present study suggest the contrary, at least insofar as adult women are concerned. It is clear that women wage earners are more vulnerable to diseases, not less. However, they fight to keep themselves on their feet through self-treatment and, when absolutely essential, resort to medical care since they cannot afford to be sick.

If the variables hypothesized earlier on as influencing susceptibility to illness and health-seeking behaviour are now referred to, an expected correlation is seen only with respect to the former. Women with a better household resource-base and access to resources are less susceptible to illness. In contrast, it is women from households with a poor resource base, with low income and no education, who exhibit positive health-seeking behaviour. A factor that could not be considered separately, namely the value placed on women by society (rather than their education and employment), seems to play the most decisive role in health-seeking behaviour.

Utilization of health care is also related to some extent to the nature of the problem. Women with reproductive tract disorders and uterine prolapse, and to a lesser extent women suffering from urinary tract infections, tend to seek medical help most often. Women suffering from problems related to menstruation do not seek medical help at all (Table 16).

A number of reasons were cited by the women for this health-seeking behaviour, the most important of all being the absence of any specific reason! More than half the women had not considered taking any action regarding their health problem, confirming their tendency to ignore or neglect health problems. Fifteen per cent were embarrassed or afraid to visit the doctor for a reproductive health problem, and about 10 per cent thought home remedies were sufficient. Other reasons given included lack of time and money, problems at home, permission withheld by the husband, or because they felt medical treatment had brought no improvement.

Most of these reasons are a consequence of the community's health culture which reflects also traditional values and biases related to women's fertility and reproduction. Menstrual problems, for instance, are not considered 'illness', and home remedies or traditional treatments are usually resorted to. Further, it is not considered appropriate for women to discuss matters related to reproductive health, especially with male doctors. The quality of health services also plays a role: dissatisfaction with treatment is a commonly stated reason, although inaccessibility is perhaps of greater consequence in influencing health-seeking behaviour.

4. Conclusions

To summarize, the burden of illness borne by the women covered by this study is enormous, and far higher than that reported from similar health interview studies. The interplay between poverty and gender discrimination seems to be the lynch-pin in any explanation of women's health problems here. Growing up in landless families, eking out a hand-to-mouth existence, children, especially girls, drop out early from school and join the labour force or manage the household while the mother engages in wage work. Girls are married early and are under tremendous social pressure to bear children immediately, a typical situation of a high mortality social group where fertility is highly valued. Inadequate nutrition together with heavy manual labour on land and low age cause high pregnancy wastage, and in turn extend the period of childbearing to the woman's entire reproductive span. It is worth noting that in a poverty group such as this, participation in the labour force increases the risk of morbidity and is not an indicator of better status but of greater deprivation.

Both the need to have at least three surviving children and the fear of health risks discourage contraceptive prevalence, contributing in turn to high fertility. With increasing age and parity women are at higher risk of obstetric as well as gynaecologic morbidity. They are also more vulnerable to general health problems. The role of overt gender discrimination is most evident in the case of reproductive tract infections in women, and injuries related to domestic violence.

The low priority accorded to women's health is reflected in patterns of health care utilization. Choices as to when health services may be sought seem to be based on a careful consideration of the value of such an investment, from the perspective of a patriarchal social setting.

For instance, women are permitted trained attendance only for the first delivery or when they are very young. Begetting the first offspring is of high significance, whereas an additional child for a woman who already has three or more children is not an event important enough for scarce resources to be invested in it, despite the fact that higher order births are more risky and may require medical attendance.

This is in direct contrast to the pattern of health care utilization in case of illness. Young women, especially teenagers, do not take any action whatsoever for their illnesses, while women in their early thirties, and wage workers take some form of action promptly. This may be because a few days' immobility in addition to loss of wages in a middle-aged woman with several dependent children is unacceptable and unaffordable from the family's point of view. The women themselves consider it imperative to take care of themselves, if only to ensure the family's survival. If a young bride without children falls ill, this is not likely to upset the family routine very much, and she is in no way indispensable. According to some of the young women interviewed, complaining of health problems and seeking medical attention were risky. Being childless, they were of little value to their marital families, and there was the fear of being sent back to their parental homes if they were seen to be 'sickly'. The husband might even remarry in such cases. Thus it seems that, in addition to constraints imposed by poverty, the main barrier to women's utilization of health services relates to how society values them. Education and awareness, and even access to money, play, if at all, a minor role.

The nature of reproductive and other health problems encountered are such that they cannot be effectively prevented without fundamental changes—not just in the poverty situation of their households, but specifically in the women's own living and working conditions, and in their relationship to men. To make an impact on women's susceptibility to disease would thus call for policies and programmes that make a perceptible dent in poverty levels, and those specifically aimed at enhancing women's access to resources.

Changing women's health-seeking behaviour seems to be a more hopeful avenue for action. Through health education and awareness-raising programmes which reach out to women (especially those in poverty groups), and through programmes aimed at enhancing their self-confidence and self-image, women have to be encouraged to initiate self-treatment or seek medical help when ill, to actively seek antenatal and delivery care, and more importantly, to feel entitled to good health and care. A number of community-based organizations have had success with such efforts, even though limited.

The commitment of the health services system to respond to women's health needs is another pressing issue to be addressed. The lack of information on women's health needs is a major hurdle in this respect. National level surveys on morbidity and mortality, and the use of health services need to include specific questions on aspects such as women's reproductive health problems, their use of health services, and factors that restrict their access to health and health services.

A minimum agenda for action would include at least two demands:

(a) a comprehensive range of reproductive health services in place of the narrowly defined maternal health care currently available; and

(b) concerted action to drastically reduce the proportion of deliveries with untrained attendance, and pregnancies receiving no antenatal or postnatal care.

The absence of specific health interventions to address the extensive reproductive health problems in women, and worse, the abysmally low proportion of women receiving health care even during pregnancy and delivery, is a sad commentary on how priorities for health services are set and implemented. Despite pious platitudes on the importance of women's well-being for national development, women's health has remained a neglected issue for far too long. It is action that is urgently needed.

Acknowledgements

Sincere thanks are due to the health workers of the Rural Women's Social Education Centre, Chengalpattu, Tamil Nadu, who carried out the health interview surveys on which this study is based. Many thanks to Viji who assisted with the data processing.

References

1. Chatterjee, Meera (1990) Indian Women, Health and Productivity. Policy, Research and External Affairs Working Paper, Washington D.C. World Bank.
2. Bhatia, J.C. (1988) A Study of Maternal Mortality in Anantapur District, Andhra Pradesh, India. Bangalore, Indian Institute of Management.
3. Registrar-General of India (1989) Sample Registration System 1988, New Delhi, Ministry of Home Affairs, Government of India.
4. Sundari, T.K. (1993) 'Can Health Education Improve Pregnancy Outcome? Report of a Grassroots Action-Education Campaign', *Journal of Family Welfare*, March.
5. Casterline, John B. (1989) 'Maternal Age, Gravidity and Pregnancy Spacing Effect on Fetal Mortality', *Social Biology*, Vol. 36, Nos. 3-4, 186–212.
6. Gopalan, C. and Nadamuni Naidu (1972) 'Nutrition and Fertility', *The Lancet*, 18 November, 1077–1079.
7. National Sample Survey Organization (1980) 28th Round Survey on Morbidity (1973–74), *Sarvekshana*, July–October.
8. National Council of Applied Economics Research (1992a). Household Survey of Medical Care, NCAER, New Delhi.
9. National Nutrition Monitoring Bureau (1980) Consolidated Report for 1975–79. National Institute of Nutrition, Hyderabad.
10. Kannan, K.P. et al. (1991) *Health Status in Rural Kerala. A study of the Linkages Between Socioeconomic Status and Health Status*. Integrated Rural Technology Centre of the Kerala Sastra Sahitya Parishad, February.
11. National Council of Applied Economics Research (1992b) Rural Household Health Care Needs and Availability. NCAER, New Delhi.
12. Indian Council of Medical Research (1982) Report of the ICMR Working Group, *American Journal of Clinical Nutrition*, 35: 1442.
13. Bang, R.A. et al. (1989) 'High Prevalence of Gynaecological Diseases in Rural Indian Women' *The Lancet*, 14 January, 85–88.

14. Dutt, P.R. et al. (1976) 'Gandhigram' in A.R. Omran and C.C. Stanley (eds.) *Family Formation Patterns and Health) An International Collaborative Study in India, Iran, Lebanon, Philippines and Turkey.* World Health Organization, Geneva, 337–44.
15. Department of Family Welfare (1989) Family Welfare Programme in India Year Book 1987–88, Government of India, Ministry of Health and Family Welfare, New Delhi, 178–181, Table C-12.
16. Registrar General Of India (1979) Survey Report on Levels, Trends and Differentials in Fertility. India, Ministry of Home Affairs, New Delhi.
17. Registrar-General of India (1988). Fertility in India—An Analysis of 1981 Census Data. Census of India 1981, Occasional Paper No. 13 of 1988, Demography Division, Ministry of Home Affairs, New Delhi.
18. Murthy, G.V.S. et al. (1987) 'A Study of Pregnancy Wastage in a Rural Area of Haryana', *Health and Population: Perspectives and Issues*, No. 10, 26–34.
19. Trakroo, P. L. and S.D. Kapoor (1990) *A Study to Identify Problems and Patterns of Acceptability and Utilization of Health Care Services by Scheduled Caste Population in Rural India.* National Institute of Health and Family Welfare, New Delhi.
20. Datta, K.K. et al. (1980) 'Morbidity Pattern among Rural Pregnant Women in Alwar, Rajasthan: A Cohort Study', *Health and Population: Perspectives and Issues*, No. 3, 282–92.
21. International Institute of Population Sciences, Bombay, and Population Research Centre, M.S. University, Baroda (1985) Baseline Survey on Fertility, Mortality and Related Factors in Rural Gujarat. December.
22. Walia I. (1988) 'Health Services and the Rural Pregnant', *The Nursing Journal of India*, September.
23. International Institute of Population Sciences, Bombay, and Department of Sociology, Marathwada University, Aurangabad (1985) Baseline Survey of Fertility, Mortality, and Related Factors in Maharashtra. July.
24. National Institute of Health and Family Welfare (1985) Levels of Fertility, Mortality, Family Welfare, and Utilization of Health and Family Welfare Services—A Baseline Report of Eight Project Districts of Madhya Pradesh. October.
25. Saramma Thomas Mathai (1989) 'Women and the Health System' in C. Gopalan and Suminder Kaur (eds.) *Women and Nutrition in India.* Nutrition Foundation of India Special Publication series no. 5, Hyderabad.
26. Division of Family Health, World Health Organization (1990) Measuring Reproductive Morbidity: Report of a Technical Working Group, Geneva, 30 August–1 September 1989. WHO/MCH/90.4, WHO, Geneva.
27. Thankappan, K.R. and V. Ramankutty (1990) 'Immunisation Coverage in Kerala and the Role of the Integrated Child Development Scheme Programme', *Health Policy and Planning*, vol. 5, no. 3, 267–73.
28. Bardhan, P.K. (1974) 'On Life and Death Questions', *Economic and Political Weekly* IX, nos. 32–34, 1293–1304.
29. Krishnaji, N. (1987) 'Poverty and Sex Ratio—Some Data and Speculations', *Economic and Political Weekly* XXII, 892–97.
30. Rosenzweig, M. and T.P. Schultz (1982) 'Market Opportunities, Genetic Endowment and Intra-Family Research Distribution: Child Survival in Rural India', *American Economic Review*, 72, 803–15.

8

Patriarchy and the Risks of STD and HIV Transmission to Women

RADHIKA RAMASUBBAN

Introduction

The focus on mother and child health as a key element in Indian health policy evolved out of what was identified as one of the strongest explanatory factors for continued high fertility, viz., the high infant mortality rates. The policy of targeting pregnant women and babies in order to sustain infant survival is likely to come under increasing strain in the coming years, as the pressures of a possible HIV pandemic open up other related issues impinging on women's health.

It is well known that seropositive mothers can pass on HIV infection to their unborn children with ease; perinatal infection is estimated to occur in 20 to 30 per cent of infants born to seropositive women. The progression of the disease, which may span an eight to ten year period in adults, is much more rapid in infected infants: 50 per cent of such infants die before they reach the age of 2 and over 90 per cent do not live to see their fifth birthday (ICMR 1991).

But the confounding issues are several. One, HIV infection has no obvious symptoms of its own but masks its manifestation through commonly encountered opportunistic infections. Its detection therefore becomes difficult in a population unserviced by extensive and good quality health care facilities, and not educated into the required changes in their health behaviour. Two, women specifically are more vulnerable to HIV infection due to penetrative heterosexual contact being an important mode of transmission. Their protection from HIV infection through this mode requires action on the part of others, viz., the use of condoms by their male partners. Three, women's reproductive physiology and the conditions under which they play out their reproductive role, add further dimensions to their vulnerability.

The above issues raise fundamental questions about state intervention in the areas of health, education and family welfare, and about individual behaviour. They throw the canvas open in ways which go far beyond the current paternalistic approach to monitoring the health of pregnant women and infants as passive agents of a family planning oriented developmental strategy. They raise questions about sex and sexuality, socialization and self-worth, gender relations, family structure and female autonomy. They bring women to centre-stage, not as passive bodies and minds to be steered by a patriarchal social and political structure; rather, the prevention and control of HIV hinges crucially on women as active and autonomous agents of their bodies and social relations.

This paper discusses some of the negative factors inherent in the conditions governing women's health, which have implications for women becoming prey to possible STD and HIV infection. According to available estimates, between one-third and one-half of HIV-positive persons in India to date are women (ICMR 1991). While many of these women belong to the particularly vulnerable group of prostitutes (commercial sex workers), a sizeable proportion belong outside this group, infected through heterosexual transmission largely within the institution of marriage. Most are in the asymptomatic phase, unaware that they are infected.

The Setting

How would women acquire the HIV virus in the first place? It has already been established that in India, as in the rest of Asia, one of the main modes of transmission of HIV is through heterosexual contact, the others being through the perinatal route, through blood and blood products and associated infected needles. The last-mentioned are the most efficient method of transmission (with a 90 per cent transmission rate), with perinatal infection coming next. Sexual transmission in fact is the most inefficient method. Yet, heterosexual transmission assumes importance in the Indian cultural context primarily due to the large size of the population and the frequency of exposure. The prevailing cultural norms of universal marriage, early age at marriage and early onset of coital activity and childbearing, as well as the prevailing demographic structure, imply that an overwhelmingly high proportion of the population comes within the sexually active age group.

What makes women particularly vulnerable in the context of the growing possibility of an HIV epidemic, is the state of their sexual and reproductive health. There are a range of biological and social factors at work here. Since infected semen remains in the vagina for a while, penetrative sexual contact is a critical route for the transmission of the HIV virus. Men therefore can infect women more effectively than vice versa. Present affliction with or past history of STDs in one or both partners, particularly those that cause genital lesions or inflammation has also been established as a risk factor for increased infectiousness or increased susceptibility to HIV infection among heterosexual individuals.

The incidence of STD prevalence in the country is high, particularly of those STDs that produce genital lesions. But it is from the preponderantly male population reporting to public STD clinics that we glean this. Most STDs are asymptomatic in women due to the complex female reproductive physiology, and in part due to women's acceptance of discomfort and suffering as part of their lot. Further, the ignorance among the general population regarding the causes, early symptoms and means of prevention and cure of STDs is abysmal. As much to blame is the low status of STDs as a teaching specialty in medical colleges and, therefore, the poor availability of trained doctors outside a few metropolitan enclaves. Finally, the inability of women to protect themselves from being infected and reinfected—if prostitutes by their clients and if wives by their husbands—due to the nature of power relations between men and women in the larger society and in its microcosm, the family, contributes to women's vulnerability.

Also prevalent among women is a range of other sexually and non-sexually transmitted/sustained infections where, again, inflammation of the reproductive tract occurs. These are caused variously by trauma to the reproductive tract arising out of the complex web of early marriage, frequent and hazardous conditions of childbirth, induced abortions, and IUD insertions. These interact with other risk factors such as anaemia, lack of access to good quality health care facilities throughout the reproductive years, lack of knowledge of early and advanced symptoms of morbidity, and poor availability of adequate water and sanitation facilities. These reproductive tract infections (RTIs) contribute to adverse outcomes of pregnancy such as foetal loss, low birth weight and prematurity, and perinatal infection. Recent evidence points to RTIs, too, as risk factors for HIV.

Quite clearly, the negative dimensions arising out of STD and HIV infection are graver for women's general and reproductive health than they are for men. Integrating an AIDS dimension into health policy requires a holistic approach, in which the aspect of women's health goes beyond looking at pregnant women alone, missing out the preceding linkages.

Inequitous feeding practices which favour boy infants and children over girl infants and children stunt physical growth and lay the basis for steady accretion of nutritional anaemia among little girls. Inequitious access to education results in girls being barely permitted to go beyond primary school if they are sent to school at all, thus leaving them bereft of any basis in education and denying them access to information about and ability to negotiate with the world outside. Early marriage of girls and onset of coital activity soon after the start of menstruation is accompanied by pressures to begin early and repeated childbearing in a state of anaemia, pelvic immaturity, lack of knowledge of sex, reproduction, contraception or symptoms of reproductive morbidity, absence of antenatal care, and economic, social and emotional subservience to the husband and family elders.

Finally, dire poverty among large sections of the population drives huge numbers of destitute women into crippling prostitution.

In the sections that follow, an attempt will be made to sketch some broad congruences between women's social status and women's health, focusing on risk factors for STDs and HIV infection within the larger context of gender roles and gender inequalities in Indian society, i.e., the social construction of women's sexuality and their reproductive role in relation to their other extra-domestic roles.

Sexuality and Heterosexual Behaviour

Research interest in sexuality and patterns of sexual behaviour is still at an embryonic stage in India and little reliable data exist on frequency of sex partner change in the general population (a factor which is of consequence to both STDs and HIV). The forces that govern sexual behaviour must therefore be reconstructed from prevailing gender relations. This has been dealt with in some detail by this author elsewhere (Ramasubban 1992). Only a brief recapitulation follows here in order to set the stage.

The cultural definition of female sexuality as all-devouring and as destructive of the woman and of others around her has been central to the organization of gender hierarchy in Indian society. Female sexuality is depicted in both major classical texts and proverbs across the country as primeval and therefore potentially more powerful than social sanctions. In the Brahminical scheme of society, women (along with *shudras*) were the lowest order—polluted, polluting, menial and subversive. Given the importance of women as childbearers, the only manner in which society could chain women's sexuality was by subordinating it to their identity as mothers. Marriage arranged at an early age, with its built-in requirement of early childbearing for the girl to be accepted by the conjugal family, evolved as an institutional solution to this problem. And within this patriarchal family, the socialization of ever newer generations of women into the passive and pliable lower order has come to be perpetuated.

The patriarchal family is the dominant family form in India and it is within its institutional framework that descent, cultural traditions, occupational skills, family reputation and aspirations, and property are sought to be nurtured. This is done under the hegemony of men who control the levers of economic, social, political and ritual power. Women given in marriage, the main transaction through which the family as an institution is renewed, are as powerless as men are powerful. Among the most grievous of their disabilities is that traditionally women neither inherit nor own/control property and are hence totally dependent on men for survival. Further, since family virtues are believed to be transmitted by blood, the purity of the blood of the woman being married—the symbol of her sexuality and her reproductive role—becomes crucial to the marriage transaction, and men define this purity. The economic protection of the woman and the protection of her purity thus takes place by and large within the monogamous family whose rules are stringently enjoined upon her. Before she is married she is under the protection of her father, brothers and other male elders. In her conjugal home this role is played by her husband and father-in-law among other male elders.

After her husband's death she must come under the protection of her son. In return for her physical, financial and emotional security a woman must continually demonstrate her adherence to the rules calculated to protect her chastity and, after her marriage, successfully play out her reproductive role by bearing sons. She thus comes to symbolize the family's 'honour', the guardianship of which overrides all other considerations.

The abstraction of the physical fact of *sexuality* into the social symbol of *honour*, requires rendering the female body—the repository of that unspeakable sexuality—powerless to perform any but the socially sanctioned tasks defined by family and caste: reproduction, housekeeping and economic maintenance. Through her reproductive role the woman is expected to secure the continuity of the family with the birth of sons and, thereby, its social identity. Through her contribution of domestic labour a woman ensures the maintenance of the household. And among the lower castes where women also labour outside the home, the woman contributes to the family's subsistence as well. Physical reinforcement of ideological controls begins early, through a combination of wilful neglect and devaluation of self-esteem. Discriminatory feeding practices begun even in infancy are complemented in childhood by denial of opportunities for physical play, thus laying the ground for chronically poor physical growth and nutritional anaemia; and denial of opportunities to go to school thus pre-empting participation in the world outside the home. The onset of menstruation marks the beginning of seclusion from the public gaze, of further restrictions on deportment even within the house and of a retreat into an inner world of shame, fear and silence about the body. It would seem that honour and purity in the cause of the family would require fearing one's body as a polluting, unclean and dangerous thing. This fear binds both the growing girl and the instruments of her socialization, her mother and mother-in-law, respectively, into a common silence regarding anything to do with their reproductive organs even as their different positions in the family hierarchy cleave them, denying them mutual support.

It is paradoxical that women must carry the burden of this shame and fear and yet play a sexually active role that can satisfy their husbands. Patriarchal family norms operate differently for men and for women. While men are expected to by and large remain within the confines of a monogamous marriage, there is social indifference to their indulging in extra-marital sex. At the base of this is the recognition of their sexuality as unbridled, and condonation of their preoccupation with it. The commonest situation for extra-marital sex is when the man has to live away from home, earning a living in the city. Other circumstances are: when the wife is menstruating, during her pregnancy and post-partum period, when she is away visiting her parents, on religious days when women fast and pray for the family's welfare, a wife's inability to bear children, her poor health, her inability to come up to the household's expectations of her domestic and/or extra-domestic labour, her inability to offer 'interesting' and 'varied' forms of sex (this is the reason given by a considerable proportion of male STD patients at STD outpatient departments of hospitals, who admit to frequenting prostitutes). In general, a wife's inability to perform her sexual, biological, social as well as status-enhancing roles to her husband's satisfaction may all become threats to effective monogamy.

Premarital sex among teenage boys, while frowned upon and sought to be avoided through early arranged marriage is, nevertheless, common (between 12 and 25 per cent of male STD patients are in their teens) (Chaudhary et al. 1988; Arora et al. 1984; Siddappa et al. 1990; Chopra et al. 1990). In patriarchal societies where pre- and post-marital chastity for women are overriding values, violation of this norm by women would require overcoming the barriers of fear, strict surveillance and threats of terrible retribution of both divine and human origin. Among the upper castes the combination of seclusion and ideological conditioning would possibly cripple any such initiatives by women, while conversely providing them with protection from outright sexual assault. Among the intermediate peasant and poorer labouring castes and tribal communities, on the other hand, where women are required to engage in farm or wage labour, violence wielded by male family elders (primarily the father or husband) might have to replace seclusion as an instrument of control.

The exposure of the sexuality of poorer women makes them vulnerable to sexual and economic exploitation and even rape by men of both upper and lower castes. Concomitantly, it may also afford opportunities for sexual experimentation. Either way, in the absence of knowledge about contraception or STDs, young girls may become victims of STDs or unwanted pregnancies and consequent illegal abortions. Dramatic stories of sexual exploitation of young girls in remote rural and forest/tribal areas break into the national press from time to time. Quack abortionists run lucrative practices in these areas where outsiders (traders, forest contractors, etc.) vie with powerful insiders in sexual exploitation of the hapless local women belonging to the poorer sections.

Generally, the patriarchal extended family provides a few spaces for women and men to express their sexuality outside marriage, yet within the family framework. There are permitted joking relationships between cousins, or with a husband's younger brother or wife's younger sister, for example. In South India where cross-cousin and uncle-niece marriages are permitted and are indeed the norm in several communities, intimacy with a potential marriage partner may not be uncommon. It must be remembered, however, that by and large men enjoy greater power within the family, and it is plausible to believe that degrees of male coercion may be at work in such relationships which women dare not reveal for fear of losing family sympathy and security.

The other dimension of this inequality is that men also enjoy greater degrees of sexual freedom *outside* the family framework, which may have serious implications for the health of their wife/other sexual partner(s) within the extended family and friendship framework. The majority of male patients visiting STD clinics as repeaters (between 30 and 40 per cent are repeaters) are found to have had their first sexual experience while in their teens, the average age being 16 to 18 years (as mentioned earlier, between 12 and 25 per cent of STD patients are in their teens, the age group below 30 years constituting between 80 and 90 per cent of all STD patients). While this first encounter is often with a prostitute, others who also figure as first-time partners are acquaintances, friends, relatives or neighbours. For subsequent fulfilment of the desire for sexual gratification (whether due to peer pressure, desire for variety, absence of wife, or her ill health, etc.), these men more often than not resort to prostitutes (the single most important source of STD infection). But having unpaid sex with friends or relatives, neighbours or casual acquaintances continues to figure in their profile, although in smaller proportion. Admittedly, our understanding of sexual mixing is largely derived from studies of patients at STD clinics. Even casual observation, however, reveals that extra-marital affairs in both rural and urban areas are much more common than is apparent.

One cannot help observing an interesting difference between northern Indian and southern Indian studies of STD patients, in this regard. In the course of a comparison of a selection of such studies one finds that in the southern Indian studies, between 65 and 92 per cent of STD male patients cite visiting prostitutes as the most important source of their infection. Between 55 and 63 per cent of these patients are married. Those citing extra-marital/pre-marital relationships within the family are a significantly small proportion (within 5 per cent) (Ramanaiah et al. 1981a and 1981b; Jeyasingh et al. 1984; Kannappan et al. 1984; Jeyapaul et al. 1985; Jeyasingh et al. 1985b; Murugan et al. 1986; Vijay Kumar et al. 1990; Meeran Saheb et al. 1990: Siddappa et al. 1990). Only from one study do we glean that non-frequent visitors to prostitutes (about 24 per cent of the STD patients studied) had sex with relatives, very often with the future spouse who was also a blood relative (Baskaran et al. 1982).

In the northern Indian studies, on the other hand, the proportion visiting prostitutes is somewhat lower—between 35 and 65 per cent. But between 11 and 21 per cent cited relatives and friends as sex partners (obviously unpaid), a study in Delhi even finding that 53 per cent of the men cited non-professional sexual contacts as against 47 per cent who traced their current infection to prostitutes. Again, a significant proportion of the women attending the STD clinics in the north Indian studies are married women (Dutt et al. 1971; Garg et al. 1980; Bhargava et al. 1981; Ganguli et al. 1983; Ganguli, Sundharam and Bhargava 1983; Arora et al. 1984; Ganguli et al. 1985; Nigam and Mukhija 1986; Chaudhary et al. 1988; Bhargava et al. 1988; Chopra et al. 1990; Meeran Saheb et al. 1990; Singh et al. 1990). In the study by Chopra et al. in Patiala, 35 per cent of the women with STDs had got the infection from friends and relatives and 20 per cent from casual acquaintances. On the other hand, 51 per cent of the men cited prostitutes as the main contact; 14 per cent cited female friends and relatives and 9 per cent cited casual acquaintances. While 28 per cent of women said they got the infection from the spouse, hardly any men reported this.

It would be difficult to explain this without resorting to a combination of observation, deduction and conjecture. Admittedly, STD patients reporting to public hospital out-patient departments are a heavily biased source of evidence. They would comprise those within access of a city, since all the hospitals are located in important towns (although a high percentage of the patients identify themselves as rural dwellers). These patients are very often among those who have come to the hospital as a last resort after doing their rounds of the quacks. They contain a heavy proportion of repeaters. Nevertheless, in the absence of the availability of wide-ranging community based studies of sexual behaviour, they do give us some clues to sexual behaviour patterns in the general population.

More than half the male patients visiting STD clinics are married (four-fifths of the women attenders are married), and up to a fourth are students or teenagers who will go on to marry (over 50 per cent of the married men have a history of pre-marital sex). There is a nearly 70 per cent representation among them of rural dwellers. They are drawn from among the poor labouring classes—agricultural labourers in the villages or unskilled workers such as coolies, rickshaw pullers, sweepers in the city—or from among the lower socio-economic groups generally, such as truck, bus and taxi drivers, policemen, etc; they are largely illiterate or primary school leavers/drop-outs and are generally among the more disadvantaged in terms of both STD awareness and access to new knowledge about HIV and the risk factors involved. This description holds across both northern and southern Indian studies.

The higher proportion of male STD patients in the southern Indian studies reporting contact with prostitutes as against contact with relatives and friends, could be a function of easier access to prostitutes in the relatively more urbanized southern Indian states. The pattern of increase in STD incidence between states, in fact, reflects the rate of growth of urban population in the different states with its concomitant feature of presence of medical facilities in these urban centres (Ramasubban 1992). Easily identifiable concentrated pockets of prostitutes exist in big urban centres and district and taluka towns and are rapidly becoming a feature of smaller urbanizing agglomerations and major inter-state highway truck-halting points. The tradition of relatively large and active concentrations of prostitutes in urban agglomerations also has something to do with the continuing cultural practice of the ancient tradition of temple prostitution in some of these regions of the Deccan peninsula. Among very destitute groups in these regions, sending daughters into prostitution is one way of coping with poverty. Generally from among the poorest of the poor, these women are pushed into this form of survival by miserably deprived natal homes where parents are unable to conform to the norm of early marriage. In other cases where parental control is minimal, or where other family members themselves engage in illicit liquor trading or paid sex, or where they are victims of violent beating or desertion by the husband, women enter into alliances with strangers who promise companionship, marriage or employment but who eventually sell them to city brothels.

In the northern Indian states, while prostitutes continue to be the single most important contact for male pre- and extra-marital sex, the relatively lower extent of urbanization could be expected to render them relatively less easily accessible to an average rural dweller. Concomitantly, the lower degree of autonomy that women in this culture region enjoy which guarantees them greater economic and social security within the extended family may, paradoxically, be conducive to men and women known to each other in the extended family network entering into sexual relationships, either through male coercion or women's submissiveness in return for protection, or even the latter's quest for intimacy in a non-authoritarian relationship.

Quite clearly, despite the overarching framework of the patriarchal monogamous family, a certain amount of sexual mixing among friends and acquaintances, neighbours and relatives would seem to be a fact both in rural and urban areas, although neither the extent nor the different patterns of such sexual behaviour that might obtain among different groups in the population have been mapped out so far. In what would seem to be a rather extreme case, a study of gynaecological diseases among women in a rural population, found, on clinical examination, the existence of pre-marital sexual activity among 46.7 per cent of unmarried girls (Bang et al. 1989). (We do not know the extent to which women of tribal background are represented in the sample, since the district concerned is a tribal area; tribal societies are furthest removed from Brahminical norms, and sexual freedom among adolescents, teenage mixed dormitories and trial marriages are socially sanctioned institutions among several tribal communities in the country.) Another survey, this time a self-administered questionnaire among educated male readers of a metropolitan English glossy (which features pin-up pictures of women as one of its attractions), revealed that almost 80 per cent had pre-marital sexual experience and 55 per cent claimed to engage regularly in extra-marital sex (quoted in Savara 1992).

But by and large, the patriarchal family with its characteristic economic and social protection of women through their subordination, constitutes the norm. This subordination makes for the vulnerability of women's reproductive health. And the degrees of freedom enjoyed by men constitute threats to women's sexual health as well. Where even the protection is missing, women's subordination and helplessness—as among prostitutes—is total.

Sexually Transmitted Diseases

The prevailing scientific wisdom is that an important determinant of STD prevalence is the existence of an STD 'core group' (the particular social group in question may differ from society to society), wherein the rate of partner change is critical enough for the STD pathogens to persist in the population. Between 40 and 60 per cent of patients attending STD clinics of hospitals in different parts of India report having picked up their infection from prostitutes. We are also aware that prostitutes, particularly in cities, may have an average of seven partners in the course of a night's work. And, given the structure and norms of the patriarchal family, for the majority of men seeking pre- or extra-marital sexual relations, paid sex with prostitutes is the principal option. All these would seem to point to commercial sex workers as the STD 'core group' in the Indian cultural context.

This variable needs to be considered in conjunction with another factor, namely, the extent to which partner change in this group is mediated by recourse to preventive and curative health care. One set of factors abetting the maintenance among prostitutes of a level of infection which exceeds the threshold in the larger society is their poverty, low level of health awareness, and fatalistic acceptance of venereal disease as an occupational hazard, as well as the lack of autonomy to seek qualified medical care and (in the event of gaining such access) to abstain from plying their trade for the duration of the treatment period. A sizeable proportion of these sex workers may be found to suffer from simultaneous affliction of up to two or even three STDs (one study found the proportion with two STDs to be 41 per cent, while a little under 10 per cent had three STDs concurrently; the rest had one STD: Kunhilakshmi et al. 1980). Again, these sex workers are powerless to negotiate the use of condoms by their clients. Among both prostitutes and their clients there is widespread ignorance about the means for the prevention of infection and reinfection and means of cure. The steadily rising incidence of reported STD cases against this backdrop may perhaps explain why the infection rate is high enough and constant enough for STDs to constitute the third most important communicable disease in India after malaria and tuberculosis.

What is worrisome in the context of the discussion here is the untargetable group: the unpaid sexual partners of those men who are STD sufferers; women who, overwhelmingly through marriage and to a marginal extent through pre-marital/extra-marital contact, constitute a large population at risk of contracting STDs and even HIV. Over the five-year period 1986–87 to 1991, there has been a steady rise in HIV prevalence among men and women attending STD clinics, reportedly from 1 to 5 per 1000 to 5 to 50 per 1000. In Bombay seropositivity rates among commercial sex workers rose from 2 per cent to 30 per cent within a span of just two years, i.e. 1988–90 (ICMR 1991). The vast numbers of prostitutes, their clients and the wives/relatives/friends/acquaintances of these clients who do not attend public STD clinics situated in cities, remain beyond the pale of statistical estimation. Epidemiological data would seem to suggest that undetected asymptomatic seropositive persons who may remain asymptomatic for 7 to 10 years play an important role in HIV transmission.

The danger of HIV transmission is not the only reason for alarm regarding the vulnerability of women to possible STD infection. The complications and sequelae of most non-HIV STDs and even other non-sexually transmitted reproductive tract infections (RTIs) commonly found among women in the sexually active age-group are so serious as to cause untold distress with even fatal consequences, given their already imperilled health, status in the family and self-worth. Bacterial infections like syphilis, gonorrhoea and chlamydia, viral infections like genital herpes, and protozoan infections like trichomoniasis all cause genital lesions/inflammation which may remain asymptomatic for long periods or cause vague and non-specific symptoms even in their advanced stages, due to the structure of the female reproductive system. For anatomic reasons, again, the diagnosis of these infections is more difficult in women (requiring internal examination and often laboratory confirmation by qualified health care providers under hygienic conditions and laboratory facilities, respectively). And social reasons may render effective diagnosis impossible. Further, the potential for the spread of infection to the upper reproductive tract is high in the case of women, mediated by nutrition and immunity. And if symptoms become manifest—itching, burning while urinating, ulcers, pain, discharge—women are most often too afraid and confused to bring this to the notice of the family and thereby pave the way for access to medical care, both because they are not supposed to have such problems in the first place and also because they are socially deemed to be the polluters, the originators of sexual problems. Male ignorance of STDs and of their own role in infecting their wives works as the most effective barrier. The movement of infection to the cervix and upper reproductive tract—fallopian tubes, uterus and ovaries—may result in pelvic inflammatory disease (PID) causing chronic and acute abdominal pain (for which they are often given analgesics by general practitioners), foetal wastage, low birth weight and prematurity, infertility, debility, and cervical dysplasia, which may lead to cancer and death.

Infertility could be an assault on a woman's already low status and self-esteem, since childbearing is a prime guarantor of protection within the patriarchal family. The presence of RTIs may also make it difficult for the sufferer to sustain a pregnancy for the full term. This may be a spur to repeated pregnancies. It also carries with it the additional danger of the inherent infection getting exacerbated with every successive pregnancy, as a previously lower RTI moves upwards to cause serious complications (Wasserheit and Holmes 1992). Since the majority of deliveries are not conducted under aseptic conditions, unhygienic delivery practices such as insertion of fingers or instruments may act to intensify the already present infection. If a woman is fitted with an IUD as a spacing device, the trauma to the reproductive tract may result in inflammation which may lead to PID; if the woman already suffers from an infection, the IUD insertion may aggravate it and push it further upward into the reproductive tract. Induced abortions—commonly resorted to—are also a contributing factor in the exacerbation of reproductive morbidity.

Syphilis, gonorrhoea, chancroid, lymphogranuloma venereum (LGV) and granuloma inguinala (GI) account for between a third to half of the STDs found in STD clinics across the country. The other widely prevalent STDs are venereal warts, genital herpes, non-gonococcal urethritis (NGU) and candidiasis. There is a large omnibus category of 'other STDs' under which chlamydia, trichomoniasis, etc.—requiring laboratory tests for their correct diagnosis—are included (Ramasubban 1992).

While men by far exceed women in the STD patient profile (Kapur 1982 and the studies cited earlier), for the medical and social reasons pointed out above, the number of male patients should be seen as an indicator of the actual (as against reported) number of female sufferers. The fact that the infected male to uninfected female route works more efficiently than the infected female to uninfected male route, underscores this further. In the case of syphilis—the predominant STD in India, accounting for around 40 per cent of all reported cases—men with primary infection may be found in sizeable numbers reporting to STD clinics given the short incubation period and painful early symptoms in males (visible genital sores). Among women, on the contrary, primary syphilis remains undetected as the lesion is in the internal genitalia and is symptomless. Overwhelmingly, among women patients with syphilis, it is the secondary and latent syphilis which are to be seen.

In a study in Chandigarh, syphilis accounted for the highest number of patients, both male and female. While among male syphilis patients 48 per cent had primary syphilis, 39.3 per cent had secondary infection and 9.5 per cent had the disease in its latent stage, among the women patients primary syphilis accounted for only 6.9 per cent, while secondary syphilis accounted for 75.8 per cent and latent syphilis claimed 13.8 per cent (Bhushan Kumar et al. 1987). The nearly 40 per cent of male secondary syphilis patients may in part be due to spontaneous healing of the primary symptoms and in part due to a recently emerging problem, namely, the inadequate and indiscriminate administration of penicillin by private practitioners (allopathic and herbalist) which causes the primary symptoms to disappear without curing the infection effectively. In another study at a predominantly women's hospital in Delhi, syphilis was found to account for 55.6 per cent of all STDs. All primary cases—4.4 per cent of the sufferers—were male, secondary syphilis accounted for 17 per cent (male–female ratio 1:2.18) (Arora et al. 1984). In yet another study, this time in Allahabad, of the women syphilis sufferers 40 per cent had secondary syphilis as against 4.4 per cent with primary symptoms. The corresponding figures among male syphilis patients were 3.3 per cent and 12.3 per cent (Singh et al. 1990). In a ten-year study in Tirunelveli, syphilis accounted for nearly 31 per cent of all STDs, and women between 21 and 30 years of age formed about 30 per cent of syphilis cases (Murugan et al. 1986).

Latent syphilis presents a strikingly high figure in the Delhi women's hospital study cited earlier, and in some studies going back to the 1970s and early 1980s the figure ranges between 38 per cent and 53 per cent. Among the highest must be the finding in a Srinagar study of a 92 per cent incidence of latent syphilis (cited in Kapur 1982).

In women, the interval from initial infection of the reproductive tract to development of complications is quite long in the case of syphilis, often years. One of the outcomes is congenital syphilis; nearly 3 per cent of women patients at the Delhi women's hospital were suffering from this condition. A review of published and unpublished studies over a 20-year period (1968–88) found syphilis seropositivity among pregnant women to range from 7 per cent to 23 per cent as determined by VDRL testing (Bhargava 1988 cited by Luthra et al. 1992). Congenital or perinatal infection is not the only adverse outcome of syphilis patients who become pregnant, although it is the most serious. Foetal wastage and low birth weight or prematurity are also outcomes. They are believed to be higher in the case of this STD than in the case of other RTIs such as chlamydia, gonorrhoea, bacterial vaginitis or trichomoniasis (Wasserheit and Holmes 1992). Indian studies have found abortions in syphilitic women to range between 27 per cent and 50 per cent (Pavithran 1988). Syphilis has also been found to be the most commonly implicated STD among HIV positive STD patients, accounting for around 60 to 65 per cent of HIV positive cases (Mathai et al. 1990; Baruah et al. 1988; Rama Krishnaiah et al. 1989).

Among the genital ulcer producing STDs that are prevalent in India, genital herpes carries long-term complications for women's reproductive health. Increasingly encountered in STD clinics around the country, it has been commonly found to be one of the risk factors related to cervical cancer. Its presence, like that of other ulcerating STDs, could facilitate HIV transmission nearly seven-fold. In order to induce transmission it is believed to require repeated exposure with predisposing factors such as trauma, or low immunity (common in people on low protein diet). The tendency of herpes to become chronic and difficult to root out and the socio-economic status of attenders at STD clinics and their partners could be risk factors in themselves. Primary genital herpes has the most negative consequences for pregnancy among the STDs in terms of predisposition to foetal death, low birth weight and prematurity; in 30 to 50 per cent of cases of infected pregnant women, congenital infection or perinatal infection could be an outcome (Wasserheit and Holmes 1992). It has been suggested that vaginal delivery may enhance the risk of neonatal infection. In a study in southern India, the proportion of primary genital herpes was found to be significantly higher in women than in men, although the prevalence of herpes itself did not differ significantly between the sexes (Jacob et al. 1989). A study of risk factors for cervical cancer found that 39 per cent of cases and 42 per cent of controls were positive for the herpes simplex virus (HSV-2) (Gupta et al. 1988, cited in Luthra et al. 1992). The infection would appear to be fairly common among women, although the precise dimensions are at present difficult to estimate.

Among the STDs that come next to syphilis in prevalence, gonorrhoea is particularly problematic for women. Almost all gonorrhoea patients at STD clinics are men. This is because the symptoms are perceptible and acute among men while in women gonorrhoea is virtually symptomless, thus pre-empting even aware and motivated women from seeking health care. Yet, the risk of infection with gonorrhoea is much higher from male to female than with the reverse route, even a single exposure carrying a risk of infection as high as 20 to 30 per cent. Further, gonorrhoea has a short incubation period and the period between the development of acute symptoms and the development of complications such as PID in women is also believed to be short. Gonorrhoea may be transmitted to the offspring by pregnant infected women, and although not as severely as syphilis, gonorrhoea is a contributing factor to low birth weight or prematurity. The role of gonorrhoea in facilitating HIV transmission is also believed to be considerable (Wasserheit and Holmes 1992). Timely treatment is therefore essential if women are to escape such complications. Yet the absence of symptoms remains a confounding factor, a factor which also serves to retain a reservoir of infection among prostitutes.

The high rates of male gonorrhoea in India—between 10 and 25 per cent of all STD patients—are probably a reflection of the considerable recourse to prostitutes by men seeking pre- and extra-marital sex that we have referred to earlier. Very nearly 50 per cent of male gonorrhoea patients are in the 15 to 24 age-group and if we were to take the 15 to 30 age-group this would account for 80 per cent of patients. A number of these patients—between 30 and 39 per cent—are repeaters (Bhargava et al. 1981; Ganguli et al. 1982). And the proportion of single men is not significantly higher than those who are married. These characteristics would seem to indicate the potential of these men to infect their present or future wives, who in turn can be expected to remain symptomless even as they function as a source of reinfection for their husbands. That 21 per cent and 53 per cent respectively, of male gonorrhoea patients in a Delhi hospital who were investigated at two different points in time, cited a nonpaid sexual contact—friend, acquaintance, generally a known person—as the source of their infection, might be seen as a proxy for how this ping-pong process might be working (Bhargava et al. 1981; Ganguli et al. 1985). A serious problem in the case of gonorrhoea (as also in the case of syphilis) is the tendency of repeaters to indulge in self-administration of drugs; the problem of drug-resistant strains is only just beginning to be recognized.

The most effective known method of controlling female gonorrhoea in the community is contact tracing of partners of male patients for prompt treatment. Given the ignorance among men regarding the mode of transmission and the balance of power within the household, men have no accountability to their wives and women have little freedom to refuse sex within marriage. Male patients at STD clinics have shown a pronounced reluctance to bring in their wives/other sexual partners for examination. The high proportion of young married women between the ages of 14 and 25 among the women patients at STD clinics—probably drawn largely from urban areas—confirms that most women begin their sex life within marriage, given the low age at marriage.

We therefore know little about the prevalence of gonorrhoea in the general population and among women in particular. One approach to identifying this has been to screen women attending antenatal clinics for check-ups or attending Ob/Gyn out-patient departments (OPDs) for non-specific symptoms like vaginal discharge or for serious problems like PID or infertility. A study in Chandigarh observed 2 per cent of the patients to be harbouring gonococcal infection while another in Varanasi found less than 1 per cent of such patients (Luthra et al. 1992; Mishra et al. 1988). There is some controversy in India about the wisdom of routinely screening all women who attend antenatal clinics for gonorrhoea, as is advocated in the U.S.A. for example. Some advocate the screening only of contacts of males with diagnosed gonorrhoea, or patients with a history of past STDs or known promiscuous persons (a survey of PID among women in after-care and state protective homes found STDs to be the most important cause: Jain et al. 1981; see also Mishra et al. 1988). It has also been argued that there is not sufficiently strong evidence in India of gonorrhoea as a cause of PID as compared with, for instance, tuberculosis of the genital tract, puerperal sepsis or post-abortive infections (Brabin et al. 1991). Certainly, the Varanasi study found that of the 14.7 per cent patients with PID, in 87 per cent of the cases the cause was abortion or some surgical procedure and not gonococcal infection.

The point, however, is that nowhere do women have easy, non-stigmatized access to good quality diagnostic and curative facilities which take into account both their sexual and reproductive health. STD clinics would tend to be avoided by women (and even by men other than the very poor), private practitioners of whatever hue being the preferred option. While most STD clinics lack the more accurate (and at present expensive) diagnostic facilities, private practitioners (of whom most are general practitioners or quacks with little or no correct knowledge of or formal training in STDs), would be severely lacking in skills. Obstetrics and Gynaecology clinics of many public hospitals, and antenatal clinics, do not have facilities for STD diagnosis. And unmarried adolescent girls are not catered to by them.

The question therefore remains an open one. The low rate of gonococcal infection in hospital based studies could be a function of the selected groups studied. Most women in India do not visit gynaecologists or attend antenatal clinics, all of which facilities are concentrated in urban areas. Those who do attend, do so only in the last trimester of their pregnancy. Again, most women do not avail of the above facilities for check-ups that are non-pregnancy related, even under the stress of acute PID. And STD screening is not a part of routine antenatal, family planning and gynaecological care. This, in fact, is one of the greatest obstacles to screening pregnant women for *HIV infection* and to counselling them if they are found seropositive. *Women* who come to antenatal or Ob/Gyn clinics for check-ups, as against, *men* attending STD clinics, could be expected to be quite a different social group—urban, with effective access to medical facilities—from the uneducated and in other ways socially and economically disadvantaged and largely rural based women whom one would expect to find as wives/other sexual partners of the male gonorrhoea patients reporting to public STD clinics.

Our inadequate knowledge about the extent of gonorrhoea in women is matched by uncertainty regarding the prevalence of chlamydia trachomitis which shares many of the features of the former and is often found to occur along with it. Chlamydia, like gonorrhoea, is to be found among women in the most sexually active age-group, it is more efficiently transmitted from male to female and may remain asymptomatic for a long period in women, detection is easier in men and reported incidence higher among them under the rubric non-specific urethritis (NSU) or non-gonococcal urethritis (NGU). Among women it is put under the general label of non-specific genital infection (NSGI). The reason for these omnibus categories is that laboratory diagnostic facilities for the range of chlamydial infections are as of now expensive and rare even in metropolitan STD clinics although the infection itself is easily curable with antibiotics.

Like gonorrhoea, chlamydia can result in PID. Chlamydia was found to be 6 per cent in acute and 29 per cent in chronic PID cases in a Delhi study of women with PID (Luthra et al. 1992). Its role in causing low birth weight or prematurity, stillbirth, abortion, post-partum fever and congenital infection is somewhat more pronounced than the adverse outcomes induced by gonococcal infection (Wasserheit and Holmes 1992). The risk of foetal or neonatal death is believed to increase tenfold if the mother has chlamydial infection during pregnancy (Schacter et al. 1975). And there is also some evidence to link chlamydia in pregnant women with the risk of infant pneumonia (Pavithran 1988). The use of IUD in the presence of chlamydial infection is believed to heighten the risk of PID and, indeed, higher chlamydial infection has been found among IUD users (1 to 15 per cent) at various family planning centres in the country than among controls (WHO 1981; Luthra et al. 1992). The reported prevalence of this discharge syndrome among 20 to 30 per cent of men attending STD clinics in the country, and the evidence that it is also to be found among sexual partners of men thus affected, particularly among those belonging to lower socio-economic groups, is a glimpse of the proverbial tip of the iceberg. Regular condom use is an effective preventive measure, as it is with all STDs. There is also growing evidence that non-ulcerative STDs such as chlamydia, gonorrhoea and trichomoniasis may also facilitate HIV transmission in the way that genital ulcer-producing STDs such as syphilis, chancroid, herpes, etc. do and that the presence of both types of STDs increase the risk of transmission at least three- to five-fold (Wasserheit and Holmes 1992).

Other Reproductive Tract Infections

Besides the STDs discussed in the foregoing account, women also suffer from a range of other RTIs—specific and non-specific inflammations—which may or may not be sexually transmitted, which are important causes of reproductive morbidity, and which may even be risk factors for cervical cancer and HIV transmission when chronic and left untreated. These are a range of bacterial and parasitic infections whose chief symptom is white discharge. Found to be a very common problem among Indian women during the sexually active years, these infections are triggered off by a range of factors such as poor sexual hygiene (due to ignorance, lack of access to adequate and clean water or clean menstrual cloths, etc.), drop in immunity, use of IUDs, induced abortions, and bacterial infestation.

Trichomoniasis and candidiasis have been found to be among the common inflammatory conditions which are sustained through sexual transmission. In a study conducted among a combined sample of women attending the STD clinic and Ob/Gyn clinic of a hospital, the most frequent causes of white discharge were found to be candidiasis and trichomoniasis—almost 60 per cent—with almost half the patients in each group being asymptomatic. An additional

13.2 per cent of patients were found to have both infections (Mishra et al. 1988). There is a wide variation in the symptoms of these infections, ranging from mild to severe and short-lived to chronic, and the extent to which discharge is regarded as a symptom of ill-health would depend on the social construction of the symptom by the sufferer. Trichomoniasis has been found to be the commonest RTI among pregnant women. If left untreated it may cause low birth weight or prematurity. Trichomoniasis infection of the baby takes place during birth and has been found as an incriminating factor in neonatal pneumonia (Pavithran 1988). Among women reporting to STD clinics, infection with an STD such as syphilis has often been found to be accompanied by trichomoniasis infestation (Jeyasingh et al. 1985a).

Transmission more often takes place from the female to male partner during sexual intercourse. In some cases the male may remain asymptomatic and contribute to recurrent infection in the female. The transmission rate is high in this range of infections—50 per cent in candidiasis, over 60 per cent in trichomoniasis and around 55 per cent in chlamydia. Trichomoniasis (and indeed each of the above-mentioned inflammatory conditions) has been found to come down considerably when barrier methods of contraception are used. In one study of trichomoniasis and candidiasis in male partners of women with the two infections, it was found that only 14.6 per cent of men using condoms developed infection while 86 per cent of those not using condoms developed it (Pradeep Kumar et al. 1990).

Even where specific pathogens are not present, vaginitis may occur. Bacterial flora may remain the same as in a healthy vagina but the number may increase several-fold and under these conditions some normally present micro-organisms may become opportunistic pathogens. Much of the vulvo-vaginitis cases reporting to STD clinics—these account for 50 per cent of all women STD patients in some studies—have been found to be due to low body resistance (Siddappa et al. 1990). How widely prevalent specific and non-specific inflammations are, can be seen from other studies as well. A community based study in Bengal found that 77 per cent of women reported symptoms of white discharge, lower abdominal pain and backache. Clinical examination and laboratory diagnosis were able to confirm the presence of non-specific inflammation among 62 per cent of women. These findings were not dissimilar to those of a hospital based study wherein only 27 per cent of women were normal; the remainder suffered from inflammation of one kind or other (both cited in Luthra et al. 1992). In the community based study in Maharashtra cited earlier, laboratory diagnosis confirmed that nearly 92 per cent of women suffered from gynaecological disorders, the average number of disorders per woman being 3.6. Among other ailments, bacterial vaginitis accounted for 62 per cent of women, and 24 per cent and 14 per cent of women, respectively, suffered from PID and trichomoniasis. Cervicitis and cervical erosion accounted for 49 per cent and 46 per cent, respectively (Bang et al. 1989).

Inflammatory conditions are also caused by IUDs. Between 30 per cent and 54 per cent of IUD users have been found to develop non-specific chronic inflammation within nine months of insertion. The complication rate is higher with duration of insertion, acute inflammation going up to 63 per cent in the case of those using IUDs for over a year (Butt et al. 1991; Anupama et al. 1989; Sarbajna 1991; Luthra et al. 1992). White discharge, menstrual irregularity and backache have accounted for nearly 70 per cent of the causes of removal. The poor service provision for follow-up—poor knowledge on the part of health workers about contraindications for IUD insertion and about frequency of physical examination—is the main factor that keeps this particular spacing method unpopular. But the estimated 5 million IUDs inserted annually give an idea of the magnitude of life-threatening morbidity faced by women who must demonstrate their fertility yet also protect themselves from its negative consequences through contraceptive technologies that cause severe trauma to their reproductive health.

By far the most commonly adopted fertility control device is induced abortion, another major cause of inflammation and reproductive morbidity, and mortality. While nearly all illegal abortions result in severe injury and sepsis, thus accounting for almost 75 per cent of maternal deaths due to this form of fertility regulation, between 25 and 50 per cent of complications—injury, sepsis, incomplete abortion, pelvic infection—are the handiwork of ill-trained, inexperienced and careless 'qualified' medical personnel who in any case are not available outside urban areas. Thus even two decades after the Medical Termination of Pregnancy Act, the legal availability of abortion remains a weak option. Poor sexual hygiene, low nutritional status and flaring up of existing cervicitis have also been found to be important factors in post-MTP complications, making for around 12 to 15 per cent of such cases (Konar 1992; Mondal 1991; Ratna Sanyal et al. 1991; M.K. Sanyal et al. 1989; Nitwe et al. 1989). The high incidence of maternal deaths due to induced abortions—legal and illegal—has been well-documented (above-cited studies; also Jejeebhoy and Rao 1992). It would suffice here to draw attention to the potential of this form of fertility regulation, as practised under the prevailing conditions of service availability—qualified and unqualified—and complicated by pre-existing health status, to set off RTIs with their attendant complications.

Conclusion

The spread of HIV in India touches some of the innermost spaces in Indian society in ways that no other infectious disease has done so far. If other areas of health and morbidity have linkages with wider social, economic and environmental dimensions that defy target-driven, wholly vertical approaches, HIV lends itself even less to a blinkered perspective.

HIV in its heterosexual transmission mode, with pre-existing STDs and RTIs as risk factors, calls into question the cultural construction of female sexuality, one of the bulwarks of the patriarchal family structure which provides the framework for the prevailing gender relations in Indian society.

The definition of female sexuality as something threatening to society and requiring male control has had several consequences for women's socialization. Growing up in ignorance, fear and shame regarding their bodies, women's subordination begins early in life, through male definition of their autonomy and overall domestic and social value. The prescription that their sexuality be channelized through early marriage and speedy demonstration of their reproductive ability, has meant denial of even school education and of exposure to information, generally, and the lowering of the age at marriage to levels that threaten their sexual, reproductive and general health.

Early onset of coital activity and the frequency and unprotected nature of this activity result in early and closely spaced births and repeated deliveries under hazardous conditions which traumatize the young female body. If due to unwanted pregnancies, women are pressurized to go through induced abortions in order to achieve the family size and gender composition of offspring desired by the husband and his kin, they may succumb to a range of RTIs—inflammatory conditions that will persist and escalate through the sexually active years—arising out of the conditions under which these abortions generally take place.

The patriarchal family with its norm of early, universal and monogamous marriage is ideally expected to constitute a secure environment for heterosexual relations. But the degrees of sexual freedom enjoyed by men may constitute threats to women's health. If men have had unprotected pre-marital sexual experience or continue unprotected sexual activity outside marriage, undiagnosed and untreated STDs may add to women's reproductive morbidity and further endanger their childbearing role either through adverse pregnancy outcomes or through infertility.

The health and family planning programmes have failed to see women outside their role as mothers, that is, they have failed to pay attention to their survival as infants, their nutritional development in childhood, their persistence through school education, their complex reproductive physiology which puts them at a disadvantage in exposure to STDs and RTIs, and the monitoring of their sexual health. Their instrumental manipulation by a family planning programme that has targeted them for sole responsibility for contraception, has left women with no choices other than questionable invasive technologies for fertility regulation. And STDs are a devalued academic discipline, thus limiting the availability of skilled medical and paramedical personnel even in big cities. The shortage of specialists and the lack of STD diagnostic skills among graduate doctors also contributes to a flourishing market for quacks. The low status of the specialty has also meant the failure of research and development to generate diagnostic technologies for detection of STDs and RTIs among women that are cheap, reliable and easy to use under Indian field conditions.

It is against this complex backdrop that HIV prevention in the context of heterosexual relations, needs to be viewed. Where women's health is so fraught with danger from the early years of life, the risk factors for HIV infection would seem to be everywhere and, therefore, difficult to encapsulate into a focused vertical programme of prevention, diagnosis and counselling for HIV alone. For HIV is the most difficult of all diseases to identify, having no specific symptoms of its own but associated with opportunistic infections which are anyway rampant and important causes of mortality. There would seem to be no easy escape to intervention strategies that take a holistic view of women's sexual and reproductive health.

The common ground for state intervention and changes in individual behaviour is education. One of the major obstacles to any strategy for improving sexual, reproductive and general health of women is that there is no way in which women may be reached regularly at all, since they are invisible in any institutional context. Health programmes to monitor children's nutrition and growth, counselling of parents to keep girls in school and defer marriage until a safe age, can be accomplished more tangibly in a school context, rather than through reliance primarily on the electronic media with no means of face-to-face follow-up, however commendable the quality of the television programmes. Enhancing the coverage and quality of school education generally, and including health and environmental education and specifically sex education for both boys and girls, could lay the basis for an informed participation by people in their own health care. It would also make for better understanding and absorption of health education in adulthood, when information tends to come through more impersonal communication channels such as television or hoardings or wall posters/writings, etc.

Self-reporting is the surest way of tackling morbidity and there is evidence that when non-formal specific education, i.e. health education, is received on a substratum of general education, it is absorbed and retained more effectively by adults than when the latter basis is missing. And in the urban context, at least, it would appear that the presence of school-going children in the household can even compensate for lack of formal education on the part of parents (Ramasubban et al. 1990). Is education then such a potent building block in making for self-esteem that it can impart the ability and confidence to evaluate and absorb even that information that is not immediately relevant to the individual concerned?

In the case of women, health awareness in the context of a growing self-awareness and general awareness of one's environment may gradually help women overcome their low self-worth, which at present prevents them from consciously and confidently constructing the symptoms of their reproductive morbidity. This may also give them the confidence to negotiate non-harmful sexual relations, such as the use of condoms and abstinence while dealing with a health problem, to seek antenatal care, etc.

Education through the media and through community and workplace outreach programmes about HIV, STDs and reproductive morbidity, and about health aspects of the micro and macro environment generally, is a necessary complementary process. Men are an equally important audience for such communications, both in their own interests and because of the role that they play in the lives of women. Men often act as a source of information for their wives. It might be necessary for men to back some services with their approval and, if need be, with active participation, in order to encourage their wives to accept these services. Male support for improving women's reproductive health is necessary also because women are not financially independent. Even where women do engage in income-earning activities, men often withdraw their household contribution (spending it on liquor and visiting prostitutes, instead), and women's earnings go into purchasing food, health care and education for the children but not health care for themselves. Finally, men must share the responsibility for sexual relations, through protecting themselves from STDs when engaging in pre- or extra-marital sex, and, through condom use again, share responsibility for contraception so that women are protected from the negative consequences of their fertility without severe trauma to their reproductive health.

References

Anupama, H., Laxmi Reddy and R. J. Srinivasan (1989), 'Can IUCD induce uterine malignancy?' *Journal of Obstetrics and Gynaecology of India* (henceforth *JOGI*), Vol. 39, No. 1 (Feb.) pp. 85–87.

Arora, S. K., R. C. Sharma and Lal Sardari (1984), 'Pattern of sexually transmitted diseases at Smt. Sucheta Kripalani Hospital, N. Delhi', *Indian Journal of Sexually Transmitted Diseases* (henceforth *IJSTD*), Vol. 5, No. 1.

Bang, R. A. et al. (1989), 'High prevalence of gynaecological diseases in rural Indian women', *The Lancet*, 14 Jan., pp. 85–87.

Baruah, M. C. et al. (1988), 'Clinical profile of persons seropositive for AIDS virus', *IJSTD*, Vol. 9.

Baskaran, S. (1982), 'Socio-psychological study of frequent visitors to STD clinic', *IJSTD*, Vol. 3.

Bhargava, N. C., D. D. Ganguli and N. L. Jaisal (1981), 'An epidemiological study of gonorrhoea in males', *IJSTD*, Vol. 2.
Bhargava, N. C., V. K. Tewari and V. K. Pandey (1988), 'STD patients: a profile', *IJSTD*, Vol. 9.
Bhushan Kumar et al. (1987), 'Pattern of sexually transmitted diseases in Chandigarh', *Indian Journal of Dermatology, Venereology and Leprology*, Vol. 53.
Brabin, Loretta, Veena Soni Raleigh and Selinah Dumella (1991), 'Pelvic inflammatory disease: a clinical syndrome with social causes', Liverpool: Liverpool School of Tropical Medicine (mimeo).
Butt, N. et al. (1991), 'Histopathological changes in fallopian tubes of women using intrauterine contraceptive devices', *JOGI*, Vol. 41, No. 2 (April), pp. 223–26.
Chaudhary, S. D. et al. (1988), 'Pattern of sexually transmitted diseases in Rohtak', *IJSTD*, Vol. 9.
Chopra, A. et al. (1990), 'Pattern of STDs at Patiala', *IJSTD*, Vol. 11.
Dixon-Mueller, Ruth and Judith Wasserheit (1991), *The Culture of Silence: Reproductive tract infections among women in the third world*. New York: International Women's Health Coalition.
Dutt, J. (1971), 'Psychosocial aspects of venereal diseases in teenagers', *Indian Journal of Dermatology, Venereology and Leprology*, Vol. 16.
Ganguli, D.D. and N.C. Bhargava, (1983), 'Genital infections due to chlamydia and mycoplasma: a review', *IJSTD*, Vol. 4.
Ganguli, D. D. et al. (1982), 'A profile of gonococcal urethritis in males', *Indian Journal of Dermatology, Venereology and Leprology*, Vol. 48, No. 3.
Ganguli, D.D., J. A. Sundharam and N. C. Bhargava (1983), 'A clinico-epidemiological study of genital warts', *Indian Journal of Dermatology, Venereology and Leprology*, Vol. 49, No. 4.
Ganguli, D. D. et al. (1985), 'Profile of gonorrhoea in males', *IJSTD*, Vol. 6.
Garg, B.R., S. Lal and B. M. S. Bedi (1980), 'Continued endemicity of Donovanosis', *IJSTD*, Vol. 1.
Indian Council of Medical Research (1991), 'HIV infection: current status and future research plans', *ICMR Bulletin*, Vol. 21, No. 12 (December), pp. 125–44.
Jacob, Mary et al. (1989), 'Epidemiology and clinical profile of genital herpes', *Indian Journal of Medical Research*, Vol. 89.
Jacobson, Jodi L. (1991), *Women's Reproductive Health: The Silent Emergency*, Washington, D.C. Worldwatch Institute Paper 102 (June).
Jain, S. et al. (1981), 'Clinicobacteriological evaluation of pelvic inflammatory disease amongst women in state protective and aftercare homes', *IJSTD*, Vol. 2.
Jejeebhoy, Shireen and Saumya Rama Rao (1992), 'Unsafe motherhood: a review of reproductive health in India', Paper presented at seminar on Future of Health and Development in India, N. Delhi (January), published in the present volume.
Jeyapaul, K. et al. (1985), 'Reasons for promiscuity', *IJSTD*, Vol. 6, No. 2.
Jeyasingh, P., T. B. B. S. V. Ramanaiah and S. D. Fernandes (1985a), 'Pattern of sexually transmitted diseases in Madurai, India', *Genitourinary Medicine*, Vol. 61.
Jeyasingh, P., T. B. B. S. V. Ramanaiah and Balasubramaniam (1985b), 'Teenagers with STDs', *IJSTD*, Vol. 6.
Jeyasingh, P. et al. (1984), 'Effect of V.D. on knowledge and attitude to sex', *IJSTD*, Vol. 5. No. 1.

Kannappan, N. N. et al. (1984), 'Level of knowledge about STD among college students', *IJSTD*, Vol. 5.

Kapur, T. R. (1982), 'Pattern of sexually transmitted diseases in India', *Indian Journal of Dermatology, Venereology and Leprology*, Vol. 48.

Khan, M. E. and Singh, Ratanjeet (1987). 'Woman and her role in the family decision-making process: a case study of Uttar Pradesh, India', *Journal of Family Welfare*, Vol. 33, No. 4 (June).

Konar, Hiralal (1992), 'Changing trends in septic abortion', *JOGI*, Vol. 42, No. 3 (June).

Kunhilakshmi, T.V., K. Vijayalakshmi and C. N. Sowmini (1980), 'STDs among the inmates of vigilance home, Madras', *IJSTD*, Vol. 1.

Luthra, Usha et al. (1992), 'Reproductive tract infections in India: need for comprehensive reproductive health policy and programs' in A. Germain et al. *Reproductive Tract Infections*, New York: Plenum Press.

Mathai, Rachel et al. (1990), 'HIV seropositivity among patients with sexually transmitted diseases in Vellore', *Indian Journal of Medical Research*, Vol. 91 (July).

Meeran Sahib, K. P. et al. (1990), 'Pattern of genital ulcers in and around Mangalore', *IJSTD*, Vol. 11.

Mishra, D., Gurmohan Singh and D. Sharma (1988), 'Unsuspected gonococcal infection, candidiasis and trichomoniasis in females', *IJSTD*, Vol. 9.

Mondal, Aftab Uddin, (1991), 'Induced abortions in rural society and need for people's awareness', *JOGI*, Vol. 41, No. 4 (August).

Murugan, S. et al. (1986), 'Pattern of late syphilis: a decade study', *IJSTD*, Vol. 7.

Nigam, Pranesh and Mukhija, R. D. (1986), 'Pattern of sexually transmitted diseases at Gorakhpur', *IJSTD*, Vol. 7.

Nitwe, M.T., S. V. Desai and V. R. Walvekar (1989), 'Teenage pregnancy: a health hazard', *JOGI*, Vol. 39, No. 3 (June).

Pavithran, K. (1988), 'Effects of sexually transmitted diseases on the foetus and neonate', *Indian Journal of Dermatology, Venereology and Leprology*, Vol. 54.

Pradeep Kumar et al. (1990), 'Trichomoniasis and candidiasis in consorts of females with vaginal discharge', *IJSTD*, Vol. 11.

Rama Krishnaiah, Y. et al. (1989), 'Clinical profile of STD clinic patients seropositive for HIV antibodies', *IJSTD*, Vol. 10.

Ramanaiah, T.B.B.S.V. et al. (1981a), 'Level of knowledge about STD', *IJSTD*, Vol. 2.

Ramanaiah, T.B.B.S.V. et al. (1981b), 'Psychosocial factors and attitudes of patients towards STDs', *IJSTD*, Vol. 2.

Ramasubban. R. (1992), 'Sexual behaviour and conditions of health care: potential risks for HIV transmission in India' in T. Dyson (ed.), *Sexual Behaviour and Networking: Anthropological and Socio-cultural Studies on the Transmission of HIV*, Liege: Derouaux Ordina.

Ramasubban, R., Nigel Cook and B. Singh (1990), 'Educational Approach to Leprosy Control: A Study of Knowledge, Attitudes and Practices in Two Poor Localities in Bombay', Bombay: Centre for Social and Technological Studies.

Sanyal, M. K., T. N. Mukherjee and A. K. Chatterjee (1989), 'MTP: a four years study in a rural medical college of West Bengal', *JOGI*, Vol. 39, No. 1 (February).

Sanyal, Ratna et al. (1991), 'Study on septic abortion in a rural medical college', *JOGI*, Vol. 41, No. 4 (August).

Sarbajna, Shankar (1991), 'Intrauterine device as a means of contraception in our population', *JOGI*, Vol. 41, No. 4 (August).
Savara, M. (1992), 'Sexuality', *Seminar*, 396 (August).
Schachter, J. et al. (1975), 'Chlamydial infection in women with cervical dysplasia', *American Journal of Obstetrics and Gynaecology*, Vol. 123.
Siddappa, K., V. Jagannath Kumar and A. K. Bajaj (1990), 'Pattern of STDs at Davangere', *IJSTD*, Vol. 11.
Singh, K.G., M. K. Joshi and A. K. Bajaj (1990), 'Pattern of STDs in Allahabad', *IJSTD*, Vol. 11.
Vijay Kumar, B. R. Garg and M. C. Baruah (1990), 'A clinical study of genital ulcers', *IJSTD*, Vol. 11.
Wasserheit, J.N. and Holmes, K.K. (1992), 'Reproductive tract infections: challenges for international health policy, programs and research' in A. Germain et al., *Reproductive Tract Infections*, N. York: Plenum Press.
World Health Organization (1981), *Non-gonococcal Urethritis and Other Sexually Transmitted Diseases of Public Health Importance*, Technical Report Series, Geneva: WHO.

Old Age

9

Widowhood and Well-Being in Rural North India

MARTHA ALTER CHEN and JEAN DREZE *

1. Introduction

1.1. Motivation

The total number of widows in India is extremely large—more than 33 million in 1991. The proportion of widows in the total female population—about 8 per cent—is comparable to that of agricultural labourers in the total male population. Among women aged 60 and above, the proportion of widows is above 60 per cent (*Sample Registration System*, 1991).

In spite of this, and the general presumption that widows are a particularly disadvantaged social group, few attempts have been made at studying the living conditions of widows in India.[1] Widows are rarely mentioned in the literature on poverty, in public debates on social policy, or even by the women's movement. While a public outcry does occur from time to time when the social marginalization of widows takes a sensational form, such as that of *sati*, there is a

---

*We are grateful to Bela Bhatia and P. N. Mari Bhat for helpful comments, to the World Institute for Development Economics Research (Helsinki) for financial support, and to the National Council of Applied Economic Research (New Delhi) and the Indian Statistical Institute (New Delhi) for logistic assistance.

[1] A major conference on Widows in India was held in Bangalore in March 1994, and the studies presented there generated a considerable amount of new evidence on the social and economic condition of widows. Much of that recent material strengthens and extends the findings of this paper, and also throws considerable light on the contrasting life-styles of widows in North and South India. The new information made available at this very recent conference could not be incorporated in this paper, but a summary of the proceedings can be found in Chen and Dreze (1994).

striking lack of public concern for the deprivations experienced by millions of widows on a day-to-day basis.[2]

This lacuna is particularly serious in view of the fact that some of these deprivations are quite severe and widespread. Poor health, evident *inter alia* in high mortality rates, is an important example. Given their large number and special vulnerability to poor health and related deprivations, widows surely deserve an important place in the study of health policy and economic development in India.

It should be added that widowhood, and the helplessness that is often associated with it, probably have an influence on the health and well-being of many people other than widows themselves. For instance, vulnerability to widowhood in old age appears to be an important motive for high fertility among Indian women (given that surviving sons are practically the only source of social support which elderly widows can count on), with adverse consequences on the health of women and children (Drèze 1990). Similarly, the children of widows are likely to be particularly exposed to ill-health, not only because the economic deprivation of their mothers would reflect on their own living conditions, but also because a helpless widow often has to turn to her children's labour as a source of economic support (Drèze 1990), with potentially devastating effects on their well-being through loss of leisure, withdrawal from schooling and exposure to health hazards (Burra 1986a, 1986b; Weiner 1991). The focus of this paper, however, will be on the well-being of widows themselves.

Even with this restricted focus, we shall not attempt to cover all the issues involved.[3] Rather, we will concentrate primarily on a few aspects of the lives of widows that have a particularly strong bearing on their health and well-being. The issue of social support will receive special attention.

1.2. Sources

The empirical material on which this paper draws comes primarily from two sources. The first is an earlier study (Drèze 1990) of widows

---

[2]There is, admittedly, a large literature on 'female-headed households' in rural India, and it is also the case that a majority of female household heads are widows. However, these studies provide a very limited basis for studying the economic and social condition of widows as individuals. See Drèze (1990) for further discussion of this point, and of the insights that can be gained into the life of Indian widows from the existing literature on female-headed households, ageing, kinship, *sati* and related subjects.

[3]For a more detailed discussion of the living conditions of widows in rural India, and of implications for action, see Drèze (1990) and Chen (1991b), on which the present paper amply draws.

in three villages situated in West Bengal (Birbhum district), Gujarat (Sabarkantha district) and Uttar Pradesh (Moradabad district), respectively. These three villages were selected on grounds of prior familiarity to the author, and surveyed on several occasions between 1983 and 1989.

The second source is an on-going study (Chen 1991b) of widows in eight villages of North India—two each in the states of Bihar (Muzaffarpur district), West Bengal (Birbhum district), Rajasthan (Udaipur district), and Uttar Pradesh (Tehri Garhwal and Dehra Dun districts). Intensive field work, including a systematic survey of all widows, was carried out in these villages in 1991. Unless stated otherwise, the figures cited in this paper (or presented in the tables) refer to this second survey, which covered a total of 262 widows.

A word should be said about contrasts across regions and between religious and caste communities. Clearly, the life of widows can vary greatly between different localities and social groups, and these diversities have to be taken into account. Our analysis focuses primarily on North India, where the data presented in this paper have been collected. For simplicity, and because each of the study villages has a large Hindu majority, we have decided to restrict the discussion to that community. We hope to investigate the status of widows in Muslim, tribal and other non-Hindu communities in a separate study.

Within the Hindu community of North India, contrasts between different castes are extremely important, and some of them will receive explicit attention in this paper. Inter-regional contrasts are also significant in some respects, but they are generally less pronounced, at least for the North Indian states we are concerned with, and they will receive somewhat less attention. Indeed, the diversities involved are perhaps less striking than the common background against which they can be distinguished. For instance, most Hindu communities in North India share a basic kinship system, of which patrilocality and patriliny are central elements. This kinship system certainly does not operate in exactly the same way in different regions, but the finer differences should not divert our attention from the existence of a shared set of practices which has very strong implications for the condition of women in general and of widows in particular. This paper concentrates more on this common background than on the subtler inter-regional differences.

1.3. Framework

The position of widows in North Indian society is strongly influenced by a set of practices that govern gender relations as a whole. It is important not to look at widows in isolation, and to recognize the pervasive links that exist between their specific situation and that of women in general.

A good illustration of this point concerns the system of patrilocal residence. Alienation from the parental home after marriage puts most adult women in North India in a position of vulnerability, but the consequences of patrilocal norms are particularly pronounced in the case of widows. This is because the social support which a widow receives in her husband's village after his death is, typically, extremely limited. As a result, many widows are deprived both of the opportunity to re-integrate in their parental home and of the support they need to live happily in their husband's village.

Similar remarks apply to the system of patrilineal inheritance (which is closely related to the practice of patrilocal residence), and to the division of labour by gender. Even restrictions on remarriage, while appearing to affect widows specifically, derive from a broader kinship system that applies to all women. The connections between the deprivation of widows and the general position of women in the North Indian society will receive sustained attention in this paper.

As mentioned earlier, social support is the main focus of our enquiry. But it is important to understand how the extreme dependence of widows on social support relates, in the first place, to the restrictions they experience in the domains of (1) residence, (2) inheritance, (3) remarriage, and (4) employment. This background will be discussed in some detail before we turn to the issue of social support specifically.

1.4. Outline

The outline of the paper is as follows. In the next section, we discuss available information on the health of widows in rural North India. More empirical evidence is needed to firmly establish the facts, but the indications that already exist do point to high rates of morbidity and mortality among widows.

Section 3 examines several basic causes of the vulnerability and dependence of widows in rural North India. Particular attention is paid to the restrictions they experience in the spheres of residence, inheritance, remarriage and employment.

In section 4, we investigate what kind of social support widows receive from relatives and the community. Household formation, inter-household transfers and intra-household distribution are the main ingredients of our analysis. The overwhelming dependence of widows on their sons clearly emerges, confirming the results of earlier studies.

Section 5 offers some concluding thoughts on the implications of our findings for action.

2. Widowhood and Well-Being

This section examines available indications (direct and indirect) of the health status of widows in rural North India. Given the general dearth of information on this subject, indirect evidence will include the findings of studies carried out in other parts of South Asia. The relevance of these findings should be cautiously considered, given the possibility of sharp regional contrasts.

2.1. Economic Background

Several authors have argued that widowhood in South Asia tends to be associated with economic deprivation (Drèze 1990; Rahman 1990; Rahman and Menken 1990; Cain 1981, 1983, 1985, 1986; Caldwell et al. 1988). Rahman (1990) compares the economic decline of widows and widowers in rural Bangladesh, and finds a much greater decline in the economic status of widows compared with widowers. The reason, he argues, is that for women access to resources is much more dependent on marital status and living arrangement than is the case for men.

Cain (1981) analyses the impact of widowhood on the economic status of women in one village of Bangladesh and three villages of India.[4] He focuses on women who become widows under unfavourable circumstances: at an early stage in their life-cycle, or without surviving male offspring. The acquisition or loss of land is taken as a criterion of economic mobility. While the author finds that the widows in the Bangladesh village suffered greater loss of land than those in the Indian villages, he also concludes that all women widowed under unfavourable circumstances are vulnerable to

---

[4]The Bangladesh village is in Mymensingh district, northern Bangladesh. Two of the Indian villages are in Maharashtra state (in Sholapur and Akola districts). The third Indian village is in Mahbubnagar district of Andhra Pradesh.

economic decline. Similarly, in her study of household coping strategies in a village in Gujarat, Chen (1991a) found that households headed by widows had, over a period of 15 to 20 years, sold or mortgaged a disproportionate share of their land.

Drèze (1990), examining National Sample Survey data for the state of Karnataka (1977–78), finds that households with a widow have somewhat lower per-capita expenditure levels than households without a widow. While the difference is not particularly striking if all widow-inclusive households are taken together, some sub-groups within this broad category do appear to experience much higher-than-average levels of poverty. This applies particularly to households consisting of a widow and her unmarried children, especially when the eldest son is still quite young.

Further findings based on a small sample of widows in Palanpur (a village in Uttar Pradesh), reported in the same study, confirm these results. In this village, nuclear households headed by a widow are observed to experience a dramatic decline in per capita income after the death of the husband.

A different type of evidence is reported by Neela Mukherjee (1991, 1992) in her study of 'villagers' perceptions of poverty' in three villages of West Bengal. This study examines how villagers themselves rank different households in the scale of economic deprivation. She finds that households consisting of a widow living alone or with her unmarried children are commonly perceived as being among the most vulnerable.

Taken as a whole, these studies have clearly brought out the high vulnerability of particular groups of widows, especially those heading households without an adult male. The economic evidence, however, tells us very little about the living conditions of the majority of widows who live as dependents in households headed by adult males. This is partly because the standard economic variables fail to capture intra-household inequalities, which may be crucial in this context.[5] The fact that the focus of this enquiry needs to be squarely on the individual, rather than on the household, is one important reason for supplementing economic evidence with the use of health indicators such as mortality rates.

---

[5] This is aside from the limitations that apply to these standard economic variables even in the absence of intra-household inequalities (see Drèze 1990, for further discussion).

2.2. Mortality Rates

Economic deprivation is likely to be reflected in high morbidity and mortality rates among widows, compared with married women in the same age-groups. To our knowledge, this hypothesis has not been tested in the case of India itself. However, a recent study of differential mortality rates among women of different marital status in Bangladesh (Rahman and Menken 1990; Rahman 1990; Rahman, Foster and Menken 1992) does bring out the expected pattern.

This study, based on data from the Matlab surveillance area in rural Bangladesh for the period 1974–82, explores the impact of widowhood on mortality among women aged 45 and above. Some illustrative results are presented in Table 1. It can be seen from this table that widows tend to have much higher mortality rates than married women in the *same* age-groups.[6] The differences in mortality rates, moreover, are statistically significant (i.e. controlling for age, widows have significantly higher mortality rates than married women).[7]

Table 1 also shows that the mortality rates for widows can be quite different depending on their living arrangements, e.g. whether they head a household or live as dependents and whether or not they live with an adult son. This particular issue was investigated in some detail in the same study. Controlling for age and physical disability, the relationship between household type and mortality risk is as shown in Table 2 (for indicative purposes, this table also gives the distribution of widows by household type in our own sample of 262 widows). Widows living alone emerge as the highest-mortality

---

[6]It is also worth mentioning that, according to the same study, the decline of life expectancy associated with widowhood is greater for women than for men.

[7]The publication on which Table 1 is based (Rahman et al. 1992) does not comment on the statistical significance of the difference in mortality rates between 'currently-married women' and 'widows', taking all widows together. Instead, the authors provide separate statistical results for the three groups of widows appearing in Table 1. Controlling for age, the difference in mortality between currently-married women and widows in the relevant group is statistically significant only for the third group ('widows living in households not headed by themselves or their sons'). However, as the same study clearly indicates, the first group ('widows heading households') is a very heterogeneous one, and essentially consists of an amalgamation of the *most* vulnerable sub-group (widows living alone) and the *least* vulnerable one (widows heading a household which includes at least one adult son). A personal communication from Omar Rahman confirms that, taking all widows together, the difference in mortality rates between widows and currently-married women *is* statistically significant.

Table 1: *Age-specific death rates of widows and currently-married women in rural Bangladesh*

Age-Group	Mortality Rate (deaths per 100 person-years)				
	Currently-Married Women	All widows	Widows heading households (a)	Widows living in households headed by their sons (b)	Widows living in households other than (a) and (b)
45–54	0.89	1.36	1.68	1.15	1.63
55–59	1.78	2.06	2.21	2.13	1.23
60–64	3.10	3.83	2.42	3.86	5.84
65–69	3.81	5.56	5.20	5.15	8.27
70–79	9.43	9.99	8.63	9.88	11.67
80+	9.38	17.50	15.04	17.66	18.52
Total	1.87	5.29	3.75	5.37	7.59

Source: Calculated from Rahman et al. (1992), Table 1(a).

Table 2: *Living arrangements of widows and mortality risk*

	Ranking of Household Types by Mortality Risk	Percentage Distribution of Sample Widows
1.	*Low mortality risk* Widows heading households with adult sons	25
2.	*Medium mortality risk* Widows living in households headed by adult sons	40
	Widows heading households without adult sons	10
3.	*High mortality risk* Widows living in households headed by 'others'	13
	Widows living alone	12
Total		100

Source: The ranking of household types by mortality risk is that found in Rahman et al. (1992). The percentage distribution of widows by household type corresponds to the Chen (1991b) sample of 262 widows, on which most of the figures reported elsewhere in this paper are based.

group. For other widows, two particular circumstances have mortality-reducing effects: (1) the presence of an adult son in the household, and (2) the position of the widow as household head. Among these widows, mortality is lowest when both of these features apply, and highest when neither of them applies.

The studies by Rahman et al. also contain interesting indications of the respective importance of household economic decline and intra-household neglect in the causation of enhanced mortality among widows. If one 'controls' for household assets (in addition to age and disability), mortality rates among widows living alone or with an adult son are comparable to those of married women. In other words, for widows in these two groups, it is the economic decline of the household that seems to be the driving force behind enhanced mortality rates. On the other hand, for widows living as dependants in households headed by persons other than an adult son, mortality risk remains significantly higher than for married women even after controlling for household assets (as well as for age and disability). This suggests that, for these dependent widows, intra-household neglect may be important as an independent source of enhanced mortality.

2.3. Regional Contrasts

There are striking heterogeneities in the incidence of widowhood in different parts of India. Some of the relevant inter-state contrasts are brought out in Tables 3 and 4. It can be easily seen that the proportion of widows in the rural female population tends to be much higher than average in the southern states (Andhra Pradesh, Tamil Nadu, Karnataka and to a lesser extent Kerala). The incidence of widowhood is comparatively low in the northern region, especially in the North-West.[8] The ratio of widows to widowers follows a similar regional pattern, taking high values (between 3.9 and 7.7) in the southern states, and much lower values (between 1.4 and 1.7) in Punjab, Haryana, Uttar Pradesh, and Jammu and Kashmir. This broad North-South contrast, with a particularly sharp divergence between the South and the North-West, deserves further scrutiny.[9]

---

[8] The state of Assam, where the 1981 Census did not take place, is excluded from the discussion of this section. So are the other states of the North-East, which have small populations and rather special demographic, social and cultural features.

[9] In this paper, 'South India' refers to the states of Andhra Pradesh, Karnataka, Kerala and Tamil Nadu, and 'North India' refers to the rest of the country.

Table 3: *Widows in rural India, 1981: Inter-state contrasts*

State	Widows as percentage of rural female population	Female-male ratio[a]	Ratio of widows to widowers in rural population	Proportion of rural Indian widows living in the state (percentage)	Average ADM (years)[b]
	(1)	(2)	(3)	(4)	(5)
Andhra Pradesh	10.5	975	4.3	10.5	5.7
Tamil Nadu	10.4	977	3.9	8.2	5.8
Karnataka	9.9	963	4.6	6.4	6.7
West Bengal	9.5	911	6.0	9.1	6.5
Maharashtra	9.3	937	4.4	9.3	5.4
Orissa	9.2	981	3.7	5.3	5.1
Kerala	8.9	1032	7.7	4.6	5.5
Madhya Pradesh	8.0	941	2.6	8.0	4.0
Himachal Pradesh	7.7	973	2.5	0.8	4.7
Bihar	7.5	946	2.5	11.1	4.9
Rajasthan	7.2	919	2.4	4.6	4.2
Gujarat	7.0	942	2.9	4.0	3.6
Uttar Pradesh	6.5	885	1.4	13.8	4.3
Jammu & Kashmir	5.7	892	1.4	0.6	5.0
Punjab	5.5	879	1.6	1.5	3.3
Haryana	4.9	870	1.5	1.1	3.9
India[c]	8.2	934	2.9	100.0	5.0

[a] Number of females per 1000 males (rural and urban areas combined).
[b] Age differential at marriage: difference between the mean age at marriage of males and females (rural and urban areas combined).
[c] Excluding Assam, where the 1981 Census was not conducted.
Source: Drèze (1990). Derived from *Census of India 1981*, and Verma (1988), Tables 3, 5 and 28. The figures reported in Verma (1988) are also based on the 1981 census. The corresponding figures for the 1991 census are still to be released.

Table 4: Incidence of widowhood in different age-groups and regions, 1981

Age-group	Widows as percentage of all rural females in the corresponding age-group and region				
	North-West	Central West	East	South	All-India[a]
0–9	0.0	0.0	0.0	0.0	0.0 (0.0)
10–14	0.04	0.04	0.03	0.03	0.03 (0.03)
15–19	0.2	0.3	0.3	0.2	0.2 (0.1)
20–24	0.5	0.7	0.9	0.9	0.7 (0.5)
25–29	1.0	1.5	2.0	2.0	1.6 (1.0)
30–34	2.1	2.9	3.6	4.3	3.2 (1.6)
35–39	3.6	5.0	6.3	7.0	5.5 (2.3)
40–44	7.9	9.6	12.3	13.7	10.8 (3.8)
45–49	10.0	14.8	18.1	19.8	15.5 (5.0)
50–54	24.1	27.5	32.2	34.2	29.4 (8.0)
55–59	20.1	30.6	32.7	40.6	30.5 (9.8)
60–64	48.7	55.3	58.1	61.3	55.6 (14.9)
65–69	44.0	59.8	61.5	66.8	57.6 (17.8)
70+	70.5	78.4	78.3	83.4	77.2 (27.8)
All ages	6.5	8.3	8.5	10.0	8.2 (2.7)

[a] In brackets, the corresponding figures for *males*.

Source: Drèze (1990). Calculated from *Census of India 1981*, Part IV-A, Social and Cultural Tables, Table C-1 (the 'all-India' column, also based on the 1981 Census, is taken from Verma 1988:87). The different regions have been 'defined as follows: North-West: Haryana, Himachal Pradesh, Jammu and Kashmir, Punjab, Rajasthan, Uttar Pradesh; Central West: Gujarat, Maharashtra, Madhya Pradesh; East: Bihar, Orissa and West Bengal; South: Andhra Pradesh, Karnataka, Kerala and Tamil Nadu. This regional division is based on Agarwal (1988).

To some extent, these regional contrasts reflect different patterns of life expectancies, especially the fact that the survival advantages of adult women vis-à-vis adult men are stronger in the southern states. With a life expectancy in the early forties, the average woman in Uttar Pradesh is comparatively well 'protected' from the prospect of widowhood. The same does not apply in Kerala, where women live on average *twenty-four* years longer than their sisters in Uttar Pradesh, and where women outlive men by a long margin.[10]

Regional differences in gender-specific survival chances, however, only explain a part of the observed North-South contrast in the

---

[10] See Verma (1988:97–8), based on the 1981 Census. For men, life expectancy is 'only' fifteen years shorter in Uttar Pradesh than in Kerala.

incidence of widowhood. Indeed, the incidence of widowhood appears to be considerably higher in the South than in the North even *within given age-groups*. As can be seen from Table 4, up to the age of about 60 the risk of being a widow is roughly twice as high for a woman of a given age in the South as for a woman of the same age in the North-West. This obviously cannot be explained by invoking the shorter life expectancies of men and women in the latter region (quite the contrary, since a shorter life expectancy for men tends to *increase* the risk of widowhood for women of a given age).

The fact that the difference between the mean age of marriage of men and women is comparatively large in the South does contribute to higher rates of widowhood in all age-groups for that region. But this can only account for a small part of the observed regional contrast since, in fact, age differentials at marriage in South India are only about one year larger than in India as a whole, and about two years larger than in the North-West (see Table 3).

A more promising explanation is that remarriage rates are lower in the South than in the North. There is, in fact, some empirical evidence in favour of this hypothesis.[11] It is, nevertheless, rather doubtful that lower rates of remarriage satisfactorily explain the much higher incidence of widowhood in the South. This is because, as will be discussed in section 3.3, remarriage rates are quite low even in the North. Also, we have to remember that, insofar as they do occur, remarriages in the North are overwhelmingly concentrated in the younger age-groups (say, below 30). Thus, if differential remarriage rates were the main factor behind the observed regional patterns, one would expect the absolute difference between the age-specific incidence of widowhood in the South and in, say, the North-West to stop widening beyond these age-groups. But in fact, this difference continues to increase well beyond, to age-groups within which remarriage rates would become negligible (see Table 4).

---

[11]See Dreze (1990). The suggestion that the incidence of widow remarriage is lower in South India than in North India may seem counterintuitive, insofar as it conflicts with the widely-accepted notion that the former region is comparatively advanced when it comes to the position of women in society. However, a substantial proportion of widow 'remarriages' in North India, and particularly in the North-West, are accounted for by ascribed leviratic unions. Higher rates of widow remarriage in the North may thus confirm rather than contradict that region's reputation for 'backwardness' in gender relations.

It seems hard to explain the North-South contrast without invoking the further hypothesis that the widows of North India, and particularly those living in the North-West, have particularly *low survival chances*. Other things being equal, this would reduce the proportion of widows in the female population, particularly in the older age-groups.

This hypothesis fits well with the results reported earlier for Bangladesh, a region which, as far as gender relations are concerned, is probably much closer to North India than either region is to South India. It also points to the possible role played by social neglect in generating high mortality rates among widows in North India. The relatively low survival chances of *women* vis-à-vis men in North India have been linked in earlier studies with various forms of anti-female discrimination, and it is not surprising that this region should also be that where the special disadvantages of *widows* appear to be particularly acute. Indeed, as will be argued later in this paper, the factors that contribute to the deprivation of widows are closely linked with more general causes of female disadvantage in North India.

3. Sources of Vulnerability

This section discusses selected aspects of the condition of Indian widows which, in our judgement, deserve to be considered as basic causes of their vulnerability. Special attention will be given to the restrictions that widows experience in the domains of (1) residence, (2) inheritance, (3) remarriage, and (4) employment.

3.1. Patrilocality

The system of patrilocal residence and patrilineal inheritance, which has the effect of isolating and dispossessing women, is a fundamental source of gender inequalities in rural North India. It also plays a crucial part in the deprivation of widows. Although both elements of this system are closely inter-related, we will discuss patrilocal residence first, and take up the question of patrilineal inheritance in the next sub-section.[12]

---

[12] Patrilocal residence and patrilineal inheritance can themselves be seen as two crucial aspects of the North Indian system of 'patrilineal kinship'. A deeper analysis of the status of women in general and of widows in particular would have to include a serious discussion of this kinshp system, as well as of the patriarchal authority structures that go with it.

Patrilocality in the narrow sense refers to the norm, prevalent in most Hindu communities of North India, according to which a woman has to leave her parental home at the time of marriage to join her husband in his own village.[13] In the broader sense used in this paper, patrilocality also refers to the drastic alienation from her parental family experienced by a married woman after her 'transfer' to her husband's family. Indeed, the departure of a married woman to her husband's home is not simply an innocuous change of residence—it marks a dramatic and irreversible change in her whole life. Once she has crossed that bridge, she literally becomes the property of her in-laws' family. Her intimate links with her parental home and its familiar surroundings are reduced to the occasional visit. In her new 'home', the life of the young bride is one of hard work and subordination, and possibly also of seclusion or even harassment.

The transfer of a young bride from her father's family to her husband's family is a crucial event not only in her emotional life but also from the point of view of her legal and social status. In particular, her customary rights to property, such as they may have been before her marriage, are considerably reduced. After her transfer to her husband's village, a woman forgoes her right of inheritance in her natal home (in the marriage ceremony of some communities, this break with the father's patriliny is symbolized by the breaking of a twig). A married woman only retains certain limited and residual rights in her parental home: she is entitled to receive gifts on specific occasions from her parents and, after their death, from her brothers; and she is entitled to visit her natal home on ceremonial and other occasions (Madan 1989).

The practice of patrilocal residence is of profound significance for widows. It means that after losing their husband they have very little freedom to 'return' to their parental home (or to their brothers). They are expected to remain in their husband's village, and in most cases they do so (unless they are childless or remarry). In our sample, the vast majority of widows (85 per cent) continued to live in their

---

[13]This definition assumes village exogamy, which is itself a nearly universal feature of marriage practices in North India. We overlook here the subtler distinction between 'patrilocality' and 'virilocality', which turns on whether or not the husband continues to live with his father after marrying.

Table 5: Widows by village of residence after husband's death

Residence	Widows	
	No.	%
Same Village:		
Deceased husband's	222	85
Parental	16	6
Other	4	1
Subtotal	242	92
Different Village:		
Deceased husband's	2	1
Parental	12	5
Other	6	2
Subtotal	20	8
Total	262	100

Source: Chen (1991b), based on a survey of eight North Indian villages (see section 1.2).

deceased husband's village after his death, whether or not he owned land or other property (see Table 5).[14]

In most cases, widows actually continue to live in their deceased husband's home. However, outside leviratic unions (which are practised only in certain communities), widows are unlikely to share a common hearth with their husband's relatives. In the study villages, only thirteen widows out of 262 reported living in households headed by an in-law, either parent-in-law or brother-in-law. Thus, while most widows continue to live in close proximity to their in-laws (e.g. in adjacent huts or rooms), very few share a common hearth with them; and, as will be discussed in section 4, very few receive substantial support from their deceased husband's relatives. Most widows are deprived both of the freedom to leave their husband's village and of the support they need to live there happily.

3.2. Patrilineal Inheritance

The inheritance rights of widows in North India will be discussed here with specific attention to *land*. A comprehensive treatment of

---

[14] An example of exceptions to this general rule is the case of a widow who used to live in her parental village at the time of losing her husband, possibly because the latter was a *gharjamai* (uxorilocal son-in-law). A *gharjamai* is a married man who is invited by his parents-in-law to come and live with them, usually because they have no sons themselves.

this subject would have to distinguish between (1) modern law, (2) traditional or customary law, and (3) actual practice. For simplicity, we shall concentrate mainly on the third notion, as it applies in the study villages. Another useful distinction to make is that between the inheritance rights of women (1) as daughters, assuming (for simplicity) the demise of both parents, and (2) as widows, after the loss of their husband.[15]

Under the North Indian system of patrilineal inheritance and patrilocal residence, women *as daughters* are rarely entitled to a share of their father's property. When she joins her husband's village at the time of her marriage, a daughter loses her status as a coparcener in her natal household. After that, she can reclaim her rights of inheritance to her father's property only under very exceptional circumstances. In the study villages, only 15 widows (6 per cent) had retained or reclaimed some inheritance rights in their parental village.[16]

If a daughter does not change residence at marriage, and her husband comes to live with her in her own village, she often retains her rights as a coparcener in her natal home. The consequence of this reversal of the normal rule of residence is that a woman acquires rights of ownership and disposal in her natal household similar to those of her brothers (if any). But this pattern is quite exceptional—it usually occurs only when the parents of the bride have no sons.[17]

As *widows*, under the traditional laws of most castes, women are widely acknowledged to have rights to their husband's share of the family land, and their entitlements are often taken into account in the event of partition. However, the rights in question are often limited—in practice at least—to use rights, as opposed to ownership rights. For instance, a childless widow who remains in her husband's village is usually allowed to use her husband's share of the family land, although she does not have the right to sell it or gift it away. After her death, her share generally reverts to her husband's family.

---

[15]As wives, women in the study villages have no coparcenary rights in their conjugal families; they only have a right of maintenance.

[16]Of the 15 widows who retained or reclaimed some inheritance from their parents, 11 are from West Bengal. The possible explanatory factors behind this high incidence of female inheritance in West Bengal need to be explored (see Drèze 1990, for a similar finding and a suggested interpretation).

[17]In such cases, the *gharjamai* (in-marrying husband) assumes the duties of a natural son (Cain 1986).

Similarly, a widow who has only daughters generally exercises use rights over her husband's share of the land until her death. If a widow has sons, she generally exercises use rights over her husband's share of the land as a trustee or guardian until her sons mature. After they mature, her sons are likely to partition the land among themselves, possibly before their mother's death. In such situations, a widow's relations with her sons determines whether or not she continues to exercise a use right over part of the family land. If she lives with one or more sons, her share is typically cultivated by her sons. If she lives separately from her sons, her share may still be cultivated by her sons or she may manage her share independently.

To exercise full ownership rights, a widow would have to assert her modern legal rights and ensure that her name is entered in the local land registers maintained by the government, or in the actual land deed. In some circumstances (e.g. if she has no brother-in-law and her parents-in-law have died, or if the partition of her husband's family's land has already taken place), a widow is more likely to have her name entered in the local land register. However, actual land deeds are seldom transferred in the name of widows, especially in places where the common practice is to change the names in land deeds only when a person wants to sell land.

Limited as they are, the accepted property rights of widows are often violated in practice. Twenty per cent of the widows in our survey reported serious conflicts with their in-laws, and the majority of these were conflicts with their brothers-in-law over land. These conflicts are primarily of two types: the brothers-in-law insist on sharecropping or managing the widow's land themselves, or they simply attempt to deprive her of her rightful share of the land (often rationalizing their claim by arguing that they spent money on her husband's funeral or on her children's maintenance). In their attempt to gain control of her land, the brothers-in-law of a widow may go so far as forcing her to leave the village, or even—in extreme cases—arranging her murder.

3.3. Remarriage Practices

Two stereotypes persist about widow remarriage in India. The first, very widespread until recently, is that widow remarriage is 'prohibited' in Hindu society. The second, currently more influential in the scientific literature, is that widow remarriage is widely practised. Reality lies somewhere between these two extreme views: while most castes (except the higher-ranked ones) do not 'prohibit' widow remarriage, actual remarriage only takes place in special circumstances.[18]

In this connection, a crucial distinction has to be made between childless widows and widowed mothers. In most communities, the remarriage of a childless widow is perceived as a fairly straightforward affair.[19] Except in the case of a leviratic union, the remarriage arrangements are the responsibility of the father and brothers of the concerned widow. The second husband is usually a widower, a divorcee, an impoverished bachelor, or a currently-married man who wishes to take a second wife (see Table 6 for some relevant information from the study villages). The marriage ceremony is simple and informal.[20] On remarrying and leaving the village of her deceased husband, a childless widow loses her entitlement to his share of the land.

Among widowed mothers, remarriage is rare. The primary reasons cited by widowed mothers for not remarrying are that they do no want more children or that they doubt whether a new husband will take good care of the children they already have (see Table 7).[21] Another frequently-cited reason is the wish to retain claim on the decased husband's land (bearing in mind that widows usually lose this claim on remarriage). Other factors that were mentioned by widowed mothers in the study villages include: the possibility of harsh

---

[18]For a detailed discussion of widow remarriage in North India, and an evaluation of earlier studies on this subject, see Drèze (1990).

[19]The remarriage of a childless widow tends to be an attractive proposition for most of the interested parties. For the widow herself, it is the only accepted path to motherhood. From the point of view of the in-laws, accepting or encouraging the remarriage and departure of a childless widow is a convenient way of regaining control over her deceased husband's land. As far as the father and brothers of the widow are concerned, it is plausible that compassion often motivates them to arrange her remarriage. In addition, among communities where brothers (or fathers) have a strong obligation to support a widowed sister (or daughter), a childless widow may be seen as a threat of lifelong liability, especially if she is anxious to leave her husband's village.

[20]In North India, the 'remarriage' of a widow is not considered as a 'second marriage', but rather as a marriage of an inferior kind (or what Louis Dumont calls a 'secondary marriage'). It is referred to by terms (e.g. *nataru* in Gujarat, *sagai* in Uttar Pradesh, *sangha* in West Bengal) which are unrelated to the words that would be used for a first marriage (*lagan, shadi, biye*, respectively).

[21]It should be added that a widowed mother cannot always assume that she will be able to take her sons with her (or even to see them occasionally) if she leaves her first husband's village to remarry. Her in-laws may object, given the notion that her sons belong to their own lineage.

Table 6: Remarried widows by marital status of new husband

Marital Status	Number and Percentage of Widows	
	No.	%
Widowed	26	72
Divorced	2	6
Currently Married	2	6
Never Married	3	8
Unknown	3	8
Total	36	100

Source: Chen (1991b).

Table 7: Never-remarried widows by reason for not remarrying

Reason	Number of widows citing Reason
No more children wanted	60
Concern about well-being of living children	37
To claim property	33
Societal pressure	2
Dislike of suitor	1
Other	27

Note: Many widows who never remarried either came from castes which prohibit remarriage or were considered too old to remarry. These two reasons for not remarrying are not included in the table. Note that some widows cited several reasons.
Source: Chen (1991b).

treatment of the widow herself by the second husband's own children (bearing in mind that a widow typically marries a widower who is also likely to be a father); the ambiguous status of a widow's children by her second husband (given that both she and he may have children from previous marriages); the fact that only widows aged below 40 years or so are considered eligible for remarriage; and uncertainty about whether a new marriage will bring happiness or security. Even among castes which have liberal attitudes vis-a-vis widow remarriage, few widowed mothers manage to overcome these obstacles and fears.

To conclude, the basic pattern in most communities is that most childless widows remarry, while most widowed mothers do not remarry. The overall probability that a widow will remarry is quite low, perhaps of the order of 15 to 20 per cent in India as a whole.[22] In the eight study villages, only 13 per cent of ever-widowed women were found to have remarried.

The extent to which low rates of remarriage reflect a deliberate choice on the part of widows themselves, rather than external restrictions or pressures, is difficult to determine. In fact, the distinction between voluntary rejection and external obstruction is itself not clear-cut, since the aspiration of widows to remarry may strongly depend on the opportunities they face, the support they can anticipate, and the 'conditioning' they have received. For our purposes, however, what matters is to note that remarriage is not a likely refuge for the majority of widows who have children at the time of losing their husband.

3.4. Employment Restrictions

One of the prominent elements of the basic patriarchal system of North India is a sharp division of labour by gender. Under this division, certain types of work are considered as male or female. For example, ploughing is almost exclusively a male task, whereas drying and storing grain are typically female tasks. Moreover, certain spheres of economic activity are often designated as male or female. In many communities, for instance, the homestead or private sphere is predominantly female; the public sphere of markets, roads and towns is predominantly male; and the intermediate sphere of fields and villages is both male and female.

These patriarchal norms are interwoven with a hierarchical social structure which considers the life-style of women as an important indicator of the status of different groups. This social-status hierarchy further restricts women's employment, insofar as an important symbol of a household's position in this hierarchy is the type of work its women are allowed to do.

Aside from the general restrictions resulting from this interaction between the social-status hierarchy and the division of labour by gender, widows face specific difficulties in seeking gainful employment opportunities. These include: lack of access to indivisible

---

[22] See Drèze (1990). As explained in that study, there is no contradiction between this estimate of 15 to 20 per cent for the probability of remarriage and the estimate of 30 per cent for the proportion of remarried widows in the *current* population of ever-widowed women, obtained by Bhat and Kanbargi (1984).

Table 8: Labour force participation rates of widows and married women (Rural India, 1981)

Age-group	Labour force participation rate[a]	
	Married women	Widowed women
10–14	18	22
15–19	23	36
20–24	24	39
25–29	25	44
30–34	27	47
35–39	28	47
40–49	27	39
50–59	22	27
60+	13	10
All ages	25	22

[a] 'Main workers' as a proportion of all women in the relevant group.

Source: Chen (1991b).

productive assets owned by the deceased husband's family (e.g. wells, ploughs and bullocks); weak bargaining power vis-à-vis male partners in economic transactions; frequent absence of a literate member in the household; limited access to institutional credit; and, particularly in the case of widows living with young children, the burden of domestic work.[23]

As Table 8 indicates, the labour force participation rates of widows in India tend to be a little higher than those of married women of the same age (this observation also applies in most individual states). But the fact remains that female labour force participation rates in India are very low for *all* women (irrespective of marital status), and that widows, despite having somewhat higher age-specific labour force participation rates, face severe employment restrictions due to the gender division of labour. Further, because widows tend to be concentrated in the older age-groups, their average labour force participation rate is lower than that of married women (Table 8).

Table 9 presents information on the primary occupations of households with at least one widow in the study villages, both before and after the event of widowhood. The table suggests some decline

[23] See Dreze (1990) and Chen (1991b) for further discussion.

Table 9: *Primary occupations of households with widows before widowhood and at the time of the interview (1991)*

Primary Occupation	Number and Percentage of Households				Difference (%)
	Before widowhood		In 1991		
	No.	%	No.	%	
Cultivation	119	53	105	40	−13
Wage labour	52	23	63	24	+1
Salaried work	0	0	44	17	+17
Animal husbandry	21	10	16	6	−4
Self-employment	16	7	14	5	−2
Domestic service	0	0	10	4	+4
Caste services	13	6	7	3	−3
Trade	3	1	3	1	0
Total	224	100	262	100	0

Source: Chen (1991b). For thirty-eight widows, there is no information on primary household occupation before widowhood.

of self-employment (farm and non-farm) after widowhood, and, correspondingly, an increased reliance on wage employment, salaried work and domestic service. In fact, the shift away from cultivation is larger than Table 9 suggests, because 'cultivation' in that table includes leasing out land, and many widows resort to leasing out due to the difficulty of continuing cultivation after the death of a husband.

The impressive expansion of 'salaried work' between the period preceding widowhood and 1991 largely reflects recent changes in the occupational structure: notably, an increased number of low-level government jobs associated with an expansion of government programmes and an increase in the numbers commuting to local towns for salaried jobs. Further scrutiny of the data indicates that salaried work is primarily an occupation of adult sons of the widows in the sample (or other adult male members of their households), rather than of widows themselves. To the extent that widows do participate in salaried work, it is mainly in the form of part-time, low-paid employment in institutions such as village *balwadis*.

The extent of remunerative self-employment among widows living in households without an adult male turns out to be strikingly restricted. This finding, which confirms the results of an earlier study of North Indian widows (Drèze 1990), illustrates the employment restrictions that result from the gender division of labour and related social norms as well as from the disadvantages that widows face as participants in the rural economy.

4. The Social Isolation of Widows

The restrictions on residence, ownership, remarriage and employment examined in the preceding section put North Indian widows in a situation of acute dependence on economic support from others. In the absence of effective forms of state-based social security measures, community support is the crucial source of potential assistance.

The extent and nature of community support can be analysed in terms of three broad determinants: (1) living arrangements (the partitioning of the village community into different households); (2) inter-household support; and (3) intra-household distribution. We need to consider, in other words, why widows live with particular persons (e.g. whether they live with their parents, or with their in-laws, or on their own), what kind of support the household they live in obtains from other households, and what treatment a widow receives within her own household. Despite their obvious interrelations, these three issues can usefully be considered separately.

4.1. Living Arrangements

A number of interesting regularities can be discerned in available studies of the living arrangements of widows in rural North India.[24] One of the clearest and most important findings is the overwhelming dependence of widows on themselves and their own sons. More precisely, the proportion of widows who live in households headed either by themselves or by one of their sons is well over 80 per cent in most samples. The vast majority of these households belong to one of three types: single widows, 'nuclear' households (widows

---

[24]See Drèze (1990) for recent empirical evidence as well as a review of earlier studies, including those of Bose and Saxena (1964), Bose and Sen (1966), Marulasiddaiah (1969), Lal (1972), Shah (1974), Cain et al. (1979), Vatuk (1981), Cain (1986), Krishnakumari (1987) and Vlassoff (1990).

Table 10: Distribution of widows by type of household and identity of household head

Household Type	Identity of Household Head							
	Self		Son(s)		Other		Total	
	No.	%	No.	%	No.	%	No.	%
Single	31	12	0	0	0	0	31	12
Nuclear	31	12	4	2	0	0	35	13
Filial Stem	30	11	76	29	2	1	108	41
Filial Joint	12	5	22	8	0	0	34	13
Other	18	7	5	2	31	12	54	21
All Types	122	47	107	41	33	13	262	100

Source: Chen (1991b). The household types are defined in the text (see Drèze 1990, for further discussion). In this table, the 'filial households' category has been further divided into two sub-groups: in 'stem' households, a widow lives with *only one* married son, whereas 'joint' households contain several married sons.

living with their unmarried children), and 'filial' households (defined as households consisting of a widow, at least one of her married sons, and possibly other persons). Very few widows live with their in-laws, married daughters, parents, brothers or indeed any relatives other than their own sons or unmarried daughters and, possibly, the nuclear families of their married sons.

As can be seen from Table 10, these common patterns clearly emerge in our own sample. In this case, the proportion of widows living in households headed by themselves or one of their sons is as high as 87 per cent; as many as 208 out of these 229 households are of the 'single', 'nuclear' or 'filial' type. The last category accounts for over half of all the sample widows.

In line with the findings of a number of earlier studies, we observe that the number of widows sharing a hearth with their in-laws is particularly small (about 5 per cent). Further, in about half of the cases where a widow does live with her in-laws, it is the widow who supports the in-laws rather than the reverse. Some examples of this situation are the following: a blind, widowed mother-in-law living with her widowed daughter-in-law; and an elderly couple who refuse to let their widowed daughter-in-law remarry because she is their only source of support.

It is, of course, not easy to determine whether the separation of a widow from her in-laws usually reflects their refusal to support her, or her own reluctance to live with them. The latter motive may be quite common, given the reportedly frequent exposure of a widow to various forms of neglect and exploitation (including sexual harassment) when she lives with her in-laws as a dependant. The important point, however, is that very few widows have the opportunity of being happily and securely incorporated in their in-laws' household.

Widows living alone deserve particular attention. Earlier studies suggest that the proportion of widows in that situation varies a great deal between different communities, but may be around 10 per cent on average for rural North India (Drèze 1990). The proportion found in the study villages is very close to that figure—about 12 per cent. A majority of widows who live alone do not have any sons. This suggests that widows seldom live alone by choice (that is, despite having sons who are willing to look after them), or because their sons refuse to look after them.

Our findings on living arrangements, and their consistency with those of earlier studies, clearly invalidate the notion that a North Indian widow who does not have adult sons is typically re-integrated in the household of her in-laws, parents or other relatives. The consequences of this residential isolation depend on the extent to which widows can count on getting regular support through inter-household transfers. This issue is taken up in the next subsection.

4.2. Inter-household Support

The dichotomy between 'joint' and 'separate' living arrangements is a sharp one in rural North India. A group of people can either live 'together in the same household' (*sajhe* in Hindi, *bhega* in Gujarati, *ekotro* in Bengali), in which case the norm is that they should pool all their resources, or they can live 'separately' (*nyare* in Hindi, *juda* in Gujarati, *prithok* in Bengali), in which case solidarity gives way to economic independence and even sometimes rivalry. Separate households, even within kin-based networks, tend to maintain a relationship of 'balanced reciprocity', involving a strict mental accounting of the goods and services that flow from one household to another and a firm expectation that every transfer will be reciprocated at some stage. Except for some specific flows of goods and services tightly regulated by social norms (e.g. ritual gifts from brother to sister, or from a married woman's family to her in-laws), unreciprocated transfers between separate households tend to be few and far between. Our observations in the study village suggest that this general pattern applies even to widows, though perhaps in a somewhat less stringent form.

Table 11 presents some information on different forms and sources of support received by widows in different household types.[25] Unfortunately, data limitations prevent us from distinguishing here between intra-household and inter-household support; *both* are included in Table 11, and the entries in the table have to be interpreted accordingly. Specifically, inter-household support as such is bound to be more restricted than the percentages indicated in the table suggest. The information on household type, however, can be used to obtain an idea about the relative importance of inter-household and intra-household support in each case. The entries in bold-face, in particular, indicate cases where support is bound to be exclusively of the inter-household type (this would always apply, for instance to widows living alone). Similarly, in the case of 'filial' households, we can be confident that an overwhelming proportion of support from sons is of the intra-household rather than inter-household type. In interpreting Table 11, it should also be borne in mind that each widow in the sample may have reported more than one source or form of support.

Taking all widows together, Table 11 suggests that the extent of inter-household support is rather limited. While a large majority of widows do receive regular support from their sons, most of this support is of the intra-household rather than inter-household type. For each of the other sources of support (daughters, parents, brothers, in-laws and 'others'), at most 15 per cent of the sample widows report regular support. The extreme rarity of support from in-laws is particularly striking.

---

[25]We concentrate here on inter-household support to *widows*, rather than to *households* that include a widow. It is possible that some households receive inter-household support by virtue of the fact that they include a widow, even though this support may not be received by the widow herself. An example is the case where one among several sons of a widowed mother agrees to take care of her in return for the right to cultivate a larger share of the family land. In this section, however, we are concerned mainly with widows who head households (e.g. single widows, or widows living with young children), so that the distinction between support received by the household and by the widow herself is not particularly crucial.

Table 11: Percentage of widows reporting different forms and sources of support

		S	D	P	B	I	O
1.	Single						
	Regular food	32	10	0	10	3	32
	Periodic gifts	19	19	3	2	0	29
2.	Nuclear						
	Regular food	40	11	14	26	6	11
	Periodic gifts	20	20	23	34	3	17
3.	Filial						
	Regular food	96	2	0	2	1	5
	Periodic gifts	49	31	1	23	1	10
4.	Other						
	Regular food	20	19	17	43	17	31
	Periodic gifts	7	13	11	19	9	17
	ALL						
	Regular food	66	8	5	9	5	15
	Periodic gifts	33	24	6	23	3	15
	Periodic exchanges	3	1	0	1	6	60
	Periodic loans	1	1	0	2	2	49

Note: The column headings indicate the source of support. S = Sons; D = Daughters; P = Parents; B = Brothers; I = In-laws; O = Others
The row headings indicate the type of household in which the widow lives, and the type of support received.

Source: Chen 1991b.

Even periodic gifts (as opposed to regular support) appear to be quite infrequent for any particular support source. It is revealing, for instance, that less than one widow in four reports periodic gifts from her brothers, despite the traditionally supportive role which brothers are supposed to play in a Hindu woman's life (e.g. through gifts at the time of major festivals) even after her marriage.

Having said this, the extent of inter-household support is obviously not the same for widows living in different types of households, and there is some evidence that the more vulnerable widows are also those who receive more support. As Table 11 shows, regular support from persons other than sons is practically non-existent in the case of widows living with adult sons, but is more frequent for widows living alone or in nuclear households. The information presented is *compatible* with the notion that most of the widows in the latter categories do receive some inter-household support from one source or another. In a sense, this is as one would expect, since many of these widows might simply not be able to survive without some external support, given their restricted ability to engage in income-earning activities. On the other hand, it is doubtful whether, even for these widows, inter-household transfers often go beyond providing the bare minimum needed to ensure the survival of the concerned widow, or to enable the supporting person to feel that he or she has fulfilled his or her 'duty'. Informal evidence from the study villages suggests that substantial economic assistance on a sustained basis (e.g. in the form of regular cash transfers) is exceptional.

On the basis of discussions with the respondents, a little more can be said about the relationships that tend to exist between a widow and various relatives.

In-laws
Most widows in our sample expected very little support from their in-laws (Table 11 confirms that support from this source is particularly rare). In fact, in-laws were quite often perceived as a source of harassment rather than of support. Common forms of harassment include sexual demands and attempts to deprive a widow of her rightful share of the land. Similar conclusions regarding the strained relationship between a widow and her in-laws have been reached in many other studies.[26]

The fact that most widows live independently from their in-laws, receive very little support from them in the form of inter-household transfers, and perceive them primarily as a potential source of harassment, contradicts the common belief that the Indian widow continues to be assimilated in her husband's family

---

[26]See e.g. Harlan (1968), Sharma (1980:53–55), Bhave (1983), Lopamudra (1983), Saraswati (1985), Dak and Sharma (1987), Krishnakumari (1987), Gulati and Rajan (1988:74), Lingam (1988:9), Ghoshal (1989), Kumari (1989), Drèze (1990).

after his death.[27] In some communities, continued assimilation sometimes does occur in the form of an ascribed leviratic union, a practice that appears to be viewed with repulsion by many widows (Drèze 1990). The general rule, however, seems to be that in-laws cannot be counted on as a source of support. The notion that the 'joint family' provides protection to widows in rural India is little more than a myth.

Parents and Brothers

A widow's relationship with her parents and brothers is somewhat more subtle. On the one hand, the practice of patrilocal residence (discussed in section 3) severs most ties between a woman and her parental home. On the other hand, a married woman does not completely cease to be a daughter or a sister. Besides the bonds of personal affection and sentiment (sometimes strengthened, rather than lessened, by forced separation), her ties with her natal home are supported by certain residual rights. She is entitled to visit her parental home, to be present at various ritual and ceremonial occasions, to move to her natal home if taken ill or at the time of delivering a child, and to receive gifts. In the early years of a woman's married life, these ties are particularly strong. But as her children grow up, and as her parents and parents-in-law die, these ties with her natal home gradually weaken (Madan 1989).

A woman's relationship with her brothers, however, remains important long after her marriage. In her position as a father's sister, she has important ceremonial roles in the lives of her brother's children. Her brother, in turn, has important ceremonial roles to play in the lives of her children in his role as the mother's brother.

Further, a widowed daughter is widely perceived to be entitled, in principle, to maintenance in her natal home if she is childless and to support if she is needy.[28] Although few widows return to live in their natal home, and while their parents and brothers often feel that

---

[27]Even as eminent an anthropologist as Stanley Tambiah assumes that 'precisely because the Indian woman is incorporated into her husband's household and joint family, she enjoys greater economic security than her African counterpart when she becomes a widow' (Tambiah 1989:416).

[28]Widows, and women more generally, commonly state that they have relinquished their share of their father's land in return for the promise of maintenance and/or support should they be widowed, divorced or deserted. Sisters tie a protective cord around the wrist of their brother during the *rakhi* festival in the expectation that their brothers, in turn, will protect and support them in times of need.

their own poverty stands in the way of the traditional norms of support, many widows do seek some help from parents and especially brothers. If a widow is particularly needy (e.g. if she has no adult sons), her brother(s) may send her regular remittances. More commonly, widows receive the occasional gift, or an annual gift (e.g. on the occasion of Diwali) from their brothers. If parents are alive and able to help, they may also be an appreciable source of support, particularly in times of crisis.

Daughters

In Hindu North India, social norms severely restrict contacts between parents and married daughters, and particularly strong stigma is attached to the flow of goods or money from a married daughter to her parents. Even a widowed mother is not supposed to seek help from her married daughters.

In the course of our survey, we had many occasions to observe the continuing strength of these traditional norms. We also found, however, that daughters often did support their widowed mothers in ways that do not openly conflict with these norms. For instance, even if they are not able (for economic, cultural or other reasons) to provide material support in cash or in kind, many daughters who live close enough to their widowed mothers provide them with various services such as caring for them when they are ill, washing their hair or clothes, or helping them to maintain or repair their homes. The survey results suggest that, when a widowed mother falls ill, daughters are the most common source of physical care whereas sons are the most common source of financial help.

Others

Many widows are able to negotiate exchanges in kind (e.g. a small amount of food) from caste neighbours. If she works for, or is the client of, a wealthy patron, a widow may receive small gifts on a regular basis. If she is on good terms with an affluent neighbour, she may also receive the odd interest-free loan. Most of the time, however, a widow's household receives little help from the village community, and is expected to fend for itself like any other.

4.3. Intra-Household Distribution

According to the traditional norms of Hindu society in North India, the life of a widow is supposed to be austere in the extreme. Fortunately, the traditional austerities have lost much of their relevance for the majority of North Indian widows, even though they can still be encountered among the 'higher' castes. However, the needs of a dependent widow remain severely neglected in many households.[29]

It is plausible that intra-household inequalities play an important part in the causation of ill-health and high mortality among widows. In fact, expenditure and mortality data provide some indirect evidence in support of this hypothesis. On the one hand, taking together *all* households with a widow, we find that per capita expenditure levels for this group are not significantly lower than for households without a widow.[30] On the other hand, mortality levels have been found to be much higher among widows than among married women in the same age-groups (see section 2). These two observations would be difficult to reconcile with the notion that the health status of a widow reflects the economic status of the household she lives in. The most straightforward interpretation of these findings, in fact, is that the extent to which a woman's needs are met in a household with a given level of per capita expenditure is much lower when she is a widow than when she is a married woman.[31]

It might be added that, as was discussed in section 2, the mortality study (Rahman and Menken 1990; Rahman, Foster and Menken 1992) finds much lower mortality rates among widows who are reported to be the 'head' of the household than among widows living

[29]Some widows have a position of authority and influence in the household; e.g. widow heads of joint families. But in 'filial' households headed by a son, the daughter-in-law tends to gain the upper hand quite quickly in the competition for authority and influence.

[30] See Drèze (1990). This finding is based on National Sample Survey data for Karnataka (1977–78); the difference in per capita expenditure levels between households with and without widows may be somewhat larger in North India than in this South Indian state.

[31]A complementary explanation could be that the incidence of poverty among households with a widow is much greater than among households without a widow, despite similar average per capita expenditure levels, due to high levels of economic inequality within the former group. The incidence of poverty may well be quite high in this group, bearing in mind that it includes a significant proportion of vulnerable households (e.g. widows with small children). However, it would be implausible to attribute all or even most of the observed contrast between expenditure and mortality data to this factor: such an attribution would imply amazingly high levels of mortality among the poorer widow-inclusive households.

as dependants in other households of a similar type (see Table 1). This finding, too, is consistent with the notion that intra-household inequalities are an important cause of high mortality rates among widows.

The literature on intra-household inequalities in rural India has, so far, concentrated mainly on the question of male-female divisions, especially those between young boys and girls. In this context, three possible determinants of intra-household inequalities have been widely discussed: (1) the 'return' which the decision-maker(s) might expect to obtain from allocating consumption to different individuals in the household; (2) the perception of what different members of the household 'deserve' to receive; and (3) the 'bargaining power' possessed by different household members engaged in a relation of cooperative conflict.[32]

Whether return, desert or bargaining power (or a combination of these) is the relevant determinant of household inequalities, one would not expect a dependent widow to receive a favourable treatment within the household. The return which a household head might hope to obtain from better treatment of a widow would, at best, take the form of improved domestic services such as child care. The perception of what a widow deserves is not likely to be very high when she is seen as an 'unproductive' dependant. And the bargaining power of a widow who lives in a situation of extreme dependence on support from other household members would also be typically very low. In these circumstances, the temptation for those who maintain a dependent widow is to confine their support to what is required by the unexacting demands of 'duty'.

The basic problem is not only that a widow often depends on other household members to survive, but also that these other household members typically *do not depend on her* for anything essential. Each of the three approaches mentioned above suggests that a widow who can contribute something important to the household (e.g. a widow who owns land, or who earns a pension, or who is gainfully employed) is much less likely to be exposed to

---

[32]On these different approaches, see Drèze and Sen (1989: Chapter 4), and the literature cited there. Note that return and desert can be important whether household decisions are seen to be taken by one maximizing individual (the household 'head') or whether they are seen as the outcome of a cooperative conflict (in which case return and desert can be regarded as particular determinants of bargaining power).

neglect than a widow who is regarded as unproductive. This observation implies, *inter alia*, that more secure property rights could play an important role in enhancing the living conditions of widows in rural India.[33] We shall return to this point in the concluding section.

These broad remarks only scratch the surface of the problem of intra-household treatment of widows, and we should not conclude without warning against the simplifications they have involved. Ultimately, the treatment a widow receives is the outcome of a decision-making process (or cooperative conflict) that is a good deal more complex than with the familiar male-female inequalities. When a widow lives with one of her married sons, for instance, the relationships between the widow and her son, between her son and his wife, and between daughter-in-law and mother-in-law could all have an important influence on intra-household distribution. These relationships are affected by factors such as duty, affection, and authority, in a way that need not fit easily into the familiar analyses based on return, desert or bargaining power. The outcome can be anything between the widowed mother taking the role of a tyrannical household head to her being at the mercy of an uncaring daughter-in-law. While there are good general arguments to explain why widows are often observed to be in a situation of vulnerability and neglect, it is also important to understand how, in some circumstances, they manage to escape that predicament. These are useful directions in which to expand the study of intra-household inequalities in rural India.

4.4. Mothers and Sons

As we saw earlier in this section, a majority of Indian widows live with one or several of their adult sons, and this living arrangement is the main form of community support they receive. The relationship between a widowed mother and her son(s) is therefore of particular importance. Some aspects of this relationship are already covered by the preceding discussion of intra-household distribution, but one particular feature deserves further attention.

---

[33] Quite a few empirical studies mention that ownership of land or other assets considerably enhance the status, treatment or bargaining power of the aged (including widows) within the household. See e.g. Harlan (1968:474), Marulasiddaiah (1969:117), Raj and Prasad (1971:156-8), Cain et al. (1979:7), Bhave (1983:6), Dak and Sharma (1987:49, 54), Wadley (n.d.). As one old man bluntly put it, 'without property, children do not look after their parents well' (cited in Caldwell et al. 1988:191).

In rural North India, the norm of co-residence of a widowed mother with at least one of her sons is still very strong. If a widow has only one son, he is not likely to take the risk of inviting the resentment of the community by rejecting this basic norm, even if this living arrangement is problematic in one way or another (e.g. because of tensions between the widow and her daughter-in-law). The same applies when a widow has several sons living together, though this is not a very common situation since the patrifraternal joint family tends to get partitioned quite rapidly after the death of the patriarch. If a widow has several sons living separately, however, the norm of co-residence loses some of its strength, since there is the possibility of each son relying on the others to look after his widowed mother.[34]

Some communities have evolved systematic ways of dealing with this potential 'free-riding' problem, for instance through the further norm that the *youngest* son should take care of his elderly parents or widowed mother (with, possibly, a standard compensation for this extra burden being provided to this son in the form of ownership of the parental house, or of a small piece of land earmarked to the subsistence needs of the parents). Otherwise, the sons may agree on a particular way to share the extra economic burden of supporting their widowed mother, e.g. by taking turns at maintaining her for a limited period of time. But these arrangements are not entirely reliable, and can break down in a number of ways; for instance, a youngest son may migrate and leave his widowed mother to be looked after by his reluctant brothers, and brothers with very unequal earning abilities may quarrel about what a fair arrangement for supporting their mother might be. The arrangements in question seem to be particularly fragile in times of hardship such as a succession of drought years, when the temptation to rely on one's brothers to take care of a widowed mother can be particularly strong.[35] In the study villages, there are several cases of a widow living on her own (often with little support from others) despite having adult sons.

[34]There is a clear allusion to this situation in the popular Bengali saying '*bhaager ma Ganga paae na*', which can be literally translated as 'a shared mother does not even get holy water' and is used in diverse contexts to refer to the problem of 'free-riding'.
[35]See Drèze (1990) and Chen (1991a) for further discussion, and some empirical evidence from drought-affected villages in Gujarat.

Having said this, it is important to note that, in some circumstances, the existence of a plurality of sources of filial support can be turned to the *advantage* of a widowed mother. More precisely, if a widowed mother is in possession of some valuable asset (e.g. a piece of land, or a pension that enables her to make some contribution to the household's income over and above the cost of her own subsistence) her sons may look at co-residence with her as an advantage rather than a burden. As a result, she is very likely to be securely integrated in the household of one of her adult sons. The credible threat of leaving the household to join one of her other sons may even strengthen her bargaining power within that household and ensure her good treatment.[36] Here again, what can make a crucial difference is the ability of a widow to gain recognition as a person who contributes to the household economy, rather than being seen as an unwelcome liability.

5. Selected Contrasts: The Influence of Caste

So far, we have concentrated on identifying common patterns in the predicament of widows in North India. A more refined analysis would also have to investigate the diversities associated with factors such as caste, class, age or area of residence. A detailed investigation of this kind is clearly beyond the scope of this paper, but the contrasts involved may be briefly illustrated with reference to the particular issue of caste.

5.1. The Sanskritization Process

There are major differences in gender relations among different castes in North India. These differences are particularly pronounced between the two poles of the caste hierarchy: at one end, the highly 'Sanskritized' upper castes; and, at the other, the so-called 'Untouchables' or scheduled castes.

Social restrictions on the life-styles of women tend to become more rigid as one moves up in the caste hierarchy. For instance, there is more seclusion of females among upper castes than among lower castes. Within upper-caste communities in North India, women are often strictly secluded and denied access to gainful employment

---

[36]This situation is not just a theoretical possibility. See Dreze (1990) and Chen (1991b) for some empirical illustrations from the study villages.

outside their homes. By contrast, lower-caste women have greater freedom to take up gainful employment. Among the many castes which constitute the vast 'middle' of the caste hierarchy, what is considered appropriate behaviour or work for women is closely linked with the family's position (both ascribed and aspired) in the social-status hierarchy (Bardhan 1985).

When particular caste groups acquire wealth, or aspire to higher status for some other reason, they often try to distance themselves from households perceived to be lower in social status by emulating the practices of higher-status households. Different terms have been used to describe this imitation of upper castes by lower castes. The most common term is 'Sanskritization', arising from the fact that certain Vedic or Sanskritic rites are confined to the upper castes. Other common terms, based on the identity of the group being imitated, are 'Brahminization' and 'Rajputization'.[37] The point here is not to argue for one term or another, but to note the 'strength of the tendency to imitate and also the main direction of the tendency' (Dumont 1980:192).

This process of imitation has very specific implications for women in general and for widows in particular. Indeed, one of the prominent forms it takes is the adoption of upper-caste norms regarding marriage and the behaviour of women. These include (1) the prohibition or disapproval of widow remarriage, and (2) the withdrawal of women from the labour market.

5.2. Sanskritization and the Life-style of Widows

Among some middle-caste groups which used to allow widow remarriage, there is an emerging trend towards prohibiting or discouraging this 'disreputable' practice, as a means to achieving higher social status. An influence in the reverse direction arises from 'modernization', social reform movements and the erosion of traditional

[37]The notion of Sanskritization is perhaps best presented in the words of M. N. Srinivas, who popularized the concept: 'The caste system is far from a rigid system in which the position of each component caste is fixed for all time. Movement has always been possible, and especially so in the middle regions of the hierarchy. A low caste was able to rise to a higher position in the hierarchy by adopting vegetarianism and teetotalism, and by "Sanskritizing" its ritual and pantheon. In short, it took over as far as possible, the customs, rites and beliefs of the Brahmins, and the adoption of the Brahminical way of life by a low caste seems to have been frequent, though theoretically forbidden. This process has been called "Sanskritization" in this book.' (Srinivas 1952: 30).

values. Under this influence, some castes have liberalized their attitude towards widow remarriage (Madan 1989). In the study villages, however, the trend towards more widespread prohibition against widow remarriage is noticeably stronger than the trend towards increased tolerance.

As far as labour force participation is concerned, a large number of widows—especially those who head households—are caught between the contradictory demands of Sanskritization and survival. On the one hand, caste norms confine them to their homesteads; on the other, they need to work in order to provide for their families. This dilemma applies particularly to poor widows belonging to an upper caste or a status-aspiring group. It is especially acute for widows with insufficient male support to meet subsistence needs, and during the period of hardship that often follows the sudden loss of a husband. The plight of widows in this predicament is not enviable: if they enter the labour force, they risk scorn, censure, and (sometimes) excommunication from their kin or caste group; if they do not seek gainful employment, their families may have to endure extreme deprivation.

In the study villages, there are marked differences in the restrictions that apply to widow remarriage and women's work among upper and lower castes. Almost uniformly, upper castes prohibit widow remarriage and do not allow women to seek gainful employment outside the household. By contrast, scheduled castes permit widows to remarry and women to seek gainful employment wherever it is available. The large number of castes which form the middle part of the hierarchy can be divided into those which aspire to higher status and imitate upper-caste norms and those which still follow lower-caste norms.

Tables 12 and 13 bring out some of these contrasts. Out of a total of 275 ever-widowed women in the eight study villages, only 36 had remarried, of which 29 were from scheduled or 'lower-middle' castes. Only six out of 95 upper-caste widows reported being engaged in wage labour, whereas a large percentage of 'lower-middle' caste widows, and an even larger percentage of scheduled-caste widows, reported wage labour as an economic activity. Further, whereas five scheduled-caste widows reported being engaged in self-employment or trade outside their village of residence, only one other widow (from a 'higher-middle' caste) reported this activity.

Table 12: *Distribution of ever-widowed women, by current marital status and caste group*

Caste Group	Not Remarried	Remarried		% of Remarried Widows to Ever-widowed
		Currently Widowed	Currently Married	
Upper Castes	91	4	2	6
Middle Castes:				
Higher	31	0	1	3
Lower	57	9	6	21
Scheduled Castes	58	10	4	19
Others	2	0	0	0
Total	239	23	13	13

Note: All six cases of widow remarriage in the upper castes are cases of leviratic union, mainly among the Rajputs in the U.P. Hills.
Source: Chen (1991b). The 'middle castes' group has been divided into the 'higher' and 'lower' sub-groups on the basis of local rankings in the study villages.

Table 13: *Percentage of widows engaged in different activities, by caste group*

Economic Activity	Upper Castes	Middle Castes		Scheduled Castes
		Higher	Lower	
Cultivation	52	13	53	31
Wage Labour:				
Farm	2	0	20	50
Non-Farm	3	0	5	24
Migrant	1	0	2	6
Animal husbandry	23	0	2	0
Self-employment:				
In village	4	3	8	9
Outside village	0	3	0	6
Caste services	0	0	6	9
Trade:				
In village	0	0	5	1
Outside village	0	0	0	1

Note: Each entry in the table shows the percentage of widows from the relevant caste group who reported the indicated activity. Some widows reported more than one activity, and some reported none.
Source: Chen (1991b).

One general lesson emerging from all this is that widows have to be treated as individuals, rather than simply as members of particular social groups (e.g. a caste or a class). While upper castes generally have a privileged social and economic status, for instance, the same does not necessarily apply to the upper-caste widow. In fact, an upper-caste widow who has no adult sons to support her and who is nonetheless prevented by caste norms from seeking gainful employment may be just as deprived as a scheduled-caste widow who does not experience these restrictions. Patterns linking the living conditions of a widow to her caste status do exist, but these patterns can be quite different from those that might apply to other members of the society.

6. Concluding Remarks

The North Indian widow tends to be a highly marginalized person. She typically receives very little support from persons other than her own children, and even when she lives with one or several of her adult sons she remains highly vulnerable to neglect (section 4). Further, her ability to engage in income-earning activities of her own is severely restricted, partly due to various patriarchal norms such as patrilineal inheritance and the division of labour by gender (section 3). The consequences of this social and economic marginalization are manifest, as far as one can tell from the limited evidence available, in poor health and high mortality levels (section 2).

The marginalization of widows in North India is consistent with the traditional perception of Hindu widows as inauspicious and potentially suspect women who, ideally, should lead a life of austerity devoted to the memory of their husband. This ideological influence, however, may be less crucial than the simple fact that widows are often seen as an economic burden. The most effective way of ensuring the social protection of Indian widows is perhaps to help them to be recognized as persons who have something important to contribute to the household economy, e.g. by protecting their property rights or by promoting their economic activities.

If we bring up this general observation in this concluding section, it is because, in the field of social security, 'incentives' are often seen—quite rightly—as a major issue. When it comes to the social protection of widows, the most important incentive effect to consider would be the possibility that state-based social security measures might 'displace' whatever support widows receive from the community. This problem should not be lightly dismissed, and it is easy to think of particular measures that are likely to have precisely that effect.[38] However, it is also important to recognize and make use of the potential complementarities that exist between state support and community support. A major source of such complementarity, discussed on several occasions in section 4, is the fact that a widow who has some economic resourcefulness of her own may well be less exposed to residential isolation and intra-household discrimination.

We have not explored, in this paper, the particular strategies that could be devised to support the livelihood of widows in rural India. The provision of pensions, the protection of land rights and the promotion of gainful employment are obvious possibilities, but the diversity of constraints that restrict the life-style of widows in rural North India also suggests that many other avenues of action can be pursued. A detailed discussion of the feasibility and desirability of alternative measures would require a study of its own, which we do hope to undertake on another occasion.[39] At this stage, our concern is mainly to contribute to a better awareness and understanding of this severely neglected problem. This is a prerequisite of effective action in this field.

Indeed, the government is unlikely to give adequate priority to the social protection of widows in rural India in the absence of public pressure. Further, an effective implementation of state-based social security measures may require a great deal of activism on the part of non-government institutions, including the women's movement. In fact, there is already a substantial scope for improving the living conditions of widows even within the existing parameters of state involvement.

This point may be illustrated with reference to the issue of pensions. In most states of India, pension schemes of some kind do exist on paper, but, with the notable exception of Kerala, they have a negligible coverage and impact. The reasons include bureaucratic indifference, inadequate financial provisions,

---

[38]For instance, a pension scheme that disqualifies widows who live with their adult sons could have the effect of discouraging the integration of a widowed mother in the household of one of her adult sons.

[39]For preliminary discussions of the scope for social security measures based on the provision of pensions, the protection of land rights and the promotion of gainful employment, see Drèze (1990) and Chen (1991b).

Table 14: Widows who never applied, applied but did not receive, and received pensions (by caste)

Status of Pension	Upper Castes		Other Castes				Scheduled Castes		Others		Total	
			Upper		Lower							
	No.	%	No.	%	No.	%	No.	%	No.	%	No.	%
Never applied	62	65	26	84	38	58	57	84	1	50	184	70
Did not receive	20	21	5	16	24	36	9	13	0	0	58	22
Received	13	14	0	0	4	6	2	3	1	50	20	8
Total	95	100	31	100	66	100	68	100	2	100	262	100

Source: Chen (1991b).

widespread corruption and limited public awareness of the opportunities involved. In the study villages, only 20 widows out of 262 reported receiving a pension, while another 58 unsuccessfully applied (see Table 14 for details). Of the 20 widows who do receive a pension, 13 are upper-caste friends of the village headman or of some other influential village elder; and three live with married sons, a fact which, according to the rules, makes them ineligible for a pension. Much can be done without delay to bring about a more ambitious, efficient and equitable implementation of these pension schemes.[40]

Similar observations apply with reference to land rights. According to the Hindu Succession Act of 1956, which is still applicable today, all the 'legal heirs' of a deceased person are entitled to equal shares of his or her property. The legal heirs, in the case of a married man, consist of his widow, his sons, daughters, and widowed mother (if he has one). As was discussed in section 3, however, these legal provisions are comprehensively violated in North India. Helping widows to assert and defend their basic property rights is another field where much can be achieved through public activism within the existing legal and policy framework, without waiting for the initiative and goodwill of the state.

We should like to conclude with a methodological remark. There is something quite astonishing about the fact that the needs of tens

---

[40] For an actual example of how collective action (led, in this instance, by widows themselves) can succeed in bringing about a radical change in the implementation of pension schemes, see Drèze (1990). See also Gulati (1990) and Nair and Tracy (1989) on Kerala's Agricultural Workers' Pension Scheme.

of millions of widows have been so consistently neglected in more than 45 years of planned economic development. The reasons for this neglect would be worth probing. One of them, evidently, is the fact that the deprivations of widows are so well hidden in economic and social statistics as they are commonly reported. The standard household-level economic variables, in particular, tell us very little about the well-being of widows as individuals. On the other hand, a careful examination of mortality data of the type reported in section 2.2 does succeed in capturing many important aspects of the problem. More generally, the combination of economic analysis with detailed information on mortality, morbidity, anthropometry and other indicators that focus on the person (as opposed to the household) has some clear advantages in this context. This is a useful direction in which to expand the informational and analytical bases of development policy and public debate.

References

Agarwal, B. 1988. 'Who Sows? Who Reaps? Women and Land Rights in India', *Journal of Peasant Studies*, 15(4):531–81.
Bardhan, K. 1985. 'Women's work, Welfare, and Status: Forces of Tradition and Change in India', *Economic and Political Weekly*, 20(50) and 20(51)
Bhat, M. and R. Kanbargi. 1984. 'Estimating the Incidence of Widow and Widower Re-Marriages in India from Census Data', *Population Studies*, 38:89–103.
Bhave, S. 1983. 'Women-headed Households in India: A Micro-study from an Indian Slum', Paper presented at the Expert Group Meeting on Forward-Looking Startegies for the Advancement of Women, ESCAP, Bangkok, December 1983.
Bose, A. B. and P. C. Saxena. 1964. 'Characteristics of Aged Population in Rural Society', *Journal of Family Welfare*, 104:33–39.
Bose, A. B. and M.L.A. Sen. 1966. 'Some Characteristics of the Widows in Rural Society', *Man in India*, 463:226–32.
Boserup, Ester. 1970. *Women's Role in Economic Development*. New York: St. Martin's Press.
Burra, N. 1986a. 'Child Labour in India: Poverty, Exploitation and Vested Interest', Social Action, 36:241–63.
_____. 1986b. 'Glass Factories of Firozabad', *Economic and Political Weekly*, 15 November (pp. 1983–85) and 22 November (pp. 2033–36).
Cain, M., S. R. Khanam, and S. Nahar. 1979. 'Class, Patriarchy and the Structure of Women's Work in Rural Bangladesh', Centre for Policy Studies Working Paper No. 43, Population Council.
Cain, Mead. 1986. 'The Consequences of Reproductive Failure: Dependence, Mobility, and Mortality among the Elderly in Rural South Asia', *Population Studies*, 40:375–88.

_____.1985. 'The Fate of the Elderly in South Asia: Implications for Fertility', Paper presented at an IUSSP International Conference, Florence.

_____.1983. 'Fertility as an Adjustment to Risk', *Population and Development Review*, 94:688–702.

_____.1981. 'Risk and Insurance: Perspectives on Fertility and Agrarian Change in India and Bangladesh', *Population and Development Review*, 73: 435–74.

Caldwell, J. C., P. H. Reddy and P. Caldwell. 1988. *The Causes of Demographic Change*. Madison: University of Wisconsin Press.

Chen, Martha. 1991a. *Coping with Seasonality and Drought*. New Delhi: Sage Publications.

_____.1991b. 'Widows in Rural India'. Report submitted to World Institute for Development Economics Research, Helsinki.

Chen, Martha, and Jean Drèze. (1994). 'Widows in India: Conference Report', mimeo, Harvard Institute of International Development; submitted to *Economic and Political Weekly* for publication.

Dak, T.M. and M.L. Sharma. 1987. 'Changing Status of the Aged in North Indian Villages' in *Aging in India: Challenge for the Society*, M.L. Sharma and T.M. Dak (eds.). New Delhi: Ajanta.

Drèze, Jean. 1990. 'Widows in Rural India'. DEP Paper No. 26, Development Economics Research Programme, London School of Economics.

Drèze, Jean and Amartya Sen. 1989. *Hunger and Public Action*. Oxford: Oxford University Press.

Dumont, Louis. 1980. *Homo Hierarchicus: The Caste System and Its Implications*. Complete Revised English Edition. Chicago: The University of Chicago Press.

Ghoshal, N. 1989. 'Socio-Economic Profile of the Widows in Varanasi City'. Unpublished dissertation, Department of Sociology. Varanasi: Vasant Kanya Mahavidyalaya.

Government of India. *Census of India 1981*.

Gulati, L. 1990. 'Agricultural Workers' Pension in Kerala: An Experiment in Social Assistance', *Economic and Political Weekly*, 10 February (pp. 339–43).

_____. 1991. 'The Female Dimension of Population Aging in Kerala State in India', Paper presented at the Expert Group Meeting on Integration of Aging and Elderly Women into Development, Vienna, 7–11 October.

Gulati, L. and S.I. Rajan. 1988. 'Population Aspects of Aging in Kerala', Mimeo, Trivandrum, Kerala: Centre for Development Studies.

_____. 1991. 'Population Aspects of Aging in Kerala, India: Their Economic and Social Context', Paper prepared for the Population Division, United Nations. Trivandrum, Kerala: Centre for Development Studies.

Harlan, W.H. 1968. 'Social Status of the Aged in Three Indian Villages', *Vita Humana*, 7:239–52.

Krishnakumari, N.S. 1987. *Status of Single Women in India: A Study of Spinsters, Widows, and Divorcees*. New Delhi: Uppal Publishing House.

Kumari, R. 1989. *Women-Headed Households in Rural India*. London: Sangam.

Lal, S. 1972. 'Some Characteristics of the Widows in Rural Society', *Rural India*, 359:205–208.

Lingam, Lakshmi. 1988. 'Women-Headed Households: Coping with Caste, Class and Gender Hierarchies', Paper presented at the 13th National Science Congress, New Delhi, 14–18 November.

Lopamudra. 1983. 'The Plight of Widows', *Social Welfare*, 2910:13–15.
Madan, T.N. 1989. *Family and Kinship: A Study of the Pandits of Rural Kashmir*. Second Enlarged Edition. Delhi: Oxford University Press.
Marulasiddaiah, H.M. 1969. *Old People of Makunti*. Dharwar: Karnataka University.
Miller, Barbara D. 1981. *The Endangered Sex: Neglect of Female Children in Rural North India*. Ithaca: Cornell University Press.
Mukherjee, N. 1991. 'Villagers' Perception of Rural Poverty through the Mapping Technique of PRA', Mimeo, London School of Economics.
_____. 1992. 'Perceptions of Poverty and Well Being: Local Views and Natural Resource Policies', Mimeo, London School of Economics.
Nandwana, Shobha and Ramesh Nandwana. 1992. 'Land Rights of Widows: A case-study from Rajasthan', Report prepared for current study on 'Widows in Rural India' (Chen 1991b).
Nair, S.B. and M. Tracey. 1989. 'Pensions for Women in the Third World: A Case Study of Kerala, India', *International Journal of Contemporary Sociology*, 26:175–87.
Potash, B., ed. 1986. *Widows in African Societies*. Stanford: Stanford University Press.
Rahman, M. Omar. 1990. 'Gender Differences in Marriage and Mortality for the Elderly in Rural Bangladesh', Paper submitted as part of Ph.D. thesis to Department of Epidemiology, Harvard School of Public Health.
Rahman, M. Omar and Jane Menken. 1990. 'The Impact of Marital Status and Living Arrangements on Old Age Female Mortality in Rural Bangladesh', Paper presented at the Population Association of America Meetings, Toronto.
Rahman, Omar, Andrew Foster and Jane Menken. 1992. 'Older Widow Mortality in Rural Bangladesh', *Social Science and Medicine*, 34(1): 89–96.
Raj, B. and B.G. Prasad. 1971. 'A study of Rural Aged Persons in Social Profile', *Indian Journal of Social Work*, 32:155–62.
Saraswati, B. 1985. 'The Kashivasi Widows', *Man in India*, 652:107–20.
Shah, A.M. 1974. *The Household Dimension of the Family in India*. Berkeley and Los Angeles: University of California Press.
Sharma, Ursula. 1980. *Women, Work and Property in North-West India*. London: Tavistock.
Srinivas, M.N. 1952. *Religion and Society Among the Coorgs of South India*. Oxford: Oxford University Press.
Tambiah, S.J. 1989. 'Bridewealth and Dowry Revisited', *Current Anthropology*, 304:413–35.
Vatuk, S. 1981. 'Old Age in India' in *Old Age in Preindustrial Society*, Stearns, P.N. (ed.). New York: Holmes and Meier.
Verma, V.S. 1988. *A Handbook of Population Statistics*. New Delhi: Office of the Registrar General.
Vlassoff, C. 1990. 'The Value of Sons in an Indian Village: How Widows See It', *Population Studies*, 441:5–20.
Vlassoff, M. and C. Vlassoff. 1980. 'Old Age Security and the Utility of Children in Rural India', *Population Studies*, 343:487–99.
Wadley, S. n.d. 'Widows: Forced Independence for Some', Paper presented at a Symposium on Widowhood, Remarriage, Divorce and Dowry in India, University of Toronto.
Weiner, M. 1991. *The Child and the State in India: Child Labor and Education Policy in Comparative Perspective*. Delhi: Oxford University Press.

10

The Indian Woman in Later Life: Some Social and Cultural Considerations

SYLVIA VATUK

When one reviews the very extensive body of scholarly literature on South Asian women that has been produced over the past two decades, it is remarkable how little detailed attention seems to have been given to the later years of life. Discussions of women's roles in India typically take little account of the way that these roles change over time, with changes in age, marital, parental and grandparental status. Indeed, a life-course perspective, such as provides the framework for the present volume, is regrettably rare in the literature on women in non-Western cultures generally. As Lamb has put it,

by assuming that participation in reproduction, motherhood, and the household is everywhere central to cultural constructions of what it is to be a 'woman', we freeze women in one stage of their lives—as sexually active and reproductive wives and mothers (1993:334).

Most accounts of the social and cultural context of Indian women's lives place women largely within the family setting, and take the point of view of the young adult woman, especially in the period before and immediately after marriage and during the early childbearing years. Discussions of women's social roles in India almost invariably focus upon issues related to the situation of the young wife and mother in a male-dominated family and social system. For example, anthropologists have written fairly extensively about such topics as the consequences for the young married woman of patrilineal descent and inheritance and patrilocal residence, about the difficult adjustment of the new bride to her conjugal joint family, the ideology of *pativrata* and its consequences for husband-wife relations in the early years of marriage, the enforcement of standards of female modesty and seclusion, the pressure placed upon young women to bear a son, and so on.[1] Recently much attention has also been drawn by scholars, activists, and the popular press to some of the serious abuses suffered by young girls and recently married women in India, especially sex-selective mortality in childhood and in the childbearing years, and violence against women, especially in the context of dowry disputes.

If older women figure at all in these discussions, it is usually in their role as villain of the piece for the young women upon whom the writers' concern is concentrated.[2] Older women—as mothers and, especially, as mothers-in-law—are described as key agents for the enforcement of 'patriarchal' social norms, socializing their daughters to accept a subordinate status, oppressing their sons' wives by forcing them to overwork and denying them adequate nutrition, insisting upon adherence to stringent standards of modesty and confinement to the home, trying to prevent the establishment of intimacy between the young couple, interfering in their reproductive decisions, and, in extreme cases of dowry abuse, even contributing to their deaths.

Seldom have scholars attempted to fathom the complexities of the older woman's lot, to try to explain her motivations, or to assess the legitimacy of the goals she is engaged in pursuing within this culturally standardized family drama. To the extent that these questions are addressed at all, the harsh treatment of the daughter-in-law by the mother-in-law is often simplistically interpreted, for example as a means by which the older woman seeks to inflict upon another what was done to her a generation before, or as a manifestation of the co-optation of women by the male-dominated system, or of a gradual process by which they come to acquiesce in their own oppression, internalize the ideology of their male oppressors and accept the role of enforcing it.

Many observers have noted that the new daughter-in-law often presents—in the mother-in-law's eyes—a serious threat to the hard-

---

[1] There is by now an enormous body of literature on these subjects. Two works that present good overviews of the place of women within the South Asian family structure are Jacobson and Wadley (1977) and Bennett (1983).
[2] Notable exceptions are Roy (1975) and Lamb (1993).

won relationship of intimacy and interdependence she has developed over the years with her son. This relationship is in many ways the most important relationship she is involved in, and she perceives its continuance as crucial to her future survival. The triangle of mother, son and son's wife has been explored to some extent by psychologically-oriented anthropologists and psychoanalysts, but again primarily from the perspective of the younger generation, and often with a focus on the male member of the group.[3] This focus on the male reflects a more general pattern in the literature: interest in the intricacies of the Indian male psyche and its development has so far outstripped scholarly interest in the female. We have numerous analyses of the traumas experienced in early childhood by the young boy, who in adult life finds himself torn between the contradictory demands of mother and wife for his exclusive attention, intimacy and loyalty. Here again, the older woman tends to be seen as a part of her son's problem, rather than as a central actor demanding of analytic attention for her own sake.

Only in the literature on widowhood in India is there some attempt to view with sympathy and concern the situation of a category of women into which fall the majority of those who are over the age of 60.[4] Widowhood is a state in which almost all women spend at least some portion of their lives if they live much beyond this age. However, all widows are not old, and there is considerable evidence that it is women who are widowed in their youth (and do not remarry) who suffer the greatest social disabilities. It is they who are at greatest risk, relative to their married peers, of poor nutrition and health, not to mention social marginalization, psychological mistreatment and emotional distress. Understandably, the fate of virgin widows and those left with the sole responsibility of supporting and raising minor children have attracted the most scholarly and welfare concern. In recent decades, with a rising age at marriage for women and reduced mortality for men in early adulthood, women widowed at a young age are of course a continually declining

---

[3]See, for example, Roy (1975), Kakar (1978), Kurtz (1992), Dhruvarajan (1989), Roland (1988).

[4]See, for example, Drèze (1990), Ullrich (1988), Tapper (1979), Vlassoff (1990), and Chen and Drèze in this volume. According to the 1981 census, 64.3 per cent of the over 60 female population was widowed. This proportion has been declining steadily in recent decades; in 1961 the corresponding figure was 75.4 (Sharma and Xenos 1992:43).

segment of the total widowed population.[5] Yet even a recent excellent and comprehensive report on widowhood in rural India does not consistently consider age, parental status, or the phase of the life-cycle during which the individual became a widow, when making generalizations about the kinds and extent of disabilities and risks to which Indian widows are exposed (Drèze 1990).[6]

The widespread absence of discussions of the older woman in the recent anthropological, sociological and psychological literature on women in India is especially surprising in view of the rapid growth of scholarly interest in social gerontology over the same period. There is increasing awareness among Indian social scientists that the Indian population is 'ageing' at an unprecedented rate and that even today the absolute number of elderly persons, if not their percentage in the total population, is enormous. Therefore the economic, health and social problems of older people in India are beginning to be recognized as deserving of special attention and amelioration. Most of the research in this field is either demographic—using aggregate national or state-level data—or sociological; studies of the latter kind are for the most part based on data from sample surveys.[7] What has come out of this body of research is unfortunately much more informative about the situation of older men than of older women. Many of the published social surveys have indeed not even included women in their samples; this is in part a consequence of the popularity of studies of government pensioners, who are, of course, overwhelmingly male (see Desai and Naik 1975, Soodan 1975, Bhatia 1983, Jagannadham and Palvia 1978). Even those gerontological studies that provide data on both sexes rarely go beyond noting certain obvious gender differences—such as the fact that old men

---

[5] For example, whereas in 1961 7.9 per cent of rural widows were under the age of 35, in 1981 the corresponding percentage was only 5.0 (Drèze 1990:28A).

[6] It would be useful, in the context of trying to assess comparatively the factors affecting the well-being of widows, to be able to separate out those widowed early in life from those widowed in late middle age or old age, who are likely to have sons who are already adult and in a position to provide some material and social support. This is not possible with census figures, but should be possible with data from micro-level studies.

[7] See Vatuk (1991) for a review of some of the most recent literature in this field. Useful overviews of the current status of the elderly in India—from a largely demographic perspective—are to be found in Martin (1990), Roy (1987), and Sharma and Xenos (1992). See also the interdisciplinary collections of essays on ageing in India edited by Biswas (1987) and Bose and Gangrade (1988).

tend to be married and living with a younger spouse whereas old women are predominantly widowed. They rarely consider in any depth the significance of the gender variable. Thus there is a puzzling failure of the two most rapidly growing social science fields in India—women's studies and social gerontology—to intersect intellectually in any meaningful way.

The Older Woman and the Life Course

When considering how a woman's social position changes as she grows older, the most useful framework is one of the stages of the life course, defined in terms of the family roles successively occupied from birth to death. Chronological age does not have great significance for most Indian women, even when they know their exact age, as many do not. And while physical signs of ageing—like greying of the hair, loss of teeth, and cessation of menstruation, for example—are of course recognized and provide visible markers of the passage of years, transitions related to the developmental cycle of the family are much more important in defining the major periods of a woman's life.

For the typical woman in India, the especially critical points of transition from one life stage to the next are her marriage (and departure from the natal home), the birth of children, their marriages (and the associated departures of daughters and arrival of daughters-in-law), the birth of grandchildren (especially the children of sons), and the death of her husband. These are events that the great majority of Indian women experience, and normally in this order. Other events whose occurrence (or non-occurrence) and timing are more individually variable include births, marriages and deaths of other members of a woman's extended family. Non-demographic events, such as the formal partition of the joint household, or the addition of new members for reasons other than birth or marriage, also precipitate crucial life course transitions.

Three broad periods of a woman's life course are of particular concern here. First, the period during which a woman's sons begin to marry, daughters-in-law join the household, and grandchildren begin to arrive. In chronological terms, these events usually commence when a woman is in her early to mid-40s, depending upon her own age at marriage, her reproductive history, and so on. I will call this period 'middle age'. A woman gradually moves from middle age into what I will call 'early old age'. During this period she typically remains fairly physically active, but has begun to withdraw from active involvement in household management as her daughters-in-law themselves approach middle age. In some cases her daughters-in-law may have separated their cooking hearths from hers, leaving her to run an independent, but much smaller household, consisting only of herself and perhaps her husband, if he is still alive. If she was in the labour force in the earlier period, a woman has probably had to decrease or cease her involvement in wage-earning activities because of age-related physical decline and has become at least partially dependent upon sons (or others) for support.

The third and final period of life is that which gerontologists have termed 'old-old age'. Though it cannot be closely tied to any particular chronological age, either conceptually or physiologically, this stage is likely to have been reached by the time a woman is in her early 70s, if not before. The old-old woman is usually a great-grandmother. She is likely to be physically incapacitated to some degree, and increasingly dependent upon others for food and shelter; she has lost a good deal of her former mobility and perhaps needs assistance even for meeting her daily personal needs. Even if she had been living on her own during early old age, she is likely again to have joined her son's (or, occasionally, a daughter's) household because she can no longer cook and keep house for herself.

The Positive Consequences of Ageing for Indian Women

Many scholars have observed that in most non-industrialized societies the passage of women from young adulthood to middle age and early old age brings positive changes, rather than the negative ones that in industrialized societies are associated with ageing (Bart 1969; Brown 1982, 1992; Coles 1990; Foner 1984). Cross-cultural studies suggest that this is especially true in societies marked by strong patterns of male dominance. Such gender asymmetry is especially characteristic of societies that trace descent patrilineally, in which productive property is owned exclusively by men and is inherited in the male line, marriages are arranged by parents rather than the young people themselves, post-marital residence is patrilocal, and the extended family is the predominant household form. The ideological concomitants of such social structural forms typically include beliefs about the need to control women's sexuality in order to be certain of the paternity of her children and the association of women's sexual modesty with the honour of the men of her family—especially her father, brothers and husband. Because of such preoccupations, it is the young woman in her reproductive years who is the primary target of male domination. Thus post-adolescent young women, especially in the early years of marriage and young motherhood are likely to be largely restricted to the domestic domain, permitted little mobility, and expected to be subservient not only to their husbands but to other elder members (female as well as male) of their conjugal extended families.

In this kind of society the waning of a woman's reproductive capacities and of her sexual attractiveness, as culturally construed, causes her to be regarded no longer as a threat to male honour. As she progresses through the life course she is consequently increasingly freed from onerous restrictions upon her activities and demeanour, gains increasing authority over other, especially junior, members of her family, and may become eligible for roles in the extra-domestic arena that provide access to wider social recognition and control over material resources than were previously available to her (Brown 1982:143–45). It is thus in middle age that a woman reaches what is in many respects the high point of her life.

The life trajectory of Indian women can be seen as conforming broadly to this widespread pattern that Brown and others have described. The powerful post-menopausal Indian mother-in-law, playing the role of matriarch to a large extended family of sons, sons' wives, and grandchildren, is a familiar image, though one that, as I have pointed out above, has rarely been subjected to very close analytic scrutiny.[8] Such a woman ideally enjoys respect, deference and unquestioned authority over others in her family—male as well as female. Freed from heavy work burdens and the need to conform to strict standards of female modesty, she is able to move about outside the confines of her home, not only in order to carry out certain necessary tasks for the benefit of her household, but also to engage in social and religious activities that interest her (see Vatuk 1980a, 1987).

---

[8] An especially sympathetic pictorial as well as aural presentation of this image, is to be seen in the documentary film *Dadi's Family*.

Within the home, the position of a middle-aged wife and mother of sons is typically one of considerable security, ease and comfort, relative to that which she occupied at a younger age and relative to that of younger women within her own household. Of course, limited economic resources may still prevent her and other members of the family from being adequately sheltered and fed. But within these constraints, the middle-aged woman's needs and desires are likely to be well attended to and accorded some priority by other members of the family. Furthermore, at this stage of life a woman is capable of acting independently with respect to many areas affecting her own well-being in a way that the young daughter-in-law in such a family is not. The fact that the middle-aged woman (whether in an extended or nuclear family household) generally controls intra-household food distribution and the allocation of many other domestic resources places her in a favourable position to obtain at least her fair share of the family's resources in terms of nutrition, clothing and medical care, as she might not have been able to do as a junior woman in the household of her husband's parents.

Old age security is something that no woman (or man) in India leaves to chance. Even the young married woman is very cognizant of the necessity of having sons to support and care for her when she becomes old. Though this is not the only reason women desire children, it is one of their important motivations (see Cain 1986; Datta and Nugent 1984; Vlassoff and Vlassoff 1980; Vlassoff 1990). Most women do, in fact, succeed in producing sons who in adulthood can provide support and the attentive physical and emotional care or 'service' (*seva*) that is every old person's hope for his or her declining years (see Vatuk 1980a, 1980b, 1982b). It is difficult, however, to state precisely how many women fail to achieve this goal. Data bearing explicitly on the question of the prevalence of 'sonlessness' among older Indian women are not readily available, and estimates of the percentage of Indians 60 years of age and above who have no surviving son vary fairly widely, between 12 and 30 per cent.[9]

However, it is clear that the great majority of older women not only have married sons, but also live with them. Evidence for this is provided in the findings from innumerable small-scale studies from all parts of rural and urban India. According to the studies I have

---

[9]See discussions of this issue in Drèze 1990 and Vatuk 1982a.

examined, the percentages of older women who are living at any one point in time with married sons range between approximately 55 and 80 per cent (see Martin 1990; Vatuk 1982a:88). Most of the rest live with other relatives, including husbands and/or unmarried children. However, if we were to examine the data on living arrangements longitudinally, tracing individual women's residential histories, we would find that much higher percentages of older women live with married sons during some period of their lives. Even if they have lived separately in early old age, it is likely that toward the end of their lives they will again rejoin a son's household. Very few old people of either sex live entirely alone, and even if they cook and keep house for themselves, they almost always live close to at least one of their offspring or another kinsman and have close relationships of interdependence with other households, of a social if not an economic character.[10] It is necessary to recognize, of course, that even if old women co-reside with their children they may not receive adequate care and attention at this stage of life, and even if their material needs are met they may suffer from loneliness and be treated with resentment and hostility.

The great majority of those older people who do live alone are widowed women. This can be explained in large part, although not entirely, by the fact that older widows are the segment of the population most likely to be without close kin with whom they could live. However, it should be stressed that, on the other hand, the vast majority of older widows, like the majority of older married women, do live with married sons or other kin. For example, according to Drèze's review of data from a number of micro-level studies, few investigators report more than 10 per cent of all widows (of whatever age) living alone (1990:116A).[11]

Young women not only try to ensure that they will have a son but, once their sons become old enough to grasp a verbal message, they begin to communicate their expectation of a later return for their nurturance. Mothers may frequently be heard explaining to their

---

[10] The issue of how 'living alone' is defined in surveys of residential arrangements needs to be raised in connection with this discussion, but I cannot examine it in any further depth here. See discussions of this in Vatuk 1982a, Marulasiddaiah 1969, Drèze 1990, and Lamb 1993.

[11] The figures range widely from 0% to 35.2% of widows living alone. Marulasiddaiah (1969) and Cain (1986), provide the highest figures, for a Karnataka and a Maharashtra village, respectively. See, however, note 10.

young sons how they expect to be repaid for all their motherly sacrifices with loving attention and care in old age. Thus boys are taught to think of the parent-child relationship not as a selfless one-way flow of goods, but in terms of long-term reciprocity enacted over the entire life course.

Women's strategies for creating close bonds with their sons are not focused only narrowly on their prospects for the distant future, but are part of a broader lifelong 'survival strategy' within the context of a patrilineal-patrilocal kinship system. Through these means, a woman aims to consolidate a closely-knit sub-unit within the family, centred upon and loyal to herself. Such a unit consists initially of herself and her sons—eventually their wives and children will be incorporated as well. Wolf has described a very similar technique employed by Chinese women, who, she says, strive to form their own individual women-centred 'uterine families' within the larger male-dominated patrilineal extended family (Wolf 1972).

The Indian Woman in Old-Old Age

As the years go by and her physical strength declines, the Indian woman inevitably begins to lose some of her ability to exert authority over younger family members. She must eventually hand over not only the labour but also the entire management of the household to her daughters-in-law, if indeed it has remained an intact unit at all. The way that this process of withdrawal occurs has important implications for her welfare in old-old age (see Vatuk 1980b). If she has been able to inculcate in her sons a strong sense of filial obligation and love, and has retained their regard for her through all of the turmoil of their early married life, and if she has earned the affection as well as the respect of their wives and has relinquished control to them gracefully, she will probably enjoy a relatively comfortable old-old age, within the constraints of the family's economic resources. If she has not been able to effectively 'invest' in these crucial social relationships, she is at some risk of neglect when the task of meeting her increasing needs becomes burdensome.[12] This is an especial danger when she becomes a widow and no longer has an

---

[12] I have discussed elsewhere (1982b, 1990) some of the intra-family tensions and strains that often lead to distress for the old-old woman (and man) in India, even when the family's economic level is sufficient to provide the necessary material comforts.

authoritative ally in the family to see that she iş kindly treated by the younger generation. The outcome of a woman's strategies for old age is of course not entirely within her own control. The 'script' for successfully weathering the transitions from middle to old age is not easy for everyone to follow, particularly when the other actors— primarily the younger men and women in the family—have their own scripts to follow in pursuing their respective and often divergent interests.

The way sons are socialized is generally effective, in the sense that in adulthood few men would be prepared to abandon or refuse to shelter an ageing parent. To do so would be to incur not only strong social disapproval but the weight of their own heavy conscience. Therefore, most men, assuming that they have the wherewithal to do so, fulfil at least their minimal responsibility to shelter and feed their parents and meet their other basic material needs. Widespread poverty, however, makes the care of a helpless older person an insupportable burden for too many families, no matter how responsible and well-intentioned their members might be. The failure of sons to adequately care for their parents in such circumstances leads in turn to an aggravation of interpersonal tensions between the generations, and inevitably erodes the affection and sense of duty that are the principal motivations for continuing to serve the needs of the old and helpless. Even among the relatively well-to-do, intergenerational tensions not infrequently cause serious distress for women in this stage of life.

A period of helpless dependency in old-old age is perceived as being fraught with risk, despite strong cultural norms for intergenerational reciprocity and filial duty. Ageing women and men in India greatly dread becoming physically incapacitated because of uncertainty about the kind of treatment they will receive from their children when they can no longer do anything for themselves. This is clear from the frequency with which in interviews they express such wishes as 'to die while my hands and feet are still working well' (Vatuk 1990; Lamb 1993).

Older Women vs. Older Men

Thus far the implicit comparison in speaking of the older woman in India has been the younger woman. However, it is also instructive to look at the older woman's situation relative to the man of equivalent age, marital and parental status. One indicator of this, drawn from data on sex- and age-specific mortality in India, suggests that in terms of health status older women are in fact advantaged in comparison with their male age-mates. After age 35, mortality rates for women are lower than those for men and life expectancy is greater (see tables in Agarwala 1985:140; Sharma and Xenos 1992:11–13, 85–88).[13] This is, of course, not surprising in the worldwide context, but it is worth remarking here in view of the fact that for the earlier portion of the life span females have a consistently higher probability of death than males. This is reflected in India's adverse sex ratio, not only in the population as a whole, but also—if we divide the population according to age—in all but the most senior cohorts.[14]

It is not clear whether the sex-differential mortality data for the 35+ age-group suggests that Indian men become subject in middle-age to some new disadvantages in terms of nutrition deficits or disease, or that women in middle-age overcome some of the biological and social disabilities that at younger ages made them more vulnerable to death than their male peers.[15] For example, the positive changes I have alluded to in females' social and family position may contribute to permitting their 'natural' biological superiority to take over, and ensuring their enhanced survival relative to men of equivalent maturity. The fact that those women who have survived through the childbearing years are already a select group in terms of their ability to resist or overcome illness must of course not be overlooked.

Older women also have certain social advantages over men in Indian society. Gerontologists have often observed that one of the central problems of the ageing individual in any society is declining physical capacity, as it almost inevitably makes it difficult to perform accustomed work roles. Unless there are alternative tasks—equally valued by society—that the older person can assume, he or she may be seen as failing to make an active contribution to the group. This

[13]Basu (1993 and in this volume) has discussed some of the implications of these and related statistics on women's health.
[14]That is, in 1991 only in the over-70 age group were there more females than males (Sharma and Xenos 1992:35).
[15]By 'biological' disadvantages I refer in particular to the greater risk of death due to childbearing. Basu (1993) discusses some of the theories that have been proposed to explain female mortality advantage in later life.

can lead to the old person being regarded as a burden, and consequently to social marginalization and even neglect.

Women, whose working lives tend to centre around the home and domestic chores, are in most societies at somewhat of an advantage over their male peers in that they are able to continue with familiar tasks well into old age, albeit at a decreased level of energy expenditure. Domestic chores are very diverse and require differing amounts of strength and skill; an older woman may continue to make an obvious contribution to the household long after she is too frail to carry out any heavy tasks. In India, the cultural pattern according to which the new daughter-in-law immediately takes over those household jobs that require strength and stamina, enables older women to make the transition to lighter work (including managerial tasks, childwatching and errands outside of the home) long before they are forced to do so by physical decline. The typical Indian woman, as she ages, therefore experiences a gradual transition in terms of kind and quantity of work, without having to assume a truly dependent role in the family until she is practically bedridden.

Even those women who have been working outside of the home, but find their ability to earn eroded by physical debility, can easily step back into a familiar and useful role upon their return to the domestic sphere. For example, poor urban parents have been reported to rely heavily upon the services of the older women in their families to care for children and carry out other light household tasks while they themselves are away at work (see, for example, de Souza 1982). Here the continuity of women's accustomed work roles, so closely associated with reproduction and the domestic domain, presents an advantage to women in middle and old age, even as it frequently works against their well-being at early phases of the life course.

Men's work does not usually allow the same kind of continuity, although this depends to some extent upon the nature of the occupation and may be less of an issue for artisans and traders than for farmers or office workers, for example. When an agriculturalist is no longer able to continue ploughing or other heavy agricultural labour, he soon has to leave farming altogether. It is often difficult for him even to retain an active managerial role once his adult sons have taken over full responsibility for the work itself. His chief opportunity to visibly contribute to the household is by assuming tasks (like babyminding) that fall within the female sphere in the traditional division of labour. Even if his basic material needs continue to be met by his sons and daughters-in-law, his adjustment to the loss of his position as the authoritarian head of the household is likely to be difficult.

Women in old age usually remain close to the centre of the family, while ageing men tend to become somewhat peripheral, spatially, emotionally and in terms of sociable interaction and decision-making. Patterns of sex segregation and female seclusion or *purdah* define the house as female space for most of the day and it is often regarded as unseemly for an adult man to spend much time at home during the day. Furthermore, especially in north India, because a man's daughters-in-law must veil from him and avoid speaking in his presence, it is awkward for them and interferes with their work if he remains in the house any more than necessary. If he must stay at home because of ill-health, he will be restricted in his freedom of movement within the house, and cannot freely take part in the casual give and take of conversation and sociability that goes on in the home when only women and children and younger males are present.

Furthermore, relationships between a father and his adult sons are rarely as close and affectionate as those between a mother and her sons. As they are growing up, boys typically learn to regard the father as a somewhat distant authority figure. While they may respect him and feel a strong obligation to provide care and support for him in old age, they are unlikely to feel the same kind of warmth and relaxed emotional closeness that they feel toward their mother. Often, in fact, this difference in emotional tone has been actively cultivated by the mother over the years, in the process of solidifying the 'uterine family' to which I have referred above. Tensions arising out of the situation in which sons replace the father as the primary support of the family—whether through work on family land, craft or business, or as wage earners—accentuate this quality of their relationship. Men's emotional distance from their sons and their inability, because of avoidance and deference norms, to establish personally close relationships with the daughters-in-law who are largely responsible for their food and care, can have a negative impact at least upon their emotional, if not their physical, comfort in old-old age.

On the other hand, older men have at least two distinct advantages over their female peers in the later years of life. For one thing, most men in old age have a wife to provide both companionship and caring attention to their needs, offsetting some of the negative aspects of their relative marginalization from productive activities and household affairs. Also, as has often been pointed out, only men in this society are likely to own and control property. Research has consistently demonstrated the extent to which ageing Indian (and other South Asian) men are aware of the importance of material assets as a hedge against neglect or mistreatment by the younger generation (see especially Goldstein, Schuler and Ross 1983; Bhatia 1983; Vatuk 1982b, 1990). On the other hand, the reality of the situation in India is such that the majority of older men in India do not in fact own substantial amounts of property or have sufficient in the way of personal income to successfully use as leverage in this way. Among the poor, this supposed advantage given to men by India's system of male property ownership and patrilineal inheritance is largely notional.

Conclusion

I have tried to present here some general remarks about the older woman in India, and to make some assessments about her overall social position. I have compared the situation of the middle-aged and older woman with that of the young adult wife, about whom we already know a great deal from the anthropological and sociological literature, and have suggested that in the Indian social and cultural context, growing older brings distinct improvements and benefits. These benefits tend, however, to dissipate when a woman reaches 'old-old age' and experiences serious physical incapacitation, particularly if—as is usually the case—her husband is no longer living. I have also made some comparisons between men and women at comparable ages and phases in the life course, concluding that in middle and old age the female disadvantage vis-à-vis males that obtains in the early years of life and in young adulthood is weakened and even reversed in certain respects.

The points I have made about the positive aspects for a woman of growing older in this society are not intended to minimize or gloss over the very real problems in terms of health and overall well-being that affect women of all ages in India. They are also not intended to dismiss the magnitude of the difficulties faced by what is in absolute terms a very substantial number of older widows. However, looked at in the perspective of the life course, I would like to suggest that gender bias is not the principal issue demanding attention with reference to the health status of middle-aged and older women. Rather, issues of poverty, of class and caste inequalities, maldistribution of medical care, and rapid social change may be of greater significance for helping us to understand why certain categories of women in these particular life stages are at greater risk than others of their peers of suffering from inadequate nutrition, disease, premature death and general distress.

References

Agarwala, S.N. 1985. *India's Population Problems*. 3rd rev. ed. New Delhi: Tata McGraw Hill.
Bart, Pauline. 1969. 'Why Women's Status Changes in Middle Age: The Turn of the Social Ferris Wheel'. *Sociological Symposium* 3:1–18.
Basu, Alaka M. 1993. 'Women's Roles and Gender Gap in Health and Survival'. *Economic and Political Weekly* 28:2356–62.
Bennett, Lynn. 1983. *Dangerous Wives and Sacred Sisters*. New York: Columbia University Press.
Bhatia, H.S. 1983. *Aging and Society: A Sociological Study of Retired Public Servants*. Udaipur: The Arya Book Centre Publishers.
Biswas, S.K., ed. 1987. *Aging in Contemporary India*. Calcutta: Indian Anthropological Society.
Bose, A.B. and K.D. Gangrade, eds. 1988. *The Aging in India: Problems and Potentialities*. Abhinav Publications.
Brown, Judith K. 1982. 'Cross-Cultural Perspectives on Middle-Aged Women.' *Current Anthropology* 23:143–48.
Brown, Judith K. 1992. 'Lives of Middle-Aged Women' in V. Kerns and J.K. Brown, eds. *In Her Prime: New View of Middle-Aged Women*. 2nd ed. pp. 17–30. Urbana and Chicago: University of Illinois Press.
Cain, Mead. 1986. 'The Consequences of Reproductive Failure: Dependence, Mobility, and Mortality among the Elderly of Rural South Asia'. *Population Studies* 40:375-88.
Coles, Catherine. 1990. 'The Older Woman in Hausa Society: Power and Authority in Urban Nigeria' in J. Sokolovsky, ed. *The Cultural Context of Aging: Worldwide Perspectives*. New York: Bergin and Garvey.
Datta, S.K. and J.B. Nugent. 1984. 'Are Old-Age Security and the Utility of Children in Rural India Really Unimportant?' *Population Studies* 38:507–509.
de Souza, Alfred. 1982. *The Social Organisation of Aging among the Urban Poor*. New Delhi: Indian Social Institute.
Desai, K.G. and R.D. Naik. 1975. *Problems of Retired People in Greater Bombay*. Bombay: Tata Institute of Social Sciences.

Dhruvarajan, Vanaja. 1989. *Hindu Women and the Power of Ideology*. Granby, MA: Bergin and Garvey.
Drèze, Jean. 1990. *Widows in Rural India*. London: London School of Economics Development Economics Research Programme.
Foner, Nancy. 1984. *Ages in Conflict*. New York: Columbia University Press.
Goldstein, Melvyn C., S. Schuler and J. Ross. 1983. 'Social and Economic Forces Affecting Intergenerational Relations in Extended Families in a Third World Country: A Cautionary Tale from South Asia'. *Journal of Gerontology* 38: 716–24.
Jacobson, Doranne and Susan S. Wadley. 1977. *Women in India: Two Perspectives*. Columbia, MO: South Asia Books.
Jagannadham, V. and C.M. Palvia. 1978. *Problems of Pensioners (in India): Socio-Economic Policy and Administration*. New Delhi: Lalita Prakashan.
Kakar, Sudhir. 1978. *The Inner World*. Delhi: Oxford University Press.
Kurtz, Stanley N. 1992. *All the Mothers are One*. New York: Columbia University Press.
Lamb, Sarah. 1993. *Growing in the Net of Maya: Persons, Gender and Life Processes in a Bengali Society*. Unpublished Ph.D. Dissertation, Anthropology, University of Chicago.
Martin, Linda G. 1990. The Status of South Asia's Growing Elderly Population. *Journal of Cross-Cultural Gerontology* 5:93–118.
Marulasiddaiah, H.M. 1969. *Old People of Makunti*. Dharwar: Karnataka University.
Roland, Alan. 1988. *In Search of Self in India and Japan*. Princeton: Princeton University Press.
Roy, Manisha. 1975. *Bengali Women*. Chicago: University of Chicago Press.
Roy, S. Guha. 1987. 'Demography of aging: Indian Experience' in S.K. Biswas, ed. *Aging in Contemporary India*. Calcutta: Indian Anthropological Society.
Sharma, S.P. and Peter Xenos. 1992. *Ageing in India: Demographic Background and Analysis based on Census Materials*. Occasional Paper No. 2. New Delhi: Government of India.
Soodan, Kirpal Singh. 1975. *Aging in India*. Calcutta: Minerva Associates.
Tapper, B.E. 1979. 'Widows and Goddesses: Female Roles in Deity Symbolism in a South Indian Village'. *Contributions to Indian Sociology* (n.s.) 13:1–31.
Ullrich, Helen. 1988. 'Widows in South Indian Society: Depression as an Appropriate Response to Cultural Factors'. *Sex Roles* 19:169–88.
Vatuk, Sylvia. 1980a. 'The Aging Woman in India: Self Perceptions and Changing Roles' in A. de Souza, ed. *Women in Contemporary India and South Asia*. New Delhi: Manohar Book Service.
Vatuk, Sylvia. 1980b. 'Withdrawal and Disengagement as a Cultural Response to Aging in India' in C. Fry, ed. *Aging in Culture and Society*. New York: Praeger.
Vatuk, Sylvia. 1982a. 'Old Age in India' in P.N. Stearns, ed. *Old Age in Preindustrial Society*. New York: Holmes and Meier.
Vatuk, Sylvia. 1982b. 'The Family Life of Older People in a Changing Society: India' in J. Sokolovsky and J. Sokolovsky, eds. *Aging and the Aged in the Third World. Part II. Studies in Third World Societies* 23: 57–82.
Vatuk, Sylvia. 1987. 'Authority, Power and Autonomy in the Life Cycle of North Indian Women' in P. Hockings, ed. *Dimensions of Social Life*. Berlin: Mouton de Gruyter.

Vatuk, Sylvia. 1990. '"To be a Burden on Others": Dependency Anxiety among the Elderly in India' in O.M. Lynch, ed. *Divine Passions: The Social Construction of Emotion in India*. Berkeley: University of California Press.

Vatuk, Sylvia. 1991. 'Gerontology in India: The State of the Art'. *Journal of Cross-Cultural Gerontology* 6:259–71.

Vatuk Sylvia. 1992. 'Sexuality and the Middle-Aged Woman in South Asia' in V. Kerns and J.K. Brown, eds. *In Her Prime: New Views of Middle-Aged Women*. 2nd ed. Urbana and Chicago: University of Illinois Press.

Vlassoff, Carol. 1990. 'The Value of Sons in an Indian Village: How Widows See It.' *Population Studies* 44:5-20.

Vlassoff, M. and C. Vlassoff. 1980. 'Old Age Security and the Utility of Children in Rural India'. *Population Studies* 34:487–99.

Wolf, Margery. 1972. *Women and the Family in Rural Taiwan*. Stanford: Stanford University Press.

11

Gender and Health: From Research to Action

ADRIENNE GERMAIN

The papers addressing gender and health issues in this volume are extremely rich and diverse. Taken as a whole they provide a valuable set of scientific and analytical perspectives on contemporary gender and health issues in India — reproductive health problems, maternal mortality, gender differentials in health status, the linkage between women's and children's health, and the health conditions of vulnerable women, such as widows. The presentation of available empirical data, the consideration of methodological issues, and the reflections on the determinants of gender differentials in health status, together provide a powerful basis for a critical examination of both action and research priorities.

This paper focuses specifically on the health of girls and women, especially those aspects of female health that clearly differ from male health. This chapter is organized around some critical questions related to analysing the nature of the problem and what approaches might be best in seeking to resolve them.

The Problem

In a paper on 'positional objectivity', Amartya Sen (1995) provides a powerful intellectual basis for understanding objective and subjective assessments of social problems, including gender and health issues. The paper discriminates between subjective and objective assessments, as well as how even objective perspectives may be influenced by the 'positionality' of the observer. In gender and health, the issue of perspectives is critically important in understanding whether inequality exists (Sen, Germain and Chen 1994). Sen's paper urges us to strive for objectivity in appraising the health status of populations and in considering equitable and effective policy alternatives.

The papers in this volume present at least two apparently competing assessments of the differential health condition of men and women. On the one hand, some postulate substantial comparative deprivation among women, while on the other hand, some argue that gender differentials are very modest and, if any, may be complex (for example, Jejeebhoy and Rama Rao in contrast to Basu in this volume). These two competing views derive in part from lack of data, uncertainty about measurement techniques, as well as divergent interpretations of 'evidence'. Most of the papers in this volume view gender inequalities as one of the major forms of social inequality. Alaka Basu's paper in this volume, however, offers a counter-interpretation: 'The South Asian female disadvantage in health and survival risks becoming the all-consuming passion of research on health differentials.... This is not warranted [because] gender differences [are] narrowing and the gender differences [are] small compared to caste, rural-urban, educational [differences].'

Other papers in this volume also offer diverse data sources and analysis, and divergent interpretation of 'facts'. Some examples are the differing estimates of the proportion of female deaths due to maternal causes by Mari Bhat and colleagues and Jejeebhoy and Rama Rao; the debate over various assessments of whether standard labour force data from national censuses may be used as proxy indicators of women's work and/or status; uncertainty on the secular trend of the sex ratio of India's population (Dyson 1984); and the debate on the significance of mortality in comparison to morbidity and disability in assessing women's health status as emphasized by Mari Bhat and colleagues or Basu, in comparison to Chen and Drèze or Sundari.

How are we to resolve what appear to be conflicting interpretations in an objective manner? Rather than argue about the magnitude and trends of gender differentials in health, it is essential to recognize certain conclusions about which there can be little debate:

(1) *Women bear the burden of childbearing*: Women bear most of the medical, emotional and social burdens and risks of contraception, pregnancy, abortion, and the delivery and care of children (Germain

and Ordway 1989). In all societies, these biological (and usually social) forces powerfully shape gender differentials in reproductive health.

(2) *Women are more vulnerable than men to reproductive tract infections.* Many sexually transmitted diseases (STDs), including AIDS, are biologically sexist in that these diseases are often more easily transmitted from male to female than vice versa. Women, it is postulated, also suffer more serious consequences from bacterial and viral STDs than do men—including infertility, increased risk of ectopic pregnancy, pregnancy wastage, pelvic inflammatory disease, and cervical cancer, among others. Women are also technologically and socially disadvantaged in protecting themselves against these diseases. Unlike the male-controlled condom, there is no widely available female-controlled technology against STDs that women can use to protect themselves. Moreover, inequity in sexual power relationships makes negotiation of condom use difficult if not impossible for many, probably most, women. Girls and women are much less often able than men to control when, with whom and under what conditions sexual relations take place. Due to their biologic and reproductive roles, girls and women are also vulnerable to the risk of iatrogenic infections (during contraceptive, abortion, pregnancy and delivery services) and to endogenous infections of the reproductive tract (Dixon-Mueller and Wasserheit 1991 and IWHC 1992).

(3) *Girls and women often have less access to food and health care than boys and men.* Where society places a lower value on the female than on the male, as documented in a number of papers in this volume, females are often given less or poorer quality food and health care than men. Many women may also deny themselves food and health care in preference to their children or husbands, as vividly described in the paper by Sundari. The comparative deprivation of girls and women may be especially severe under circumstances of resource insufficiency but may exist even under circumstances of resource abundance, as described by Kishor.

(4) *Girls and women are more subject to gender-related violence than men.* Gender-based violence may take many forms, ranging from the 'mysterious' category in the census called 'burns' (Mari Bhat et al. in this volume) to sexual demands on widows (Chen and Drèze in this volume). The burning of wives, called 'dowry deaths', due to inability

of brides and their families to meet the pecuniary demands of grooms and their families, has attracted much media attention in India. The consequences of the threat of violence against the physical and emotional health of women are severe and often neglected or underestimated.

(5) *Women shoulder a triple workload.* Most women in India face the multiple demands of productive work, household maintenance, and childbearing and rearing. The triple burden often leaves many poor women with persistent fatigue or chronic pain. Workload, together with the common practice of women being given less food or food of poorer quality, may result in significant nutritional deficiencies, especially iron deficiency anaemia.

(6) *The sex ratio in India is very low in comparison to other national populations.* Whether the sex ratio is worsening or stable is currently under debate (for example, see Dyson 1994). This debate obscures the fact that India's sex ratio is severely skewed: 930 women per 1000 men is one of the lowest in the world. Most agree that the deficiency in women should be corrected, irrespective of decennial trends.

While it is estimated that a woman who reaches age 35 has better survival chances than a man, it is important to remember the girls lost unnecessarily before they reach age 35; the unnecessary suffering of those who survive to age 35 and beyond; and the precarious plight of the women who do survive, especially the 60 per cent of women over age 60 who are widows (Chen and Drèze in this volume).

Goals

This paper proposes five goals based on the particular biological and social roles females play in reproduction, and the consequences that these roles and sex discrimination have on their health. The goals are to enable girls and women to:

(1) grow up healthy;
(2) experience sexuality and reproduction with dignity, safely, and free of disease, disability, pain, violence or death;
(3) manage their own fertility by conceiving when desired, safely terminating unwanted pregnancies, and carrying wanted pregnancies safely to term;
(4) bear and raise healthy children when desired; and
(5) experience healthy life in the post-reproductive years.

Basic Health and Social Issues

It is generally agreed that female disadvantage begins at birth, in India as well as in many other countries. If the goals specified above are to be achieved, the social practices leading to gender differentials in health, as well as the special demands of the female's biological role, should be met. The paper by Jejeebhoy and Rama Rao provides an unusually rich review and synthesis of available data on reproductive health and, importantly, recognizes that reproductive health needs to be broadly defined beyond maternal mortality. Data on sexual health, chronic diseases specific to women, and work-related health issues remain, however, still to be incorporated. Ramasubban's and Sundari's papers add to our understanding of some of these issues. Figure 1 summarizes the health problems specific to females that should be addressed.

HEALTH PROBLEMS SPECIFIC TO FEMALES

1. *Related to Sexuality and Reproduction*
   STDs: conventional STDs
                                       HIV
   Reproduction: preventable infertility (due to STDs, tuberculosis, etc.)
                                       contraceptive safety and efficacy
                                       pregnancy
                                       abortion
                                       delivery
                                       post-partum malnutrition, especially anaemia
   Gynaecology: iatrogenic infections
                                       prolapse
                                       hygiene and endogenous infections
   Menopause
   Cancers of female organs: breast
                                       cervical
                                       ovarian
                                       uterine
2. *Gender-based*
   Discrimination in health care and nutrition, including anaemia
   Physical violence
   Emotional intimidation
   Commercialized sex
3. *Work-related*
   Chronic fatigue or pain
   Specific occupational hazards

Figure 1

Professor Sen (1995) emphasizes the important role that *perceptions* play in making objective health assessments, pointing out that various actors may perceive 'health' differently. Perceptions of women's health—its dimensions, its importance, its causes—vary widely among women themselves, family members, the community, health professionals, researchers, and policy makers.

The papers in this volume themselves illustrate well how perceptions can influence understanding of particular health problems and policy decisions. For example, Basu recognizes gender differences and discrimination, but concludes that the differences are narrowing and are relatively modest. Kishor shows, on the contrary, how various forms of development can actually *worsen* female health. Mari Bhat et al. argue that maternal mortality has declined to 555 per 100,000 and imply that we may assume the trend will continue. Others would instead argue that this mortality level, even if correct, is still extremely and unacceptably high. Some limit their concern for women's health to maternal mortality. By comparison, Jejeebhoy and Rama Rao's review uses an expansive definition that encompasses morbidity, social behaviours and other factors that determine women's health. Chen and Drèze and Vatuk examine the micro-level social and human realities that lie behind macro-data.

To reconcile such divergent perspectives and to understand their implications for public policy, the socio-economic context of female disadvantage must be carefully assessed using a gender lens. At least three major aspects have been discussed:

Poverty: Several studies examine in some depth regional, state, and class differentials in health status (see the papers in Das Gupta, Krishnan and Chen 1995). They pay less attention to the feminization of poverty and the important ways in which poverty constrains women's access to social services. These include, among others, lack of cash and the opportunity costs of women's time. We need to learn much more about the coping strategies of women in poverty.

Discrimination: Especially, but not only, among the poor, as Basu suggests, women are constrained from achieving their health potential by such restrictive practices as seclusion, kin relationships, and differential access to services, education and employment opportunities, among others. Chen and Drèze, Sundari, and Kishor show that these differentials are powerful also amongst the richer groups in the society.

Women's status: Several papers debate techniques for defining and measuring women's status. For example, Shiva Kumar attempts to create an index using several variables as proxies for women's status. These individual elements of composite indicators tend to be interrelated, and their reliability has yet to be clearly demonstrated. Similarly, Basu uses conventional measures of employment, which do not include a range of women's productive work. Basu's discussion of the concept of women's 'bargaining position' recognizes the complex realities of women's status.

While more work is needed to develop valid measures of the feminization of poverty, discrimination and women's status—note that there is a burgeoning literature on the subject—it is important not to let such measurement issues obstruct health research and action.

Premises for Action

To clarify perceptions about women's health and the context which affects it, it is important to specify the underlying values and justifications for attention to women's health. There has been a strong tendency to adopt rather narrowly defined cost/benefit criteria in allocating health resources. In the case of women's health, most actions to date have been justified as means to control fertility or to improve child survival. In this paper, I propose the following premises for action:

(1) *Women's health should be an end in itself not just a means to achieve other ends.* Dilemmas arise when women are seen largely or solely as means to other ends. For example, it is sometimes suggested that the children of working women may suffer from their mothers' absence from the home. Are we then to conclude that mothers should not work? Or should we provide child care services? Health policies that emphasize maternal-child health and family planning do not meet the needs of older women or, often, young people aged 5–16. Chen and Drèze illuminate the plight of older women and widows whose needs are not well served by existing programmes. Recognizing women's health as an end in itself requires serving women throughout their lives. It also requires development of a better balance between the quantity and quality of services offered.

(2) *Women have multiple needs and responsibilities.* Several papers (including Basu, Sundari, Jejeebhoy and Rama Rao) underline the

importance of improving services. The major need is to ensure that national programmes provide at least minimum services routinely and efficiently with respect for the women. Examples include integrating health and nutrition programmes; clarifying the appropriate roles of various levels of health personnel, especially fostering the appropriate involvement of lower levels of personnel; and setting appropriate goals (e.g., is it appropriate and necessary to achieve hospital delivery for all pregnant women as some suggest, or is it most beneficial to assure attendance by a trained person at home or at the local health centre level, with strong referral and transport facilities for emergency cases?). Several papers in this volume highlight the failures of current, narrowly vertical programmes and some warn against adopting a similar strategy for AIDS prevention. What is needed is to learn from existing integrated efforts and to assess their possible application in large-scale health programmes. Several papers also assert that more domiciliary services are needed to provide care to women who otherwise could not have it because they are too poor, opportunity costs are too high, their movement is too restricted by norms of seclusion, and they are constrained by myriad other factors.

(3) *Investments in women's health can have beneficial ripple effects*. Kerala's experience underscores the value of giving priority to women's health services, and to the training and development of female health workers (Kabir and Krishnan 1994). While Kerala is distinct, its experience does provide very important lessons and insight regarding how investments in women's health, broadly defined, can have powerful beneficial ripple effects into social advancement, fertility reduction and labour productivity.

(4) *Women's social disadvantage should be reduced* to prevent poor health and to create effective demand for health care and fertility control. Chen and Drèze also point out that investment in girls' and women's health, and in improving other aspects of women's status, will affect fertility levels, as well as child survival, through changes in reliance on sons for old age security.

These premises for action will require modification in deeply held social values, existing budget allocations, standard programme strategies, and the 'conventional wisdom' of the health and family planning field. Many recognize that advocacy and political action for women's health will be essential. These basic premises point toward action and research priorities as presented in the next section.

Action and Research Priorities

The suggestions below are not meant to be comprehensive. Rather, they are indicative of actions needed from the point of view of women's health, in the context of overall health planning and development. The proposed list of priorities begins with research, but research is not the only priority. Rather, it is essential that action be taken even though existing data and research are incomplete. Action programmes themselves provide excellent opportunities for learning. If research and documentation efforts are built into action programmes from the beginning, research and action can be effectively integrated, an iterative process, with synergistic impact.

Research: From women's perspectives, and more generally, it is essential to examine the human realities behind macro-level data. Disaggregation of gender-specific data by subregion, urban/rural, age, caste, and other social categories would also be helpful. Excellent examples of the insights gained are provided by the Chen and Drèze paper. At the same time, Jejeebhoy and Rama Rao have clearly identified important areas of women's reproductive health for which neither micro- nor macro-data exist, e.g., induced abortion and sexually transmitted diseases (see also Ramasubban). The Government of India's expressed concern about AIDS prevention and control could provide an excellent opportunity to begin to investigate the latter systematically.

We need to know much more about women's perceptions of their own health, their utilization of the full range of health services (from ayurvedic to allopathic), and their service preferences. At the same time, we need to examine much more closely our understanding of the determinants of women's health and gender differentials in health. The variables referred to in several papers—such as age at marriage or education—are relatively easily quantifiable. Other crucial variables, such as 'status', gender-based power relationships, 'custom and culture' remain weakly understood 'black boxes', though they are very often invoked as major determinants of women's health.

Services: The central question is: are the current emphases of health services appropriate and are such services delivered in such a way as to meet women's needs? Special attention is needed on neglected issues, including safe abortion, sexually transmitted diseases including AIDS, and contraceptive safety.

Broad Social Action: Ultimately, as Jejeebhoy and Rama Rao and others suggest, reductions in the morbidity and mortality among girls and women depend upon changes in broader social structures which restrict girls' and women's ability to value and maintain their own health, their status and their rights. In the shorter term, advocacy for increased attention to girls' and women's health is required.

Changes in Male-Centred Social Attitudes: Many health problems that are specific to girls and women are the result of gender discrimination and ultimately derive from male-centred social attitudes and behaviours, whether from spouses or policy-makers. Changes in male attitudes and behaviours are urgently needed. The first step is to recognize that these are central to girls' and women's health disadvantages. We can then move forward to reduce gender differentials and to meet the special health needs of women consequent to their sexual and reproductive functions.

References

Das Gupta, Monica, T.N. Krishnan and Lincoln C. Chen (eds.). 1995. *Health, Poverty and Development in India*, Bombay: Oxford University Press.

Das Gupta, Monica, T.N. Krishnan and Lincoln C. Chen. 1995. 'Introduction' in M. Das Gupta, T.N. Krishnan and L. C. Chen (eds.), op. cit.

Dixon-Mueller, Ruth and Judith Wasserheit. 1991. *The culture of silence: reproductive tract infections among women in the Third World*, New York: International Women's Health Coalition.

Dyson, Tim. 1994. 'The Demography of the 1991 Census' in M. Das Gupta, T.N. Krishnan and L.C. Chen (eds.), op. cit.

Germain, Adrienne and Jane Ordway. 1989. *Population control and women's health: balancing the scales*, New York: International Women's Health Coalition.

International Women's Health Coalition. 1992. *Reproductive tract infections in women in the Third World: national and international policy implications*, New York.

Kabir, M. and T.N. Krishnan. 1994. 'Social Intermediation and Health Change' in M. Das Gupta, T.N. Krishnan and L.C. Chen (eds.), op. cit.

Sen, Gita, Adriene Germain and Lincoln C. Chen (eds.). 1994. *Population Policies Reconsidered: health, empowerment and rights*, Harvard University Press.

Sen, Gita, Adrienne Germain and Lincoln C. Chen. 1994. 'Overview' in G. Sen, A. Germain and L.C. Chen (eds.) op. cit.

Sen, Amartya. 1995. 'Objectivity, Health and Policy' in M. Das Gupta, T.N. Krishnan and L.C. Chen (eds.), op. cit.

Index

abortion (or MTP), 122, 129–30, 145–46, 214, 234–35
adolescence, 4, 131, 133–34; adolescent marriage/childbearing, 123, 133–35
age, and women's health, 177, 186–87, 190, 192, 194, 195, 197, 205, 206
age at marriage, 66–68, 133, 183, 215, 216
ageing, see older women
age–specific mortality, 100, 107–10, 112, 166
AIDS, 10, 147; see also HIV infection
Andhra Pradesh, 99, 105–107, 115–16
anaemia, 122, 129–30, 133, 138–40, 171, 177, 214
antenatal care (ANC), 135–41; see also pregnancy

Bangladesh, 12, 105–107, 116
'BIMARU' states, 57–59, 62, 65, 67, 68, 69, 73, 78, 77, 79, 80, 82, 83, 84, 86, 87
birth weight, 122, 215
breast-feeding, 143–44

caste: and contraceptive prevalence, 201; and gender discrimination, 35–36, 70; and reproductive health problems, 186–87, 190, 191, 198; and utilization of health care services, 203, 205
cause of death, 97, 129–30; accidents, 100, 158; pregnancy related, see maternal mortality; suicide, 100; violence, 100, 158; surveys of (SCD), 110, 113, 116, 117, 119, 158, 159

Census of India (various years), 21–25, 56, 58, 59, 61, 62, 63, 65, 68, 69, 74–75, 146, 161, 162
childbearing, frequency, 144, 185
childbirth, see pregnancy and childbirth
child care, 89
child marriage, 2
child mortality, 5–7, 11, 21, 186: due to HIV, 212; neonatal, 20–21, 122, 131, 134; perinatal, 20, 122, 127, 131, 139; post-neonatal, 21, 127; gender differentials in 19–54, 161, 163, 167, 175–76; related to parity, 188; state-wise variations, 21–23; district level data, 24–26, see also infant mortality
child survival, 88, 90, 161, 162
childhood, vulnerability of females in, 4, 5–7
chlamydia, 231–32
community/collective action (by women), 85–86, 88
contraception, 122, 144–45, 180, 199, 200–202; leading to health problems, 9, 198, 214, 225, 234
convalescence, 165
cultural norms/institutions, 157, 167, 207, 213–14, 216

death rate, 4, 11, 97; see also mortality rate
demographic factors, 20, 179, 183–87
district level data, 24–26, 43–48
dowry payments, 32, 155
dummy-variable regression, 104, 108

Index

economic activity, women's 155–57, 163–64, 165, 168; *see also* employment

economic/socio-economic status: and contraceptive prevalence, 201; and gender discrimination, 36–38, 171–72; and health, 178–79, 182–83, 189–91, 195, 196, 204; of widows, 249–50

education, women's, 14–15, 189–90, 192, 194, 195, 201–202, 203, 204, 205; *see also* literacy

electoral participation (women's), 86–88

employment/occupation, women's, 155–7, 161, 163, 168–69, 182, 187, 190, 192, 194, 197, 199, 203; and well-being of children, 63–65

Family Planning/Welfare Programme, 123

female infanticide, 1–2

fertility levels/rates, 7, 8, 97, 99, 101, 104, 105, 120–21, 133, 166, 170, 180, 183–86

gender bias/discrimination, 1, 6, 19, 120, 133, 179; in allocation of food, 26–28, 29, 215, 217; in allocation of medical care, 28–29; cultural basis of, 29–30, 32–34; economic basis of, 29–32; impact of economic growth/development, 39–42; impact of demographic change, 42–43; impact of socio-economic status, 34–39; religion and, 34

gender differentials: in child mortality, 19–54, 169; in health and survival, 154–72; model for explanation of, 43–48; *see also* sex differentials

gender relations, 10

gender roles, effect on health, 8–9; 153–72

genital herpes, 227–28; *see also* sexually transmitted diseases

gonorrhoea, 228–31; *see also* sexually transmitted diseases

gynaecological disorders, 142–43

haemorrhage, 129–30, 188

health care expenditure/services, 28–29, 81, 82, 133, 165, 179; women's utilization of, 204–207, 208–10; *see also* antenatal care

health problems, women's: general, 191–95; reproductive, 194, 195–200

health status of married women (Tamil Nadu study), 182–200

heteroscedasticity test, 103

HIV infection, 212–38; heterosexual transmission, 213, 214; use of condoms, 213; women's vulnerability, 214

housing, 182–83

hygiene during childbirth, 142

immunization, 137–38

income, women's access to/control over, 168, 179, 180

income and wealth distribution, 78–80

infant mortality: rates, 127–28, 132, 139; relation to birth interval, 144; relation to female education/literacy, 59–63, 131; relation to health services, 59; relation to maternal mortality, 118–19; relation to position of women, 55–90; relation to state domestic products, 55–58

infertility, 122, 142, 146, 225

Integrated Child Development Services (ICDS) Programme, 123, 139–40

intranatal stage, health care, *see* pregnancy and childbirth

Kerala, 7, 57–62, 64, 65, 67, 68, 69, 72, 73, 74, 77, 78, 79, 80, 81, 82, 83, 84, 85, 86, 87, 90, 177, 202

kinship structures, and gender discrimination, 33–34, 35

labour force participation, women's, 11, 30–31, 180; non-wage contributions, 32; *see also* employment, income

life expectancy, 158, 175

literacy: and gender discrimination, 38–39; women's, and infant mortality, 59–63; *see also* education

Manipur, 7, 55–90
maternal advancement, index of (IMA), 71–73, 74–75; relation to infant mortality rate, 73, 76–77, 79
Maternal and Child Health Programme, 123
maternal mortality, 8, 11, 97–121, 122, 123–27, 129–30, 134, 146, 166, 176; model for estimation of, 101–105; regional variations in, 167
morbidity: abortion related, 145; contraception related, 145; data, 176–77, 180–81; pregnancy related, 142–43, 187–91; regional variations in, 167; see also under reproductive health
mortality levels/rates, 4, 12, 19; male, 158–60; in rural areas, 116–17; regional pattern, 116, 118–20; among widows, 251–53; see also child mortality, infant mortality, maternal mortality, sex differentials in mortality

National Sample Surveys, 97, 105, 114–15, 176
nutrition/malnutrition, 133, 134, 138–40, 159, 170–71, 176–77

occupation, see employment
older women, 11–13, 289–304; see also widows

parity, 188, 190, 192, 194, 195, 205
patriarchy, 216–23
patrilineal inheritance, 259–61
patrilocality, 257–59
policy/policy-making, 13–15, 88–90, 212
political participation (women's), see electoral participation
poverty, see economic status
pregnancy and childbirth, health care during, 135–42, 167; place of delivery, 176, 202–204; problems during, 187–91; see also maternal mortality, morbidity
pregnancy wastage, 176, 186–87, 188

programmes, health, 14, 147; for future action, 313–16
prostitutes/prostitution, 213, 218, 219, 220, 221–22

religious composition of population, 69–70
reproductive health: fertility-related aspects of, 122–48; problems/morbidity, 7–8, 9, 10, 181, 194–200
reproductive tract infections, 232–35
reproductive years, vulnerability of females in, 7–11

Safe Motherhood Initiative, 97
Sample Registration System (SRS), 21–23, 107–109, 112, 114–15, 119–20
sanitation, 81, 83–85, 183
Sanskritization, 35, 37, 41, 280–81
sati, 1, 2, 245
sepsis, 129–30, 142
sex differentials: in exposure to illness, 168–71; in illness outcome, 160–67; in mortality, 5–6, 11, 100–101, 104, 105, 107–10, 112, 120, 166; see also under gender differentials
sex, extramarital, 218, 220, 229
sex, premarital, 218, 220, 229
sex ratio, 32, 97, 120
sexual behaviour, 215–23
sexual exploitation, 218–19
sexually transmitted diseases (STDs), 10, 122, 146–47, 213, 214, 215, 218–21, 223–32, 233, 235–36, 238: see also AIDS
Sharda Act (1936), 2
'Sisterhood Method', 99–100
social inequalities, 13
social reform movements, 2
socio-economic development, and gender discrimination, 34–39
socio-economic status, see economic status
sons, dependence on, 12; preference for, 161; see also under gender bias
Sri Lanka, 105–107
syphilis, 226–27; see also sexually transmitted diseases

Tagore, Rabindranath, 2–3
Tamil Nadu, 10, 180–207
tetanus, 137–38, 142
toxaemia, 129–30
traditional birth attendants, 141–42
tuberculosis mortality, 158

water, 81, 85, 183
widows/widowhood, 11–13, 165–66, 245–86; employment, 264–67; incidence in different age groups, 255–57; life-style, 280–83; position in household, 274–80; regional contrasts, 253–56; remarriage 261–64; social isolation of, 279; sources of support, 269–74; vulnerability of, 257–67
women's position, roles, 1, 10, 154–72, 216–18
World Health Organization (WHO), 9, 99, 158, 196